Single Mothers in an International Context

Feminist Perspectives on The Past and Present Advisory Editorial Board

Single Mothers in an International Context: Mothers or Workers?

edited by

Simon Duncan and Rosalind Edwards

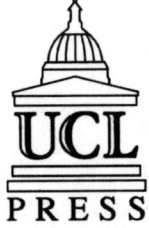

UCL
PRESS

Selection and editorial material © Simon Duncan and Rosalind Edwards 1997

First published in 1997 by UCL Press

UCL Press Limited
1 Gunpowder Square
London EC4A 3DE
UK

and

1900 Frost Road, Suite 101
Bristol
Pennsylvania 19007-1598
USA

The name of University College London (UCL) is a registered
trade mark used by UCL Press with the consent of the owner.

British Library Cataloguing-in-Publication Data
A Catalogue Record for this book is available from the British Library.

Library of Congress Cataloging-in-Publication Data are available

ISBNs: 1-85728-790-8 HB
         1-85728-791-6 PB

Typeset in 10/12 pt Linotron Times
by Wilmaset Ltd, Birkenhead, Wirral.
Printed and bound in Great Britain by SRP, Exeter.

Contents

List of Figures

List of Tables

Acknowledgements

We would like to thank Graham Crow for his detailed comments on the Introduction to this book and suggestions for the Afterword, as well as support for our joint research project on lone mothers' uptake of paid work. Thanks also to Alison Chapman at Taylor & Francis for bearing deferred manuscript delivery dates with equanimity.

Chapter 1

Introduction:
A Contextual Approach to Single Mothers and Paid Work

Simon Duncan and Rosalind Edwards

Single mothers caring for dependent children are an important and increasing proportion of the population in industrialized countries. In all countries they overwhelmingly outweigh the number of single fathers. Single motherhood is a gendered position, shaped by notions of appropriate relationships between men and women and the roles of mothers and fathers. In some countries single mothers are seen primarily as mothers; in others, they are seen primarily as workers; and sometimes they are seen as an uneasy combination of the two. Similarly, in some of these countries single mothers are characterized by poverty and dependency on state benefits, while in others their income levels are closer to the average and they are more likely to have paid work. This edited collection aims to explore these international variations. It describes the varying situations for single mothers along this mother–worker continuum for eight exemplary case study countries, exploring how these situations have developed, and with what effects in terms of single mothers' lives and uptake of paid work.

Many collections of comparative material concerning single motherhood concentrate on national welfare regimes and policies. Indeed, within the comparative body of work concerned with welfare state regimes single motherhood is often used as 'a litmus test, or indicator, of gendered social rights in different welfare regimes' (Hobson, 1994: 171; see also Millar, 1995). (We return to this point below.) Such analyses adopt an explicit or implicit stimulus – response causal model, whereby national policy is presumed to be the dominant context for single mothers' uptake of paid work. The assumption is that if a social policy stimulus is changed, single mothers will respond in an appropriate and uniform way. For example, it may be presumed that reducing the state benefit levels available to single mothers will force them to take up paid work, or less punitively, that increased provision of publicly funded child care will encourage them to do so. Such a simplistic causal approach tends to ignore social processes in local labour markets and neighbourhoods, and to play down single mothers' own understandings and capacities for social action

– albeit within the constraints of gendered and stratified socities. Indeed, in general, comparative policy analysis has tended to focus around theoretical or 'league table' descriptive secondary work. There has been very little primary cross-national intensive research on social processes, exploring informal structures, subjectivity and action (see Chamberlayne and King, 1996, for an exception).

Furthermore, edited collections often lack a coherent underlying conceptual approach, and thus end up presenting little more than a number of juxtaposed case studies from an ad hoc variety of countries. In contrast, this comparative collection is guided by a multi-layered context–action model for understanding the various dynamics and processes by which single mothers are positioned as mothers and/or workers, and by which they are constrained or enabled in combining motherhood and paid work. The selection of the case study countries is conceptually informed, therefore. The countries represented in this volume provide archetypes of the ranges of welfare regime categorizations, and within this a range of specific policies towards single mothers. The authors of the chapters in this book address both structural forms and the subjectivity of single mothers themselves in each national case, paying attention to the variety of social and material contexts in which single mothers are situated and which structure opportunities and constraints for taking up paid work.

Each chapter thus follows a common analytic structure which sees opportunities and constraints operating at four contextual levels: dominant and alternative discourses about single motherhood; state welfare regimes and policies; gendered and stratified labour markets; and neighbourhood resources and supports. Readers therefore are able to examine how this structure of opportunities and constraints for single mothers' uptake of paid work empirically operates for each country. Furthermore, readers are also able to make comparisons across countries for themselves at any one contextual level.

We now elaborate further on the underlying conceptual model for understanding single mothers' uptake of paid work which guides the structure of each chapter, and discuss the ways in which the four contextual levels interlock to produce the overall social contexts that present opportunities and structure constraints for single mothers.

Single Motherhood: Terms, Definitions and Characteristics

Following an introduction, section 2 of each chapter discusses national trends in the prevalence and characteristics of single motherhood. Such a task raises issues around terminology and definitions. Although this book is entitled 'Single Mothers in an International Context', 'single' is not a term that is uniformly used by the various authors to refer to all mothers living with dependent children and not living with a spouse or partner. In the British social policy context, as we note in chapter 3, single motherhood tends to be used specifically to refer to never-married mothers, and 'lone motherhood' is the generic term covering divorced, separated and widowed, as well as never-married, mothers. In their chapter on Australia, McHugh and Millar use the nationally prevalent generic term 'sole mothers', where again 'single' refers to the specific never-married category. Elsewhere, in other publications, authors have used still other denominations, such as Hobson's (1994) adoption of 'solo mother' as a political strategy to denote the strengths of women 'flying' as mothers on their own.

Moreover, single motherhood (in its generic sense) is not an unproblematic household structure or family type; as Millar (1994) points out, it is a set of social relations. In different national contexts there can be wide variations in the definition of what constitutes the generic category of single motherhood according to the age cut-off signifying 'dependency' of children, whether mothers living in households with other adults such as friends and relatives are included, and even whether cohabiting mothers are included, and so on (see Roll, 1992). Such variations significantly affect estimates of levels and trends in single motherhood and bedevil demographic cross-national comparisons. Nevertheless, within comparative studies there is a convergence towards a definition of single motherhood that focuses on the situation where a mother lives with her dependent children, either alone or in a larger household, but without a spouse or partner (Millar, 1994).

Whatever the definition used, in this section authors are concerned to show the variety of characteristics and circumstances, in any one national context, of the women who form the generic category of single, lone or sole mothers. Thus, within the limits of national data collection, authors provide analyses of structured and material divisions within the generic group, and between single mothers and partnered mothers, around routes into single motherhood, race/ethnicity, income levels, living standards, uptake of paid work, and so on. Single motherhood may be a genereic family form, but at the same time it is both varying and variable within countries as well as between them.

Discourses Around Single Motherhood

Single motherhood is not an apolitical situation, but one suffused with political and moral evaluation. Having set out the (more or less) 'objective' facts about single motherhood, section 3 of each chapter considers the ways the situation is framed within dominant and alternative political and popular discourses around single motherhood, and particular groups of single mothers, as well as around families and motherhood in relation to paid work in general.

Through assigning meaning and causes to actions, discourses both name and make sense of social relationships and behaviour, and instruct us how we should think of and react to aspects of the social world. In other words, the sort of social world we see, and how we understand it, can depend on the lens of the discourse that guides our search and shapes our perceptions just as much as it depends on the actual 'facts' of the situation we scrutinize.

The dominance of a particular discourse or set of discourses around single motherhood in each national context not only affects how the situation of single motherhood is understood, but also what should be done about it. Furthermore, political rhetoric on single mothers, based on particular ideological stances about the welfare state and the nature of 'the family', can also influence the constitution of, and changes to, policy. (And in turn, policies towards single motherhood and families in general interact with popular and political perceptions to provide another reference point for the formation of discourses.) So, for example, in the USA and Britain, New Right discourses around the nature of the welfare state, as well as of 'the family' and relationships between men and women, and the threat to these provided by single motherhood, have gained prominence. As such, they have shaped quite different policy developments to those in, for example, Sweden, which has been shaped by discourses that have alternative concepts of the nature of the welfare state and gender roles, and which place single-mother households as merely another, unthreatening, form of family. Other chapters show other developments.

Thus, examination of the development and patterns of national discourses is important in that these provide another context, in terms of both influencing popular everyday perceptions and state policies, in which single mothers must negotiate their lives, including decisions to try for paid work or not.

State Welfare Regimes and Single Mothers

Section 4 of each chapter moves on to analyse the way national policies position single mothers within the context of the overall welfare state regime. They may be positioned as essentially home-makers who care for children, or essentially as paid workers, or perhaps as a variety of uneasy combinations of the two.

The comparative analysis of welfare state regimes as systems of stratification, as developed by Esping-Andersen (1990), has been both immensely influential and heavily criticized for being gender-blind. Various alternative classificatory systems have been produced that attempt to place gender relations in a more central position, with varying success in providing analytic accounts of different systems of gender inequality (see Sainsbury, 1994; Duncan, 1995, 1996).

In this book, authors assess the overall thrust of welfare policies in each national case, either drawing on Esping-Andersen's categorization or more gender-aware versions. They provide an evaluation of the ways policies towards single mothers enhance or constrain their opportunities to take up paid work. For example, Ireland typifies a 'strong breadwinner' welfare regime, where policies position women primarily as mothers in home-maker roles and single mothers are excluded from paid work; Germany is a typical 'conservative' welfare regime, but here single mothers are expected to move into paid work after their children reach a certain age; the USA typifies a 'liberal' welfare regime, where policies ostensibly give mothers a 'choice' on whether or not to take up paid work, but lack of child care provision on the one hand, and minimal and stigmatized welfare benefits on the other, place single mothers in a difficult position; while Sweden typifies a 'social democratic' system, where state policies treat all women, including single mothers, as autonomous citizens and workers. Other countries occupy more transitional positions.

National contrasts in single mothers' uptake of paid work are associated with differences in social policy, and as we have pointed out, this has been seen as dominant in comparative discussions of the issue. However, the nation state is only one of several contexts for single mothers' actions: local labour markets, and neighbourhoods or social networks may also be important. Sections 5 and 6 of each chapter turn to these levels of analysis.

Single Mothers in Labour Markets

Section 5 of each chapter is concerned with labour markets. In order for single mothers to take up paid work jobs have to be available. Furthermore, the supply of jobs within any one country often varies markedly between local labour markets.

Within a national context there is remarkably persistent horizontal and vertical occupational sex segregation, with women concentrated in particular sectors, often in particular occupations, and at lower status levels, for less time, and in less secure and lower paid jobs (OECD, 1994). (And for women from minority ethic groups, sex segregation can interact with racial segregation to provide even more limited opportunites.) Thus in many countries most 'women's jobs' cannot provide single mothers with an independent income.

But more than this, spatial and gendered divisions of labour mean that different amounts and types of jobs are available to women in different areas (Massey, 1995). In addition, women – and mothers in particular – often have limited job search areas because of their domestic and child-care responsibilities. This limitation can be even more severe for single mothers. So even if single mothers want to take up paid work, and even if state polices provide support for this, they may not be able to do so within a particular area.

Furthermore, there are entrenched historical and cultural regional social expectations about whether women, especially mothers, should work for a wage or primarily be home-makers. These regional discourses about women and work will interact with the nature and amount of jobs made available by spatially divided labour markets, leading to sub-national variations in single mothers' uptake of paid work. Nonetheless, perhaps because of the dominance of national state policy in the literature on single mothers, this crucial context remains underexplored.

Single Mothers in Neighbourhoods: Social Support and Subjectivity

Section 6 of each chapter explores the constraints and opportunities provided by the neighbourhood contexts in which mothers live, and their own under-standing of their identity as mothers and/or workers.

The local setting is a particularly important and relevant part of single mothers' lives – a socially structured factor in the background of opportunities and constraints that are built into single mothers' daily routines. Single mothers' neighbourhood support networks represent local structures of interaction, giving them access to resources, or being resources in themselves, both through organized groups and other personal ties. Localized networks of kin and friends can be significant materially, including providing single mothers and child-care support in contexts where there is little publicly funded provision available (such as Ireland and Britain). Yet the way that single mothers' support networks may vary according to locality and social group – affecting their ability to take up paid work – has received little attention in comparative work (for an exception see Cochran et al., 1993).

Social networks and support imply people in groups; groups that will define experiences and situations in common as well as individually. Thus as well as providing material support, single mothers' social networks are significant in terms of their own subjectivity. Local social attitudes towards mothers who work and towards single motherhood can play a role in single mothers' decisions about taking paid work, in terms of shaping their identity as mothers and/or workers, quite apart from national policy and labour market structures. Such neighbourhood norms may be similar to or differ from dominant national discourses.

Integrating single mothers' own perceptions and sense of belonging within analyses of the structural contexts of their lives allows them to be seen as 'creative, reflexive agents both constrained by and enabled by, as well as creating, the social conditions in which they exist (Williams, 1996: 3), rather than assuming they will simply respond to national benefits and services in uniform ways. Indeed, social policy research generally needs to pay as much attention to social action and people's sense of identity as it does to analysis of policy and welfare states if it is to fully understand social welfare processes (cf. Williams, 1996).

The Structure of the Book

As we have said, this collection represents more than a series of ad hoc case studies from a variety of countries. Rather, each national example represents a particular position, at the level of state welfare regimes, in single mothers' characterization as mothers who care for children and/or paid workers. This can be envisaged as a continuum between home-based motherhood and work-based motherhood. In the former, single mothers are supported as mothers. In the latter, policy support is provided for mothers to take paid work and single mothers are supported as workers. The continuum thus takes into account understandings of women's, especially mothers', roles in relation to those of men. (As we have argued, such policy characterizations are not necessarily uniformly reflected in single mothers' understandings of themselves as mothers and/or workers and in their decisions about taking up paid work. A continuum constructed at this level may well look quite different).

We begin with the Republic of Ireland where, as McLaughlin and Rodgers show in chapter 2, the influence of nationalism and Catholicism has resulted in a high value being placed on the traditional male-breadwinner family form, and policies for single mothers position them firmly as mothers rather than workers.

We then move along the continuum to a more ambivalent set of state welfare regimes, ranging from a lack of support to women either as mothers or as workers, through the regimes which support mothers at home but expect single mothers to work.

The British welfare regime, which we discuss in chapter 3, is not clear as to whether women should be mothers or workers. There has been a specific move towards treating single mothers as workers, but little in the way of supportive provision to back up this course of action. Similarly, the US welfare regime, addressed by de Acosta in chapter 4, positions single mothers as workers, but again provides little support for this.

The Japanese welfare regime's stance towards single mothers is driven by notions of a 'Japanese-style welfare society', stressing mutual family aid and employment as a citizenship obligation. As Peng shows in chapter 5, policies support the traditional male-breadwinner, two-parent family at the same time as they require single mothers' economic self-reliance. Single mothers' uptake of paid work is also a policy aim under the Australian welfare regime in recent developments. However, in chapter 6 McHugh and Millar argue that while schemes have been initiated to support single mothers in seeking paid work, other policies do not adequately support their actual employment.

The situation in Germany is also contradictory. Despite a state welfare regime that supports home-based motherhood for women, as Klett-Davies discusses in chapter 7, single mothers are largely expected to take up paid work while still being positioned as wider family dependents.

The final two case study chapters move us to countries where a range of policy provisions are more coherent in supporting all mothers as workers. In France, as Lefaucheur and Martin explain in chapter 8, longstanding worries about declining birth rates have led to policies supporting both motherhood and paid work, including those for single mothers. Finally, Sweden has long been held up as a state welfare regime that enables all mothers to be workers, with no distinctions for single mothers. Nevertheless, in chapter 9 Björnberg suggests that economic and political change is threatening single mothers' position.

In conclusion, in the Afterword, we critique the dominant 'black box', categorical approach to single motherhood. In contrast, the chapters in this volume show the variability and differences in single mothers' uptake of paid work between and within national policy regimes. Drawing on these case studies, we comment on the implications of such variations for theory, research and policy concerning single mothers as mothers and/or workers.

References

CHAMBERLAYNE, P. and KING, A. (1996) 'Biographical approaches in comparative work: the Cultures of Care project', in Hantrais, L. and Mangen, S. (Eds) *Cross-National Research Methods in the Social Sciences*, London: Pinter.

COCHRAN, M., LARNER, M., RILEY, D., GUNNARSSON, L. and HENDERSON, C. R. (1993) *Extending Families: The Social Networks of Parents and Their Children*, Cambridge: Cambridge University Press.

DUNCAN, S. S. (1995) 'Theorising European gender systems', *Journal of European Social Policy*, **4**, pp. 263–84.

DUNCAN, S. S. (1996) 'The diverse worlds of European patriarchy', in Garcia-Ramon, D. and Monk, J. (Eds) *Women of the European Union: The Politics of Work and Daily Life*, pp. 74–104, London: Routledge.

ESPING-ANDERSEN, G. (1990) *The Three Worlds of Welfare Capitalism*, Cambridge: Polity Press.

HOBSON, B. (1994) 'Solo mothers, social policy regimes and the logics of gender', in Sainsbury, D. (Ed.).

MASSEY, D. (1995) *Spatial Divisions of Labour*, London: Macmillan.

MILLAR, J. (1994) 'Defining lone parents: family structures and social relations', in Hantrais, L. and Letablier, M-t. (Eds) *Conceptualising the Family*, 4th Ser., Cross-National Research Papers, London and Paris: ESRC/CNAF.

MILLAR, J. (1995) 'Mothers or workers? Policy approaches to supporting lone mothers in comparative perspective', in Bortolaia-Silva, E. (Ed) *Good Enough Mothering? Feminist Perspectives on Lone Motherhood*, pp. 97–113, London: Routledge.

OECD (1994) *Women and Structural Change: New Perspectives*, Paris: Organisation for Economic Co-operation and Development.

ROLL, J. (1992) *Lone Parent Families in the E.C.*, Brussels: EC Commission.

SAINSBURY, D. (Ed.) (1994) *Gendering Welfare States*, London: Sage.

WILLIAMS, F. (with PILLINGER, J.) (1996) 'New thinking on social policy research into inequality, social exclusion and poverty', in Millar, J. and Bradshaw, J. (Eds) *Social Welfare Systems: Towards a New Research Agenda*, Bath Social Policy Paper 4, Bath: University of Bath/ESRC.

Chapter 2

Single Mothers in the Republic of Ireland: Mothers not Workers

Eithne McLaughlin and Paula Rodgers

1. Introduction

Under the 'male breadwinner' typology of welfare regimes developed by Lewis (1992) and Lewis and Ostner (1994), the Republic of Ireland (hereafter Ireland) is characterized as a 'strong' variant, in which women's status as citizens has historically been, and continues to be, resolutely focused on their family status as home-workers (wives, mothers and daughters). Ireland's welfare regime has also been examined by McLaughlin (1993) in terms of the extent to which it embodies the characteristics of a Catholic corporatist welfare regime, a variant of Esping-Andersen's conservative corporatist welfare regime. This chapter can be seen as bridging these two approaches, given the close relationship between Catholic corporatism and restrictions on women's economic, social and reproductive rights. Conroy Jackson (1993), McLaughlin (1993), and more recently Yeates (1995), have indeed demonstrated that a central theme in the development of Irish social policy has been management of mothers' – and hence women's – social and reproductive rights. In turn, as Conroy Jackson, Yeates, and others, have argued, analysis of the position of single mothers is central to understanding the position of welfare regimes in Lewis and Ostner's typology, since such 'deviant' cases illuminate the extent to which the material, political and ideological structures of social policy as premised around 'normal' (male-breadwinner/non-employed mother) households.

The term 'single mothers' is here used to denote all mothers rearing children without a co-resident father. The term 'unmarried mother' is used when it is necessary to distinguish between women who have borne their children outside marriage and women who have become single mothers as a result of marital breakdown or widowhood.

Analysis of single motherhood can examine, firstly, how social policies structure the choices and options of single mothers, and secondly, the political and social construction of single motherhood in its historical context. (This includes examination of women's own efforts to create and change the political and social construction of single motherhood.) The latter is essential if we are to understand how 'single mothers' as a category is a product of the gendered historical development of social welfare (Yeates, 1995: 3). In section 2 of this chapter, the prevalence and chararacteristics of single mothers in Ireland are documented, drawing particular attention to the very considerable rise in both marital breakdown and births outside of marriage in the second half of the 1980s. The majority of mothers in two- and one-parent families are not in employment, and section 3 documents the way all women have been encouraged to adopt a private-sphere role, and the importance of nationalism and Catholicism therein. Section 4 describes the contemporary welfare regime, noting some recent changes to the social security system. Section 5 discusses employment rates among women and recent social policy changes which have begun to incorporate single mothers into active labour market policies. In section 6 we draw on the very limited material available on the experience of single motherhood in Ireland, and it should be noted that the experiences of single mothers in areas outside Dublin have not yet been researched. The final and concluding section comments on the extent to which further reform towards a 'single-mothers-as-workers' model might be expected or desired, and discusses the importance of understanding the development of national welfare regimes.

2. Single Mothers in Ireland

The prevalence of single motherhood

Before the mid-1980s Ireland, like the southern Mediterranean and central European countries, had comparatively low levels of single motherhood. But during the later 1980s, a rapid rise in single motherhood resulted in Irish levels which are now about average in European terms (Roll, 1992; Millar et al., 1992). Ireland shared with Portugal the distinction of being the two European countries whose relative positions changed most during this time. Estimates of the extent of single motherhood in Ireland are problematic however, since different sources (the Census of Population, Labour Force Survey, Continuous Household Survey, and statistics on Social Security recipients) produce different estimates.

The best estimate of the number of single mothers is assumed to be that from the Census of Population. However, the Census reports in terms of single-parent families with children under 16, rather than 18; nor does the Census count single mothers who are living with their own parents as separate family units. Table 2.1 shows the number and proportion of single-parent households according to Censuses from 1981–91, and the proportion headed by mothers. The Census reported 90,906 single parents in 1991, of whom 83 per cent were single mothers (Courtney, 1995: 60) and the rise in the numbers of single-mother families was particularly dramatic between the Census of

Year	Single-parent households			Single-mother households		
	N	% of all families	% increase	N	% of all single parents	% increase
1981	29,658	5.7	–	23,684	80	–
1986	36,353	7.2	123	30,568	84	29
1991	90,906	7.9	250	75,337	83	246

Source McCashin (1993) and Courtney (1995)
Table 2.1   Number of single parents, Census of Population: Republic of Ireland, 1981, 1986, 1991

1986 and that of 1991. McCashin (1995) reports that single-parent families were 7.1 per cent of all familes with at least one child aged 15 or less in 1981, 8.6 per cent in 1986 and 10.7 per cent in 1991.

Routes into single motherhood

Although widowhood has been declining as a route into single parenthood, and even though divorce was not legal in Ireland,[1] marital breakdown remains a very important route into single motherhood. The overall 'widowhood rate' has been declining over a long period, falling from 163 per 1,000 in 1971 to 139 in 1981 (McCashin, 1993: 30). Because of the absence of divorce, legal separation is a more important route into single motherhood than in other countries. Table 2.2 shows that, as in other European countries (Ermisch, 1990), there was a very significant rise in marital separation during the 1980s in Ireland – a rise of 570 per cent between 1979 and 1991.

Year	No. separated	Rate per 1,000 married persons	% 1979 rate
1979	7,600	6.1	–
1986	37,200	28.6	468
1991	46,700	34.8	570

Source McCashin (1993: 32), estimates derived from Labour Force Survey and Census of Population data.
Table 2.2   Estimates of marital breakdown: Republic of Ireland, 1979, 1986, 1991

Another indicator of the rise in separation is the increase in the number of recipients of the 'Deserted Wives Benefit' (see next section for an explanation of social welfare benefits), which almost quadrupled between the late 1970s and the late 1980s, rising from 3,147 to 12,124 (Millar et al., 1992: 20). By 1990, the numbers had risen again to 16,000 – a rise of over 50 per cent in just four years (Fahey, 1995: 226). As Millar et al. point out, it is important to note that the lack of divorce in Ireland 'cuts off' one route *out* of single motherhood

11

– remarriage – which means that single motherhood may be a more permanent
and long-term state in Ireland than in other countries. This in turn may partly –
and paradoxically – account for the very dramatic increases in single motherhood which Ireland has experienced.

There has, however, also been a dramatic increase in the number of non-
marital births. As a proportion of all births, these have risen by 900 per cent
between 1958 and 1992 (see Table 2.3), with most of the increase concentrated
in the 1980s.

Year	% of all births	% 1958 rate
1958	2	
1961	2	0
1973	3	150
1980	5	250
1990	15	750
1992	18	900

Source Flanagan and Richardson (1992); Cherish (1974); McCashin (1993); Magee (1994).
Table 2.3   Non-marital births as percentage of all births: Republic of Ireland, 1958–92

As in other countries, the rise in non-marital births is made up of both a
decrease in marital births, and an increase in non-marital births. Between 1980
and 1991 marital births declined by about 40 per cent (McCashin, 1993: 33),
partly as a result of some increase in age at marriage and delayed onset of
childbearing (Flanagan and Richardson, 1992: 8), and partly as a result of
legislative changes which increased the availability of contraceptives (see next
section).

In the European context, the Irish rate of birth outside marriage has been
low, but relatively speaking it has increased more than in other countries. Over
the past 30 years, the increase in the proportion of non-marital births in Ireland
has been the third highest in Europe, exceeded only by Denmark and the
Netherlands (Flanagan and Richardson, 1992; 8).

The ratio of non-marital to marital births tends to be greatest among
younger age-groups. Thus, 32 per cent of first births in 1991 (16 per cent in
1981) occurred outside of marriage, compared with 17 per cent of all births
(Fahey, 1995: 225), with the group of women having their first birth being
younger on average than the group of all women giving birth. In 1992, over
66 per cent of extra-marital births were to women under 25, and 89 per cent of
all births to women under 20 were outside marriage, compared with 50 per cent
in 1980 and 24 per cent in 1972.

The 1986 Census of Population showed that unmarried mothers
amounted to 16 per cent of total single-parent families, while widows/
widowers accounted for 24 per cent, and separated people for 60 per cent. But,
as pointed out earlier, the Census of Population does not count never-married
mothers living with their own parents as separate family units. This is of

considerable signficance, since as Flanagan and Richardson (1992: 37) found, over half (57 per cent) of all unmarried mothers, and almost three-quarters of teenage unmarried mothers, lived in their parents' homes (at least at the time of birth). Thus in 1986, although there were 12,000 women receiving the Unmarried Mother's Allowance, only 6,000 unmarried single-mother families were counted in the Census (McCashin, 1993).

Alongside the rise in non-marital births has been a decrease in adoption (McCashin, 1993: 35). The number of adoptions in the 1970s was in the range of 1,000 to 1,500 per annum, but declined to 590 in 1991. As a proportion of non-marital births, the adoption figure was 6.7 per cent in 1991, compared with 41.4 per cent in 1978 and 86.2 per cent in 1968 (ibid.). The high rate of adoption in the past was largely involuntary as single women were strongly 'persuaded' by both statutory and voluntary sector (Church) agencies to give up their babies for adoption (see next section).

Characteristics of single mothers

Because of the undercount of unmarried mothers in the Census, it is difficult to get an accurate picture of the characteristics of all single mothers in Ireland (McCashin, 1993). Nevertheless, Millar et al. (1992) believe that in terms of characteristics such as sex, age and number of children, Irish single mothers are probably not very different from single mothers in other countries, apart from the duration of single motherhood pointed to above. As regards the number of children, single-parent families tend to have fewer children than two-parent families. The median family size is about 2.3 for couples, 2.0 for single fathers and about 1.5 for single mothers (Millar et al., 1992: 16). Unmarried mothers usually have young children (73 per cent aged under five), while widowed mothers have older children (60 per cent aged 10–14). Nearly two in three of all single parents are in the age range 30–49 (63 per cent); about one in five 20–29 years (22 per cent); just over one in ten are aged 50 or more (13 per cent); and only one in a hundred are aged 15–19. In comparisons, nearly two in three unmarried mothers (62 per cent) are aged 20–29 years; just under one in three (30 per cent) are aged between 30 and 49 years and just under one in ten (8 per cent) are aged 15–19 (ibid.: 18).

Single mothers' employment rates

Significant differences in economic activity rates by marital status meant that half (51 per cent) of single women were working in 1988, compared with 23 per cent of married women, 37 per cent of separated women and 7 per cent of widowed women. Direct examination of the employment status of single mothers is difficult because the Labour Force Survey only gives information on the employment status of heads of households. It is therefore only possible to identify those single parents who are also heads of household, which excludes unmarried mothers living with their own parents (although see the Household Budget Survey data given below). In these terms, 37 per cent of single mothers who were also heads of households were economically active in 1989: 18 per cent were employed on a full-time basis, 7 per cent on a part-time basis, and 13 per cent were unemployed. In contrast, 55 per cent of single fathers were in full-time employment (Roll 1992: 18). Although the proportion of married mothers in the labour force (31 per cent) was somewhat lower than the proportion of single mothers (35 per cent), the two groups' *employment*, as opposed to *activity*, rates were very similar – 17 per cent of married mothers and 18 per cent of single mothers were in full-time employment.

In the European Union as a whole, single mothers have higher levels of both economic activity and employment than mothers in two-parent families – with three exceptions: *Ireland*, Netherlands and the UK. In six of the twelve Member States at the end of the 1980s, over half of single mothers were in full-time employment (France, Italy, Luxembourg, Denmark, Greece and Portugal). Although there is clearly considerable variation of employment rates of single mothers across countries, as Millar et al. (1992: 54) point out, it is difficult to draw direct comparisons and interpret these statistics. This is due to the nature of the national policy environment around single motherhood; that is whether single mothers are treated as mothers or workers. However, participation rates of single mothers, as of other mothers, are related to the age and number of their children, as well as to subnational cultures which vary by geography, class, ethnic identity and so forth (see below and sections 5 and 6). Variation in employment rates by age of children and low levels of child-care provision suggest that we should expect employment rates of single mothers in Ireland to be low, and lower than in other countries. In Ireland, only 14 per cent of single mothers with children under two were employed, with 23 per cent of those with children aged between three and six, and 33 per cent of those with children aged 6–15 (Millar et al., 1992). Given that the growth of single motherhood has been relatively more recent in Ireland than in other countries, and that therefore relatively high proportions have young children, this in itself would be expected to depress the overall employment and activity rates of single mothers in Ireland compared with other countries.

Particularly low employment rates can be found however among umarried single mothers. The Household Budget Survey of 1987 (a survey undertaken every seven years) showed that almost 90 per cent of unmarried single-mother households had household heads who were not economically active, and contained no economically active persons. The corresponding figures for widowed and separated single-parent households were 59 and 65 per cent respectively. In contrast only 2.3 per cent of two-adult households with two children contained no economically active persons (McCashin, 1993: 44). The particularly low employment rates of unmarried single mothers is probably the result of the three related factors of low educational attainment, social class background and (relatively young) unmarried motherhood. Thus, unmarried single-parent households had by far the largest proportion of household heads in the lowest socio-economic groups (as measured by the Central Statistical Office's classification) at 88.5 per cent, compared with, for instance, 10.7 per cent of two-adult two-children households (ibid., 45). On the other hand, it is also unmarried single mothers who are most likely to have very young (pre-school) children, and this, as pointed out above, would further reduce their likelihood of employment.

Income levels

Low levels of employment among all women in Ireland, especially mothers, mean that single mothers are heavily dependent on welfare payments. Although rates of welfare payments are somewhat higher in Ireland than in the UK, they are not high in relation to many other West European countries. Furthermore, rates of benefits for families with children tend to be low (taking into account their expenditure needs) compared with those for people without children. As a result many single mothers experience poverty.

Using the 1987 Household Budget Survey, McCashin (1993) found that unmarried single parents had a disposable income of £80.70 a week, separated single parents £110.30, and widowed single parents £133.07. Standardizing this data in per capita equivalent terms, unmarried single parents had the lowest average incomes, followed by separated single parents, then two-parent families with two children and finally widows. Using 50 per cent of average incomes as the poverty line, unmarried single-parent households had the highest risk of poverty – 35 per cent – followed by large two-parent families with four or more children. Using the measure, 28 per cent of separated single parents and 14 per cent of widowed single parents were in poverty (see also Callan et al., 1989, and Nolan and Farrell, 1990, for similar findings). Richardson (1992: 81) showed that the income and expenditure of unmarried mothers compares unfavourably with that of married mothers and the former's receipt of Unmarried Mothers Allowance was not providing unmarried mothers with incomes comparable to those of mothers with husbands. A number of studies of single mothers' experiences have concentrated on poverty and the management of low incomes and these are discussed further in section 6 below.

In summary, single motherhood rose remarkably in Ireland in the second half of the 1980s and early 1990s, both because of marital breakdown and increases in births outside marriage. The majority of single mothers (like married mothers) are not in employment, rely on welfare benefits of various sorts and a significant proportion experience poverty. The extent to which this situation is the result of generally high levels of unemployment and poor employment opportunities for women as a whole in Ireland, or the structure of the welfare system itself (i.e., the availability of benefits for single mothers not in employment, and poor provision for part-time work within benefit provision), and/or the more general policy environment (including issues such as child care and the ideological construction of motherhood), is unclear. The latter two issues form the focus of the next two sections, and we turn first to the historical and ideological development of policies towards mothers, and single mothers, in Ireland.

3. The Development of Discourses Around Single Motherhood in Ireland

To understand both the current dominant and alternative discourses surrounding single motherhood, it is necessary to review attitudes to the family and motherhood in general. Dominant discourses can be identified through the historical development of social policy towards both mothers and single mothers, and such a discussion inevitably involves the position of mothers in the Irish Constitutions of 1922 and 1937, and the intertwining of the Catholic Church and state enshrined in the latter. Both dominant and alternative discourses are evident in general population attitude surveys, in the attitudes of single mothers themselves, and in public debates surrounding recent referenda on family matters. In addition, the voluntary sector, lobby groups and academic feminists have all offered analyses of the nature of women's, and mothers', positions in Ireland. Many of these explain the current position as having its roots in nationalism, and argue that the ideology of nationalism has been the major factor in shaping women's position in Ireland. Feminist views in Ireland are by no means a unified set of perspectives however. We turn first to a consideration of the historical development of social welfare in Ireland, and the discourses within it concerning motherhood and single motherhood.

The pre-war development of social welfare in Ireland

Neither the development of the Irish welfare regime generally, nor the social construction of single motherhood specifically, can be separated from the country's experience of colonialism, nationalism and post-colonial Anglo–Irish relations (Burke, 1987; Breen et al., 1990). The pervasive influence of Britain on the development of Irish social policy prior to, and following, independence has been widely noted (Cook, 1983; Burke, 1987; Conroy Jackson, 1993; Curry, 1993) and is often described in terms of the extent of importation of British social policy into Ireland. However, the legacy of colonialism goes beyond 'importation' to the much more complex ways in which that legacy has structured the relationships between people, Church and state within Ireland. This has had fundamental implications for the development of social welfare in Ireland, and in particular the categorization of women as non-employed mothers.

The nineteenth-century Poor Law

The Irish social welfare system remains today much more rooted in nine-teenth-century principles of sexual difference, and in the separate roles and unequal positions of men and women, than in other European systems. The origins of this 'gender categorical approach' (Yeates, 1995: 5) can certainly be traced to the importation into nineteenth-century Ireland of the British Poor Law, through the 1838 Poor Law (Ireland) Act (Burke, 1987), and from which social welfare and social services systems subsequently developed. As Yeates (ibid.) points out, it could be argued that the British Poor Law has had a stronger contemporary role in Ireland than in Britain. For instance, Ireland has retained a local structure of social assistance (in terms of payment and administration – rates and entitlements are set nationally) whereas Britain moved away from this aspect of the Poor Law inheritance to a national system. Significant for single motherhood is the Poor Law principle that women were 'deserving' and entitled to relief only if they could prove that their husbands had failed to provide for them or had been absent for more than 12 months. Unmarried mothers, having no husbands, had a more 'automatic' right to Poor Law relief in the workhouse, but on the other hand, had no legal rights to their child – from whom they were often separated. Under common law a child born outside marriage was said to be *filius nullius*, a 'child of no one' – neither parent was the guardian nor had any rights to custody over the child.

The Irish workhouse system came under intolerable strain during the tragedy of the Great Famine (1845–49)[2] and in 1847 the most 'deserving' of single mothers – widows – were separated from the less deserving and granted the right to 'outdoor' relief (i.e., relief while living in their own homes). The pressures of the Great Famine, however, meant that such rights were rapidly extended to other groups of women and men. In the case of mothers, and as a development of the deserving/undeserving categorization of mothers, entitle-ment to outdoor relief rested on a hierarchy of more and less legitimate reasons for husbands/fathers' failures to provide (e.g., disability, desertion, and so on). Orphan girls and single women in the Workhouse (institutions for the poor not eligible to receive relief at home) were assisted to emigrate to other British colonies, while single Irish women living in England who became pregnant were forcibly returned to Ireland to the workhouses (Burke, 1987), where they joined other unmarried mothers:

> Throughout most of the nineteenth and approximately half of the twentieth century many unmarried mothers, when rejected by the community, found refuge in the workhouse. Even there among society's misfits and rejects they were stigmatized.
>
> (O'Hare, 1983: 3)

Despite entitlements for 'blameless' mothers to outdoor relief and the 'assisted' emigration of single childless women, women outnumbered men in the workhouses by three to one in the latter half of the nineteenth century, and many of these were unmarried mothers.

In the early part of the twentieth century, in common with most other European countries, Britain, and hence Ireland, began to develop social insurance systems. The 1911 National Insurance Act consolidated the wage system, reinforced the concept of husbands/fathers as family breadwinners (Fraser, 1984), and removed some men from the scope of social assistance. It had little impact on mothers without husbands. Following constitutional independence from Britain in 1921, the Poor Law was expanded and there was little development of social insurance (e.g. by 1926, only one in five of the Irish labour force was insured against unemployment (Yeates, 1995: 9)). Some social insurance expansion took place in the 1930s, and significantly for single mothers, the 1935 Widow's and Orphan's Pension Act was prompted by a concern to upgrade the status of deceased (male) breadwinners' dependants (one in three recipients of home-based social assistance were widows). This concern was consistent with the wider political and social welfare changes occurring at that time, which culminated in the replacement of the 1922 with the 1937 Constitution. The latter involved the inscription of sexual difference and the writing into a national constitution of an exclusively private sphere role for women to an extent unparalleled across the rest of Europe. The roots of this uniqueness lie in the conjunction of Catholicism and nationalism.

Catholic corporatism and constitutional nationalism

During the nineteenth and early twentieth centuries Catholicism had come to be part of the definition of 'Irishness' itself in the culture and politics of nationalism. The binding of a religion into nationalist political activity and identity is, of course, far from unique to Ireland. But the particular experience of colonialism over several centuries in Ireland meant that Catholic social teaching played a prominent role in the establishment of the independent state set up in the 1920s. Initially the 1922 constitution of the new 'Republic' was influenced (from within and without) by the Irish suffrage movement and 'first-wave' feminism (Ward, 1983), and accordingly gave equal rights and opportunities to 'all citizens' (Owens, 1983). However, an integral element of Irish nationalism (as in most other forms of nationalism), with its emphasis on the renewal of the post-colonial Irish 'race', was the notion of sexual difference and the importance of women's role as mothers and home-makers in the private sphere (Meaney, 1993). This nationalist emphasis on women as mothers had co-existed with more radical republican ideals of liberty and equality in the pre-independence era. But, following independence, constitutional nationalism joined forces with the Church on family issues and maternalist policies, and the 1922 Constitution was replaced by the 1937 Constitution containing a suite of linked social and economic policies designed to fix women firmly in the private sphere.

The 1930s has been described as the decade in which the De Valera Republican Government and the Catholic Church joined forces to confront the 'Unmanageable revolutionaries' of feminist republicanism, and to clarify 'once and for all' the role and rights of women in Irish society (Ward, 1983). Articles 40 and 41 of the 1937 Constitution of the Irish Republic and the associated Social Welfare Code (Donnelly, 1993) prescribed a private-sphere role for women. Article 40 qualified equality before the law by allowing the state to have 'due regard to difference of capacity, physical and moral and social function' between women and men. More specifically, Article 41, citing the importance of the work that mothers do in raising the next generation, stated that no married woman should be obliged by economic necessity to work outside the home. Throughout the 1930s, policies were implemented to remove women, especially mothers, from the economic sphere. For example, the Land Commission, set up to redistribute land in the new post-colonial era, refused women the right to inherit land. In 1932 a marriage bar banned the employment of married women as civil servants. The 1933 Conditions of Employment Act allowed the government to prohibit female employment in any form of industrial work and to set quotas for particular sectors.

The Irish Catholic Church's position on these matters, expressed in the powerful Catholic Social Movement of the 1920s and 1930s, derived from the Roman Catholic Church's enunciation in the late nineteenth and early twentieth centuries, of a set of corporatist principles. While this was thus not specific to Ireland it was arguably most influential there. Catholic corporatism generally favoured a social and moral order based on small-scale capitalism, family property, small businesses and farms – an order with particular resonance in colonial and post-colonial Ireland. Central to Catholic corporatism were the principles of subsidiarity, family solidarity and social consensus (McLaughlin, 1993: 206). Although there was no commitment to redistributive and egalitarian social policies in Catholic corporatism, neither was it held that the state should preside over extreme inequalities or manifest social injustices, so that Catholic corporatism was able to embody both liberal and social-democratic welfare principles (ibid., 207), as indeed it has done in Ireland since 1921.

While in Catholic corporatist thought the state may, and indeed should, spend on social welfare, it should not deliver social welfare, this being properly the responsibility of other subsidiary organizations. The Irish Church was thus able to retain and consolidate its own authority and influence through the voluntary associations it operated in the fields of health and social welfare (Peillon, 1982). The latter were more numerous than in other Catholic European countries because during the nineteenth century, the Catholic Church had been permitted and used by the British colonial administration to develop a social welfare infrastructure for the native population. As a result, in early twentieth-century Ireland, the Church was not only the moral guardian of constitutional nationalism, but also in effect 'a state-in-waiting' – with the means and structures to occupy a key role in the formation and delivery of social welfare provision (McLaughlin, 1993: 208).

The success of the Catholic Social Movement in the 1920s and 1930s, and the leading role the Church already had in the provision of education and health services and assistance for the poor, meant that the social services in Ireland subsequently developed little beyond those which emerged in the late nineteenth century. This has had particular implications for mothers, and other carers, because it led to a general failure to develop pre-school or after-school child-care services, or social-care services targeted at disabled or infirm older people needing help with the activities of daily living (Glendinning and McLaughlin, 1993; Lynch and McLaughlin, 1995). The absence of publicly funded child-care services in particular continues to have major implications for the position of single mothers.

McLaughlin describes the Church–state consensus of the 1920s and 1930s as resulting in the creation of:

> a theocratic state by legislating a set of principles that ensured state activities remained within the parameters set by Catholic social teaching . . . [these principles] gave recognition to the 'holy trinity' of the family, Church and nation and outlined a series of social policy principles which were intended to re-establish and reinforce traditional gender relations by removing women from public life.
>
> (1993: 210)

Although women's groups fought against Articles 40 and 41 of the 1937 Constitution, and won back the guarantee of political participation 'without distinction of sex' which had been in the 1922 Constitution, they failed to reverse the economic and social policy clauses. The 1937 Constitution also banned divorce, while the sale, advertising and importation of contraceptives were legally prohibited under section 17 of the Criminal Law Amendment Act 1935.

The post-war development of social welfare

The 1940s and 1950s: continued application of the breadwinner principle

In common with other countries after the Second World War, the social insurance system was extended, in Ireland's case through the 1952 Social Welfare Act. However, Yeates (1995) and Conroy Jackson (1993) stress the continuity between pre- and post-war welfare in Ireland due to the consistent application of the male-breadwinner model. The 1952 development in social insurance again benefited and was targeted at men, with more men moving off social assistance than women. Between 1935 and 1970, for example, the proportion of social assistance recipients who were women increased from 57 to 68 per cent (Yeates, 1995: 12). Conroy Jackson (1993) therefore argues that the immediate post-war period did not constitute a landmark in social policy terms for Irish women. The reasons for this, however, do not lie solely within the provisions of the Social Welfare Act itself, nor even the extent to which distinct policy approaches such as universalism, selectivity and gender-categorical approaches, were, or were not, adopted. They have as much to do with, firstly, differences in labour markets between Ireland and other European countries in the post-war period and, secondly, the unity of purpose of Catholicism and nationalism in the post-independence state, so evident in the 1920s and 1930s, and which continued to set the direction of social welfare development in the post-war period.

Firstly, Ireland 'missed out' on the first period of economic prosperity experienced by Western societies in the 1950s and early 1960s (Kennedy, 1989). National income expanded at less than 1 per cent per annum, and net industrial output by 1.3 per cent during the 1950s; industrial employment, already low in Ireland, fell even further (by 14 per cent). In addition, government attempts to redress Ireland's poor economic and employment performance were consciously geared towards the twin objectives of promoting economic development and the reproduction of male-breadwinner/female-home-maker familial relations (Pyle, 1990; see also section 5 below).

Secondly, and equally important, was the continuing influence of Catholicism on the development of Irish social welfare. This is particularly well demonstrated by the fate of the Mother and Child Scheme in the late 1940s and early 1950s. This scheme would have provided a universal and compulsory health service for mothers and children funded out of taxation, and free at the point of provision. The scheme was opposed by some of the medical profession (as was the NHS in Britain), but also by the Catholic Church – which argued that the scheme would extend women's reproductive rights through instruction on 'sex relations' and the provision of 'gynaecological care' – interpreted as encompassing provision for contraception and abortion (Barrington, 1987: 210). The ensuing political controversy, which involved the resignation of the Minister for Health and the collapse of the government in 1951 (Coogan 1993: 649), ended with the adoption of a substantially watered-down Mother and Child Scheme as part of a means-tested health service, which accorded greater weight to selectivity, voluntarism and 'individual' (i.e., family) responsibility (Yeates, 1995: 18).

The impact of second-wave feminism in the 1960s and 1970s

The 1960s and 1970s were important decades in Ireland, as they were in other European countries, in terms of the development of the women's movement, which began to articulate demands that women be entitled to social welfare in their own right, and that discrimination in the labour market be outlawed. The growing influence of second-wave feminism, together with Ireland's entry to the European Community in 1973, and a movement towards left-of-centre Catholicism post-Vatican II, laid the seeds for some degree of reform.

1970 saw the establishment of the Commission on the Status of Women (renamed in 1995 the National Women's Council of Ireland), which has since provided some institutional apparatus and considerable impetus for reform (Smyth, 1993). Meanwhile, single-issue lobbying groups pointed up the contradiction between the 'punishment' model still used by the Catholic Church in relation to 'fallen women', and the Constitution's statement of the value of motherhood. Unmarried mothers in the 1950s and 1960s were often 'confined' (sometimes for many years) in special 'homes' run by Catholic religious orders and 'encouraged' to give up their babies for adoption. In 1970 a major conference was held on the position of single mothers – the Kilkenny Conference on the 'Unmarried Mother in the Irish Community' (Cherish, 1974: 34). The subsequent 1974 conference on 'The Unmarried Parent and Child in Irish Society' was introduced by Mary Robinson, then President of Cherish (a secular voluntary organization formed to promote and protect the interests of single mothers and their children), and now President of the Republic of Ireland.

However, single mothers presented the Irish Government with a problem because the reverence for motherhood in the Constitution referred of course to married motherhood – as was more obvious in the associated male-breadwinner/female-home-maker model of the social welfare and taxation systems. The Constitution was clear that the family unit should be nurtured and given every support intact, and the government therefore regarded themselves as caught in a difficult position: by offering more support to single mothers, they might be accused of undermining the sanctity of marriage and the traditional family unit, and therefore of contributing to a breakdown in family values. The result was an ambiguous position for single mothers: they were accorded certain priority in their role as 'mothers' because as such the Constitution demanded that they be provided for, but they also presented a threat to dominate social and moral codes:

> these children [of unmarried mothers] were regarded as representing a threat to the social structure of marriage.
> (Patrick Cooney, TD, cited in Cherish, 1974: 6)

However, the Catholic Church, reacting to the introduction of the 1967 Abortion Act in Britain (which indirectly provided those Irish women who could afford to travel access to abortion facilities), was anxious to see that single women who proceeded with a pregnancy rather than terminating it, would be 'rewarded' in some way (Conroy Jackson, 1993). The result was the introduction of a range of benefits for single mothers which were presented as expressions of the Constitutional commitment (Article 41) to provide the material means which would allow mothers to stay at home rearing their children rather than attempting to find paid work (Millar et al. 1992: 56). More generalized demands by the women's movement for women's access to social welfare in their own right, and hence a reduced or absent role for the male-breadwinner principle, were thus responded to through reform which firmly retained sexual difference and the male-breadwinner principle as the basis of provision. Similarly, there was no change in the strategic role the Church occupied in the delivery of education, health and social services.

The range of status-based benefits targeted at the various categories of single mothers which were introduced included a Deserted Wife's Allowance (1970), a Deserted Wife's Benefit (1973), Prisoner's Wife's Benefit (1974) and, most significantly of all, Unmarried Mother's Benefit (1973). Through these benefits single mothers who were not 'blameless' widows, gained entitlements in their own right within the mainstream, centralized, social welfare system, rather than the previous Poor Law-inspired system of locally administered social assistance. No time limits were imposed on receipt of any of these benefits – the assumption was that recipients should be full-time mothers for all of their children's lives (i.e., up to age 18) (McCashin, 1993: 59).

Through the introduction of Deserted Wife's Benefit, Ireland became unique in social welfare terms in defining one specific kind of marital breakdown as an insurable contingency in the same way as unemployment, sickness, etc. (McDevitt, 1987). The uniqueness of Ireland's recognition of this form of marital breakdown was, however, made possible by one of Ireland's other unique features – the absence of divorce legislation. This meant that the size of the risk was assumed to be much less than would be the case in countries with divorce. In addition, Deserted Wife's Allowance and Benefit were in fact targeted at two different groups: a) older wives, and b) younger wives only in so far as they were mothers, since women under 40 had to have at least one dependent child in order to qualify. Only women who had been 'deserted' by their husbands were eligible – those women who had separated (or divorced in other countries) were not. Husbands must have left the home for a minimum time of three months. The 'deserted' woman must not receive maintenance from the husband, but had to prove that 'reasonable' efforts had been made to secure maintenance.

The nature of the new provision posed a number of problems. Firstly, 'desertion' was difficult to prove. It required social welfare officers to make judgements about the nature and cause of marital breakdowns, a process which not unexpectedly resulted in a high number of refusals and appeals. The courts were given the responsibility of reviewing evidence about people's personal lives in the course of appeals against failed claims. Secondly, the system continued a principle of unequal treatment for 'deserving' and 'undeserving' single mothers – the 'deserving' being those women who had been abandoned by their husbands and the 'undeserving' those who had agreed to separate and who participated in the breakdown of the marriage. Yeates therefore argues that the emergence of the category of desertion in its own right in the 1970s benefits (as opposed to its earlier administrative use as a way of determining eligibility for social assistance), not only strengthened the male-breadwinner model by institutionalizing different categories of single mothers, but also 'sexualized' social welfare in so far as women applicants had to prove their sexual and moral innocence as a precondition of claiming their rights to state support (Yeates, 1995: 23).

The tension between the women's movement's increasingly vocal discourse of equal rights for women and a state built upon the male-breadwinner/ female-home-maker model was also evident in the difficulties surrounding Ireland's entry to the European Community at this time. In 1973 the Irish Government sent a delegation to Brussels to seek to obtain a derogation from Article 119 (equal pay) of the Treaty of Rome upon its imminent membership of the European Community. The demand was refused by the other Member States, and the Irish Government reluctantly and slowly had to introduce limited measures towards implementation of the various Equality Directives – a process which has extended over the whole of the 1970s, 1980s and early 1990s (Mahon, 1995) (for further discussion, see section 4 below).

New divisions in the 1980s and 1990s

During the 1980s and early 1990s, women's groups have increasingly turned to EU institutions and legislation in their political efforts to reform social policies, especially those in the area of reproductive rights (Mahon, 1995). At home, too, the Supreme Court has begun to make some interpretations of the 1937 Constitution which support liberalization. Thus it was Supreme Court decisions in the early 1970s and in 1985 which permitted the use and sale of contraceptives in Ireland, while a Supreme Court decision in 1992 overruled a High Court judgement that a 14-year-old girl could not travel to Britain for an abortion, confirming that Irish citizens, as EU citizens, had the right to travel to avail themselves of medical services in other countries. However while the Catholic Church has increasingly given its blessing to state efforts to resolve economic problems by applying modified neo-liberal economic principles, it has been less prepared to condone any liberalization of state policies which it views as threatening to family life (McLaughlin, 1993: 225). The result is that conservative and liberal social forces, and increasingly Church and state, have clashed over the status of women in Irish society. It is this conflict, rather than mass unemployment, poverty or any other of the crises which have beset the post-colonial Irish state, which has in recent decades threatened to traumatize Irish society and destablize the state.

In the early 1980s constitutional referenda on abortion (1983) and divorce (1985) both resulted in victories for the conservative options. Meaney claimed that the Constitutional amendments following from the 1983 abortion referendum, recognizing the 'equal right to life of the unborn child', showed:

the extent to which women only exist as a function of their maternity
in the dominant ideology of southern Ireland.

(1993: 3)

In relation to divorce, opinion polls prior to the 1985 referendum had
suggested a clear majority in favour of permitting divorce. However anti-
divorce campaign groups – many sponsored by the Church (e.g. 'Family
Solidarity') – used statistics about the poverty of single-parent families in the
USA as an example of what could happen to Irish women if divorce were
introduced. It is also true that the referendum took place at what appears to
have been the early stages of a very considerable shift in public attitudes
throughout the 1980s and the early 1990s (the same period in which there was
such a considerable rise in single motherhood).

Ten years after the first divorce referendum, in a second referendum on 24
November 1995, 50.4 per cent voted in favour of the introduction of limited
divorce legislation, and 49.6 per cent against. Again there had been vigorous
anti-divorce campaigning, much of it involving various Catholic groups, and
both the Pope and Mother Theresa urged the people of Ireland to reject
divorce legislation. The legislation which was proposed in the referendum was
limited to couples who had been separated for four years, where there was no
prospect of reconciliation, and where adequate financial provision had been
made for spouses and children (scheduled to take effect from February 1996).
The narrow 'yes' vote was subject to judicial review by the Supreme Court
which has since decided to uphold the referendum result.

Turning to more general attitudes on gender roles and family life, Fine-
Davis' (1988) studies looked at attitudes from 1975 up to 1986. A noticeable
shift towards more egalitarian attitudes was in evidence by 1986 (see Table
2.4). The item which showed the greatest shift was 'Being a wife and mother
are the most fulfilling roles any woman could want' – 70 per cent of people
agreed with this in 1975 compared to just 39 per cent in 1986.

Fine-Davis (1988: 92) argued that as more and more married women and
mothers enter the workforce, the already increasing acceptance of maternal
employment will grow further. However, the gap between men's and women's
attitudes has also grown. The continued absence of supportive social policies,
such as publicly funded child-care services, means that women may find it
difficult in practice to combine employment with mothering large families.
Some degree of resolution may occur through reductions in fertility and indeed
fertility in Ireland has halved over the past 25 years – compared with a decline
of one-third in the whole of Europe. Irish fertility levels by 1992 were only
fractionally higher than in the UK, and lower than in Norway and Sweden.
However, attitudinal studies do continue to show both Irish women and men
continuing to place a very high value on family life and child rearing, and it is
unclear how much 'resolution' will be achieved through reductions in fertility.

In summary, despite the real divisions which exist at the level of discourse,
Irish people, especially Irish women, have been 'voting with their feet'

Statements	1975	1986
	(% agreeing)	
Being a wife and mother are the most fulfilling roles any woman could want	70	39
The husband ought to have the main say in family matters	50	25
It is bad for young children for their mothers to go out to work	68	46
Women should be more concerned with housekeeping and bringing up their children than careers	59	38
Women with children should not work outside the home if they don't need the money	55	49
When there is high unemployment, married women should be discouraged from working	65	51
Women who do not want at least one child are selfish	*	48
Women should take care of running their homes and leave running the country to men	*	22
Working mothers can establish just as warm and secure a relationship with their children as non-working mothers	*	65

Note * not asked in 1975
Source Fine-Davis (1988)
Table 2.4 Public attitudes to the family and women's position: Republic of Ireland, 1975 and 1986

throughout the 1980s and early 1990s. As section 2 showed, rates of marital breakdown and the proportions of births outside marriage have risen dramatically in the late 1980s and early 1990s, while overall fertility levels have decreased markedly, and support for a 'mothers *and* workers' approach has grown.

Contemporary feminisms

As previously discussed, dominant discourses surrounding motherhood and mothers' role in Ireland have their roots in nationalism-Catholicism. Whether the ideology of nationalism is inherently anithetical to equality for women remains a prime focus for debate between Irish feminists. Meaney (1993) argues that the intertwining of concepts of sexual and national identity are common to all former colonized countries. She draws comparison between colonizers' attitudes towards colonized people and those of the same societies' treatment of women. The characteristics alleged (by their colonizers) to be characteristic of colonized people – passivity, a need for guidance, romantic, unruly, incapable of self-government – have, it is argued, been transferred on to women in ex-colonized countries. In claiming independence, a subject people aspire to a traditionally masculine form and model of power, and so after colonization, colonized peoples (in practice, men) impose strictly differentiated gender roles. In the Irish case, the symbolic importance of 'Mother Ireland' means that 'We have apostrophised the country itself as mother' (Mary Holland writing in *The Irish Times*, cited in McWilliams, 1993: 83).

Women are not merely regarded as symbols of the nation but are objects within the power struggle, becoming part of the territory to be won over and ruled (Meaney, 1991: 7). As such, control of women's bodies and the governance of their sexuality are especially critical in nationalist struggles and in post-colonial 'new state' establishment:

> Women's sexuality is used as a pawn in men's power games, and classically so in struggles over 'ownership' of national territory. Trojan women, constantly reconstructed. Symbols, functions, and instruments of the nation, guarantors of its legitimacy, reproducers of its destiny, targets and prizes for its enemies. Women's bodies are national property. . . . As I understand them, through the prism of the history and contemporary reality of the state I inhabit, feminism and nationalism are antagonistic practices.
>
> (Smyth 1994: 16, 33)

It would be wrong to suggest that all Irish feminists are of the opinion that nationalism and feminism cannot co-exist. Feminism in Ireland is not homogenous and tensions and contradictions exist within the movement (McWilliams, 1993: 93), with divisions very often focused around whether the modern feminist 'interrogation of nationalism' (Meaney, 1993) involves an implicit or explicit devaluation of motherhood and other caring work. Whatever the 'truth' of nationalism in the past, others argue that it is possible to integrate feminist and republican nationalism in Ireland's future. Certainly it is true that feminists in Ireland must respect the value that women themselves, as well as men, have and do attach to motherhood and family (McWilliams, 1993). However, Irish women increasingly appear less than impressed by 'a rhetoric of martyrdom in the name of a manifestly male common good', and are refusing to be the keepers of a national culture which reduces them to silent symbols (Smyth, 1994: 32). The election of Mary Robinson as President, a woman who has consistently opposed the conservative version of Irish womanhood, indicates that that version no longer holds the same appeal (Meaney, 1993: 5). Coulter (1994) sees it as a sign of rebirth of the women's movement, while Smyth regards it as:

> A positive vote for a new force capable of breaking the strangle-hold of the historical narratives of Ireland and Irishness. It was a vote for disruption and disturbance of the myths on which we have fed ourselves for longer than we now want to remember. . . . Exploding myths and shibboleths, she allows us to break free of constraints and to set about re-creating ourselves.
>
> (1992: 62, 73)

4. The Contemporary Irish Welfare Regime

There have been some changes in the nature of the social welfare system which reflect the growing rejection of Catholic nationalism's views on motherhood, as discussed in the last section. This can also be seen as representing a weakening of the 'strong male-breadwinner'/'Catholic corporatist' welfare regime in which women's status as citizens is focused on their family status as home-workers.

Single parents are provided for in a range of ways in the Irish social welfare system: as families with children; as poor families; and as single parents specifically (Millar et al., 1992: 40). As families with dependent children, single parents receive Child Benefit, which is paid in respect of all children regardless of family income. Rates are lower for the first three children than for the fourth and subsequent children, and since single parents tend to have fewer children than two-parent families, most receive the lower rates. In terms of tax allowances however, single parents receive double the single person's tax allowance, to 'make up' for the absence of a partner. As poor families with actual or potentially low wages, single parents may be eligible for Family Income Supplement (FIS) (similar to the UK's Family Credit). However, this has not proved successful in terms of encouraging single parents into employment. In 1990, for example, there were 6,500 recipients of FIS, of whom only 123 (2 per cent) were single.

Single parents benefits

As single parents specifically, three main forms of support are available: the Lone Parents Allowance (LPA), introduced in 1990 and received by 25,000 families with dependent children in that year (equivalent to 6 per cent of families with at least one child aged 15 or less in the 1991 Census); the Deserted Wife's Benefit (DWB), received by about 8,000 families with dependent children in 1990; the Widow's Benefit (a contributory pension), received by about 7,800 families with dependent children in 1990 (Millar et al., 1992: 38). The introduction in 1990 of the new LPA, which lifted many single mothers out of the previous array of 'women's benefits' and placed them into a new 'unified' category of single parents – that is, including lone fathers – was part of the incomplete and slow implementation of the EC 1979 Equal Treatment Directive in Ireland. The LPA was designed to bring together and replace the previous Unmarried Mother's Allowance, payments for lone fathers (widowers and deserted husbands), the Prisoner's Wife's Allowance and the Widow's Non-contributory Pension and Deserted Wife's Allowance. The benefit only applies to those with dependent children, is not available to cohabitees and is means tested. The LPA goes some way to ensuring that parents are not discriminated against on the basis of the cause of their single-parent status (McCashin, 1993: 62), but the eligiblity criteria are different for those who are separated: these single parents must have been separated for at least three months, have made reasonable efforts to get maintenance from their spouse and must not be receiving adequate maintenance.

The retention of maintenance as, in principle, the first 'port of call' for separated single parents (which in effect means separated mothers, given the differences in employment rates of mothers and fathers), together with the retention of benefits for widows and deserted wives without dependent children, and the fact that single parents, widows and deserted wives do not have to register as available for employment in order to receive social welfare benefits, all signify the extent to which the state continues to regard marriage as the main means of economic survival for women. In the absence of a husband, the state will step in as surrogate financial provider. Such provision is then framed in one of two ways: firstly, while women have dependent children it is assumed that they will be at home full-time; and secondly, it is assumed that women who have had dependent children in the past (and hence have been at home full-time) will not have the capacity to support themselves later in life, in the event of marital breakdown or death of the spouse.

Child-care provision

As discussed above the assumption that mothers in Ireland will not be in paid work is also obvious in the lack of publicly funded child-care provision. Ireland still has little publicly funded child care and non-publicly funded child-care provision is scarce (especially outside middle class areas) as well as expensive. Workplace creches are a rarity – only 240 Irish children were known to be in workplace creches in the late 1980s (Daly, 1989). Philips and Moss found that 2 per cent or less of under-three-year-olds received publicly funded services, and just under half of children between three and school age were in pre-primary or early primary schooling (usually for very short periods per day). They go on to point out that:

> In Ireland there are not publicly funded 'outside school hours care' facilities. . . . Ireland and the UK are the only countries with government policies which do not consider children of employed parents to be a priority group for admission to publicly-funded services.
>
> (cited in Millar et al., 1992: 60)

Disincentives

A number of studies have also shown that there are disincentive effects in relation to paid employment from the nature of social welfare payments (WRC, 1992; Magee, 1994; NCOPF, 1995). DWB and Widow's Benefit (i.e., provision for ex-married women who no longer have dependent children) are not means tested, and therefore the level of earnings of recipients of these benefits does not affect their welfare benefits. However, the LPA is means tested so that income from employment is taken into account when benefit payment is made. There is an income disregard of just £6 per week and an earnings disregard of £6 per child per week, which combined gives a minimum earnings disregard of £12 per week for single parents on LPA. In addition, 'reasonable allowance' may be made for the costs of working, such as child-minding and travel costs (Millar et al., 1992; 61), though whether these provisions are widely known to single mothers is debateable. In September 1991, only 9 per cent of those receiving LPA were receiving reduced payments, indicating possible receipt of income from employment.

In recognition of these possible disincentive effects, the budget of January 1994 introduced two significant changes: an increase in the income disregard to £30, and a reduction of LPA by 50p (rather than a pound) against any further £1 earned; clearer and enhanced provision to off-set travel costs to and from work, and child-minding expenses against earned income. These represent clear improvements in faciliating part-time paid employment among single mothers. At the lowest levels of gross pay the impact will greatly improve the financial gains from part-time employment for single mothers on social welfare. These positive steps in relation to facilitating combinations of paid part-time work with benefit receipt for single parents seem to suggest that government may be gradually moving away from policies which prevent women from taking up employment:

> policy is now shifting towards facilitating, if not encouraging labour market participation.
>
> (McCashin 1995: 181)

However, McCashin's recent study (1995: 138) showed that single mothers on the whole still perceived that they would be worse off financially if they were working, and suggests that the changes are neither fully understood nor widely known.

The overall context remains one where, notwithstanding adjustments to means-tested benefits to allow some earnings, and the gradual extension of active labour market provision to single parents as well as unemployed people:

> Ireland's policies, viewed comparatively, [remain] somewhat extreme in their assumption and re-enforcement of dependence.
>
> (McCashin 1993: 82)

This is due to the lack of affordable child care, the poor labour market status of women generally compared with men, the assumption of non-participation in the labour market for mothers generally in the fiscal system, and eligibility for social welfare payments without time limit for all single parents without requirements to register for paid work.

5. Lone Mothers in Labour Markets

Women's employment and national employment policy

Ireland has the lowest rate of economic activity in the European Union for mothers with dependent children in two-parent families – just 31 per cent in 1989. This compares with rates of over 60 or 70 per cent in most other EU countries (Roll, 1992: 18). Given the explicit policy aim of reducing mothers' employment accompanying the 1937 Constitution (see section 3 above), this is not surprising. Both social and economic policy in the post-1937 era were consciously geared towards the twin objectives of promoting economic development and the reproduction of male-breadwinner/female-home-maker familial relations (Pyle, 1990). Given that the Irish state opted for an export-led development strategy in terms of economic policy (Breen et al., 1990), and that this usually involves increases in the use of female labour, efforts had to be made to prevent an increase in the participation of women in the labour force. Accordingly, economic and social criteria for evaluating proposed industrial projects and for awarding financial incentives were developed, and included an explicit statement regarding the preferred gender composition of the work-force of incoming projects. Industrial Development Agency reports from as late as the 1970s stressed that the IDA wished to fund proposals which would employ at least 75 per cent men (McLaughlin, 1993: 226). This policy is one reason why the proportion of the labour force who were women rose from 9 to only 15 per cent between 1946 and 1961 (Yeates, 1995: 13).

In the 1970s and 1980s, Ireland's membership of the European Union forced the gradual and reluctant abandonment of such policies. The marriage bar was removed, relatively weak employment equality legislation was introduced, and a maternity allowance for employed women was finally introduced in 1981. By the late 1970s the policy of attempting to influence investors' workforce composition in favour of men was under great pressure and was effectively abandoned (Pyle, 1990). These changes were associated with an increase in women's, and especially married women's, labour-force participation: married women's participation increased from 7.5 to 19.5 per cent between 1971 and 1984, with a much bigger increase among younger married women (25–34 year olds), from 8.8 to 26.9 per cent (Fine-Davis, 1988). Nevertheless the legacy of five decades of discouragement of women, especially mothers, from working outside the home is that by 1988, less than one-third (31 per cent) of Irish women were in the labour force (Millar et al., 1992: 31), while 53 per cent were classified in the 'home duties' category. Single mothers of course share this constrained position, as discussed in section 2, with low levels of employment.

Mothers and workers? The introduction of active labour market measures

Attempts to improve employment rates among single mothers in recent years have included changes in the social security system to promote part-time work among single mothers – noted in section 4 above. In addition, in July 1993 the Minister for Social Welfare announced a number of measures to enhance the educational opportunities for single parents and subsequently their employment chances. However the extent of these measures was small in terms of public expenditure, with £100,000 made available in 1993–94 and £200,000 in 1994–95, to fund projects specifically designed to help young single parents get back into education (Magee, 1994). Another step has been the allocation of vocational training opportunities to single parents over the age of 21 (who did not previously qualify), while single parents who enter higher education may now retain their social welfare payments – a provision which had previously been available to registered unemployed claimants only. There is therefore a very recent gradual drawing together of active labour market policies for single parents with those for unemployed people. However it is unclear how successful this strategy can be, given the absence of public support for child-care services and more general attitudes favouring full-time motherhood. As McCashin says:

> the role of the social security system per se in shaping the labour market decisions of single parents must be set in a wider familial, social and institutional context. The potential inefficiency of the labour supply effect of the poverty trap in Ireland is best considered, therefore, not merely as a technical issue affecting the tax/benefit/ social security nexus, but as a wider issue concerning the social and institutional obstacles facing lower income women with children in their attempts to take up paid employment.
>
> (1993: 97)

Sub-national labour markets

The most important sub-national differences in labour markets occur between urban and rural areas (see also the discussion of urban/rural differences in section 6 below). Unemployment rates are generally higher in Ireland than in most other European countries (e.g. unemployment rose from 6.9 per cent in April 1979 to 16.7 per cent in April 1988), but unemployment seems to be a particularly significant feature of the experience of younger urban single mothers in Ireland – which is also the group of single mothers which has increased most (see below). On the other hand, it is easy to underestimate unemployment and underemployment in rural areas because of traditional inadequacies in counting and defining work on and in family enterprises, and no studies have been undertaken of the experiences of single mothers in rural Ireland.

In terms of urban women's experiences, employment rates fell from 42 per cent to 37 per cent among unmarried women delivered in the National Maternity Hospital in Dublin in just two years. In 1988, 37 per cent of unmarried mothers delivered in the National Maternity Hospital in Dublin were employed, 55 per cent unemployed, and 7 per cent in education (Donohoe et al., 1990: 23). In 1986 the figure for employment had been 42 per cent. Both Donohoe et al.'s and O'Hare's (1983) studies showed that never-married mothers were heavily concentrated in the semi-skilled and unskilled manual groups, and thus particularly vulnerable to unemployment. In O'Hare's study, 55 per cent of unmarried mothers belonged to the semi- and unskilled manual groups, compared with 25 per cent of women nationally, according to the 1981 Census of Population. It is this group of young, single, usually never-married, low-skilled mothers in urban areas, which has been the focus of recent government policy initiatives around education and employment.

6. Single Mothers in Neighbourhoods

Urban–rural differences

Single motherhood is probably a very different experience in urban than in rural areas in Ireland. Although no studies have been undertaken of the experiences of single mothers in rural areas (and indeed very few studies of rural women's experiences in general), it would be reasonable to assume that neighbourhoods containing very few single mothers, especially those in more traditional and conservative rural areas, are experienced as less supportive than those with more. It is clear that a considerable divide has developed between rural and urban areas in rates of single, especially unmarried, motherhood. Table 2.5 shows the extent of urban–rural variation in births outside marriage,with all those local government areas having above average rates also containing conurbations and cities, while those having low rates being primarily rural. O'Hare (1983) also found urban–rural differences in cohabitation and numbers of previous non-marital births. Higher proportions of women from the Eastern and Southern Health Board areas, containing the large conurbations of Dublin and Cork respectively, were cohabiting and/or had had previous non-marital births than in other health board areas.

In addition, attitudinal studies have found the biggest differences in attitudes in relation to gender roles and family issues to be between rural and urban groups, with rural groups, as well as older people, showing more traditional attitudes. Fine-Davis (1988: 92) argued that as more and more married women and mothers enter the workforce, the already increased acceptance of maternal employment will grow, but clearly this will not be an

	% of total births
Areas above national average	
Dublin County Borough	32.6
Limerick County Borough	29.5
Waterford County Borough	24.0
Cork County Borough	21.6
Dublin Belgard	16.6
Wicklow	16.1
Tipperary SR	15.9
D'leary Rathdown	15.6
Wexford	15.6
Louth	15.5
Galway County Borough	14.9
Areas below national average	
Monaghan	6.4
Galway County	6.5
Mayo	5.7
Roscommon	4.7
Leitrim	0.3
National average	14.6

Source Magee (1994: 5)
Table 2.5   Regional variations in births outside marriage: Republic of Ireland, 1990

'even' process given urban–rural as well as male–female attitudinal differences. The importance of such differences was underlined by the recent referendum on divorce. Although the national verdict was very slightly in favour (50.4 versus 49.4 per cent), 26 out of the 40 parliamentary constituencies are thought to have voted against divorce. The strongest 'yes' vote was in Dublin, where areas of high unemployment and urban deprivation (containing high proportions of single-mother families) appeared to have returned particularly high 'yes' votes. The narrowness of the overall result demonstrates the divide that now exists between urban, especially working-class, and rural conservative Ireland.

Single mothers' own views

A number of studies of single mothers' experiences have been undertaken in Ireland but these studies have usually taken place in Dublin, predominantly in large public housing estates where single mothers have become a significant visible group (see e.g. WRC, 1992). The growing concentration of single mothers in urban areas of poor environmental quality is partly the result of a reduction in recurrent expenditure on public housing (McLaughlin, 1993: 221). Recurrent expenditure fell from 8.4 per cent to 5.8 per cent between 1971 and 1981, and capital spending halved between 1982 and 1987. The deterioration in housing conditions experienced by those at the bottom end of the housing market in recent years in Ireland has thus disproportionately affected poor women. and even within this group, low-income single mothers have experienced the worst disadvantage as they are given low priority status by local authorities and are allocated the worst public authority housing.

Poor housing together with low weekly income, caused by low employment rates and low social security benefit levels, mean that most studies of single mothers in these areas are dominated by single mothers' experiences of poverty. The 'Parenting Alone in West Tallaght' study, for example, found that two-thirds of single mothers had debts which were causing them serious difficulty and worry, while 63 per cent felt socially isolated and 35 per cent said they were finding it impossible to make ends meet (WRC, 1992: 20). McCashin's 1995 study also found that levels of personal consumption were very low and that most single mothers could not afford things which many other people take for granted such as books, a weekend away, new clothes, and a social life. Such feelings are well described in one single mother's words (a widow with nine children, and an income of £110 per week):

> Being frightened every time a stranger pulls up outside the door. A strange car means trouble, and trouble means money.
> Being labelled a waster, or a sponger, especially when it is said to the kids.
> Planning bank raids in my head.
> Feeling irritable.
> Feeling inadequate.
> Planning every detail of my life, the fridge, the money, yet knowing the smallest thing can throw it off balance.

However, McCashin's recent study (1995) also highlighted positive elements in the experiences of single mothers (in Coolock, Dublin):

> Women were virtually unanimous in their view that poverty and deprivation were the worst aspects of being a lone mother. However they placed their difficult financial circumstances in the context of their lives as a whole. Lone motherhood also brought with it the experience of greater independence. Separated women placed great emphasis on the freedom and independence they enjoyed. . . . Single women also experience a distinct sense of independence . . . they see their single status as something to be appreciated and not lightly to be given up. . . . The accounts of their involvement with their children show that the children are accepted into a loving, welcoming context, that they are extensively involved in caring for the children, and that they see this as an important and enjoyable task. [Though] they also acknowledge the physical and emotional demands that their children make on them.
>
> (McCashin, 1995: xiii)

None of the single mothers in McCashin's study reported overt discriminatory behaviour against them and their children in their neighbourhood, though a small number referred to some possible instances where they might have been treated differently as a result of their status. The majority had very good relationships with their own families of origin, receiving gifts and cash support, as well as some babysitting services if they and their family of origin were living nearby. Although very few of the single mothers were in paid work, almost all had a positive orientation to paid work, although this was regarded as subordinate, or subject, to the needs of children. A desire to further establish independence strengthened women's positive approach to work or to training – in this case, independence from their own parents and family, and independence from benefits. But against this single mothers had to weight up what they saw as the needs of their children to have a considerable amount of care directly from them, and the difficulties of obtaining substitute child-care services reliably and cheaply (and without undue dependence on their families of origin).

The need for appropriate, high-quality, inexpensive child-care services, together with work and training patterns which facilitate continued considerable inputs of child care from the mother herself, has emerged from most studies of single mothers in urban Ireland. A recent report on teenage parents (Magee, 1994) found that many teenage mothers find it difficult to move out of a situation of dependency on welfare because a lack of state subsidized child care means they cannot access training, still less paid work. Another study indicated that the majority of single mothers would like to enter training courses to improve their employment opportunities, but a large number of them (29 per cent) could not do so due to child-minding responsibilities (WRC, 1992). A report on the experiences of women in a small working-class neighbourhood in Dublin also commented on the difficulty that single parents have accessing employment: in addition to the shortage of jobs, a serious lack of creche and child-care facilities prevent women from having access to work (O'Neill, 1992: 45).

Single mothers' attitudes to paid work reflect a more general increase in Irish women's positive attitude towards employment for mothers. This has not occurred to the same extent among men. In 1987, Ireland was one of only three European countries where a majority of married men preferred their wives not to work (Gardiner, 1992: 72); one of the others was Germany, see chapter 7, this volume). In addition, single mothers, like married mothers in Ireland, continue to place a high value on motherhood and family life. Ireland is still strongly child-centred: a European study by Harding in 1989, for example, found that 51 per cent of the Irish sample favoured a family of four or five children (cited in Gardiner 1992: 70) and 46 per cent believed that 'women who do not want at least one child are selfish'. The result is that there has been some shift in women's own views away from a 'mothers not workers' towards a 'mothers *and* workers' approach. However, both married and single mothers find it difficult to translate that approach into practice in the absence of supportive social policies.

7. Conclusions

Summary

Since the late 1980s, Ireland has experienced a rapid rise in single motherhood. By 1991, one in ten families with children under 15 were single-parent families, and 83 per cent of these were headed by single mothers. The rise is partly the result of increases in marital separation and partly a rise in the proportions of births occurring outside of marriage, with the latter heavily concentrated among younger women. In terms of sex, age and number of children, Irish single mothers are not very different from single mothers in other countries, but they do differ in two important respects. Firstly until 1996 the absence of divorce cut off an important route out of single motherhood (i.e. remarriage). Secondly employment rates among single mothers are low, though they are almost equally low for mothers in two-parent families (at about 18 per cent working full-time). Both of these factors mean that single mothers in Ireland experience high probabilities and rates of poverty.

The policy environment surrounding single mothers has been deeply affected by the approach taken to motherhood generally. The 1937 Constitution prescribed a 'private' sphere for mothers and married women, and was accompanied by economic and social policies structured around the male-breadwinner/female-home-maker model, despite considerable resistance from Irish feminists. The reasons for this are complex and much debated. It may be partly the result of the nature of the integration of post-independence Ireland into the global economic order, itself structured by Ireland's economic relationship with Britain. It is also in part due to the historical legacy of the 'gender categorical approach' of the nineteenth-century Poor Law, which Ireland shared with Britain. It is also, however, the result of the development of Irish nationalism and the special nature of the role played by the Catholic Church in the development of the Irish welfare regime, both before and after constitutional independence from Britain in 1922. The Church has remained a key political actor in the development of social policies, and in addition delivers many social welfare provisions. This has had particular implications for mothers because of the lack of development of child-care services.

Ireland's membership of the European Union in the early 1970s, together with the development of second-wave feminism, led to a number of important, if incomplete, economic and social policy reforms. These included the introduction of special status-based social security benefits targeted at the various categories of single mothers who had until the 1970s relied on social assistance – deserted and prisoners' wives and unmarried mothers. These benefits were available without time limit or requirement to be available for work.

The 1980s and 1990s have been a time of considerable upheaval in social attitudes to gender roles and family issues in Ireland, with growing divisions evident between men and women and urban and rural areas. Unmarried motherhood is low in rural compared with urban areas and it is is difficult to say whether women in rural areas share the increasingly common positive attitude to mothers' employment evident in the general population. Irish women as a whole seem now to be attempting to reconcile a positive attitude to employment with the traditional high value attached to (relatively) high fertility, motherhood and family life. More liberal attitudes to family issues such as divorce and contraception culminated in the narrow vote in favour of the introduction of limited divorce legislation in 1995. On the other hand, maintenance has been retained as the first 'port of call' for separated single parents, publicly funded child-care provision remains nearly non-existent, and there have been only limited reforms to social security benefits so as to encourage some degree of part-time, but not full-time, work among single mothers.

Not surprisingly, Ireland continues to have the lowest employment and economic activity rates for mothers in two-parent and single-parent families in the European Union, though some of this is attributable to the presence of young children in a high proportion of households coupled with the absence of pre-school child-care provision. Employment is particularly low among unmarried younger single mothers in urban areas. This group has recently been targeted by some limited measures designed to enhance educational and training opportunities (and hence future employment rates). However, the absence of publicly funded child-care services continues to make the uptake of such opportunities difficult and the majority of single parents continue to live in poverty. Single mothers themselves, however, weigh this deprivation against the gains they experience in terms of personal independence. Most single mothers, in urban areas at least, see paid work as an important route to yet further independence, but wish to combine flexible forms of work with a relatively high child-care contribution by themselves, and limited use of high-quality, inexpensive substitute child-care (which, as pointed out above, is rarely available).

Mothers and workers? The potential for reform

Both McCashin (1995) and Millar et al. (1992) argue that it would be inappropriate for Ireland to attempt to move quickly towards a model based on single mothers as workers, and that further development of the current 'mixed model' system would be better. Both argue that to require all single parents to register to seek employment before they could receive any benefits in a country with high levels of unemployment and scarce job opportunities (particularly for women) would be a retrograde step. Clearly high levels of unemployment set considerable constraints on any attempts to move from a model based on single mothers as full-time mothers to one based on single mothers as workers. Equally it would be wrong to move to an employment-based system until the necessary supports were in place – pre-eminently child-care provision. Finally, rapid movement to an employment-based system would be problematic in so far as it would not take into account the impact that Ireland's history and past social welfare regime has had in forming mothers' attitudes. Thus most women positively value staying at home full-time while their children are young, and working part-time and in other flexible ways when their children are older, as shown clearly in McCashin's recent study (1995).

This is not to deny the evidence that single parents have a higher standard of living in countries where they are more likely to be employed than in those where they have relied heavily on social welfare (Bradshaw and Millar, 1991; Hardey and Crow, 1991; Millar et al., 1992). However, the labour market in Ireland differs greatly from that of other EU countries, and as a result, enthusiasm for employment-driven approaches in social welfare need to be tempered by realism. For all of these reasons, further development of a mixed model which would facilitate real choice on the part of single mothers – allowing women to make their own judgements about how their children should be reared, while increasing job, education and training opportunities for those who wish to access them – would be more appropriate in Ireland than attempts to import the approaches some other countries have adopted to single motherhood (see, e.g., chapter 9, this volume, on Sweden).

Understanding and evaluating welfare regimes

In terms of understanding the development of welfare regimes, the case of Ireland is instructive in that it highlights the way historical links between countries and the practice of 'regime shopping' have been important aspects in the formation and development of gendered welfare regimes in Europe. This leads to the question of the extent to which any one country's welfare regime can be regarded as a purely national product (cf. Yeates, 1995: 33). It would be wrong, however, to conceptualize processes of importation and exportation in terms of 'backward' countries retaining 'old-fashioned' or 'traditional' social welfare systems, which they had imported from other countries' earlier welfare regimes, where the latter have since reformed or abandoned such exported systems in favour of new more 'progressive' systems. This is wrong partly because what constitutes 'progressive' and 'regressive' welfare regimes is far from clear. At one end of the continuum of welfare regimes and their organizing principles lies universalism, which is assumed in some sense to be the opposite of gender-categorical systems, lying at the other end of the scale. Universalism however can often hide and subsume the significance of gender within apparently gender-neutral terms and models, and the failure of apparently universal and 'weak' male-breadwinner systems to deliver gender equality has been widely noted (Langan and Ostner, 1991). Meanwhile, gender-categorical and 'strong' male-breadwinner systems, such as that of Ireland, 'up-front' premises of sexual difference, and, as a result, may be seen by some women themselves to value the social reproductive work of mother-ing, philosophically if not materially, in a way that other systems do not. Given these complexities, evaluations of welfare regimes must take into account the extent to which these two extremes are capable of (a) responding to womens' changing definitions of themselves and (b) accommodating differences between women in terms of their aspirations, values and goals.

Secondly, the 'backward/progressive' and 'importer/exporter' views of cross-national social welfare development ignore the way in which the formation and development of modern nation-states and their social welfare systems has depended on the positions of the various nation-states within the global economic order. This is significant for two reasons: first, the different positions of nation-states in the global, or even European, economic order imply very different opportunities for employment for men and women (mothers or not). In the case of Ireland, this also means low levels of employment. Secondly, different experiences of colonialism, neo-colonialism and imperialism affect the ways in which gender is incorporated into 'national' social welfare systems. 'Maternalist' policies have been fundamental to the formation of all modern European nation-states (Koven and Michel, 1993), in different ways and with different manifestations in different countries. But in the case of Ireland, the creation of nationhood came considerably later (the 1920s) and as the result of politically violent struggle. 'Mother Ireland' is the outcome of all these factors.

Notes

1 In November 1995 a referendum was held on whether provision should be made for divorce and this was carried by a narrow margin; see section 4 below.
2 Prior to 1845, about one-third (2.3 million, according to the Poor Law Commis-sioners of 1835) of the 8 million Irish population were dependent for survival on a single staple crop – the potato. This rose to nine-tenths of the population in the extreme west. Over a quarter of the Irish population at this time spent part of the year in a state of semi-starvation. Famine was a regular occurrence (e.g. in 1800, 1817 and 1822) but the famine of 1845–49 was the worst because crop failure was more extensive and over time a higher proportion of the population had become totally dependant on the potato. While increasing volumes of cereals and meat were exported from Ireland, about 1 million died of starvation. Famine deaths and emigration reduced the population by 25 per cent in the six years 1845–50, and 'as a direct result of the famine the population of Ireland was almost halved in twenty years' (Kee, 1976: 258).

References

BARRINGTON, R. (1987) *Health, Medicine and Politics in Ireland: 1900–1970*, Dublin: Institute of Public Administration.

BRADSHAW, J. and MILLAR, J. (1991) *Single Parents in the UK*, London: HMSO.

BREEN, R., HANNAN, D., ROTTMAN, D. and WHELAN, C. (1990) *Understanding Contemporary Ireland: State, Class and Development in the Republic of Ireland*, Dublin: Gill & Macmillan.

BURKE, H. (1987) *The People and the Poor Law in Nineteenth Century Ireland*, Littlehampton: WEB.

CALLAN, T., NOLAN, B., WHELAN, C., HANNAN, D. and CREIGHTON, S. (1989) *Poverty, Income and Welfare in Ireland*, Dublin: The Economic and Social Research Institute, General Research Series, Paper no. 146.

CARNEY, C. (1994) *The Cost of a Child*, Dublin: Combat Poverty Agency.

CHERISH (1974) *Report of a Conference on the Unmarried Parent and Child in Irish Society*, Dublin: Cherish.

COMMISSION OF THE EUROPEAN COMMUNITIES (1993) *Mothers, Fathers and Employment 1985–1991*, Brussels: DG V. B. 4, Equal Opportunities Unit.

CONROY JACKSON, P. (1993) 'Managing the mothers: the case of Ireland' in Lewis, J. (Ed.) *Women and Social Policies in Europe. Work, Family and the State*, Aldershot: Edward Elgar.

COOK, G. (1983) 'The growth and development of the social security system in the Republic of Ireland', *Social Studies*, 7, 2, pp. 127–42.

COOGAN, T. P. (1993) *De Valera: Long Fellow, Short Shadow*, London: Hutchinson.

COULTER, C. (1994) *The Hidden Tradition: Feminism, Women and Nationalism in Ireland*, Cork: Cork University Press.

COURTNEY, D. (1995) 'Demographic structure and change in the Republic of Ireland and Northern Ireland' in Clancy, P., Drudy, S., Lynch, K. and O'Dowd, L. (Eds) *Irish Society: Sociological Perspectives*, pp. 35–89, Dublin: Institute of Public Administration

CURRY, J. (1993) *The Irish Social Services*, 3rd Edn, Dublin: Institute of Public Administration.

DALY, M. (1989) *Women and Poverty*, Dublin: Attic Press.

DONNELLY, A. (1993) *Gender and the Law in Ireland*, Dublin: Oak Tree Press.

DONOHOE, J., FITZPATRICK, A., FLANAGAN, N. AND SCANLON, S. (1990) *Unmarried Mothers Delivered in the National Maternity Hospital 1988*, Dublin: Department of Social Administration and Social Work, UCD and Social Work Reseach Unit, National Maternity Hospital.

ERMISCH, J. (1990) *Single Parent Families: The Economic Challenge*, Paris: OECD.

FAHEY, T. (1995) 'Family and household in Ireland' in Clancy, P., Drudy, S., Lynch, K. and O'Dowd, L. (Eds) *Irish Society: Sociological Perspectives*, pp. 205–34, Dublin: Institute of Public Administration.

FINE-DAVIS, M. (1988) *Changing Attitudes to the Role of Women in Ireland: Attitudes Towards the Role and Status of Women 1975–1986*, Dublin: First Report of the Second Joint Committee on Women's Rights.

FLANAGAN, N., and RICHARDSON, V. (1992) *Unmarried Mothers: A Social Profile*, Dublin: Department of Social Policy and Social Welfare, UCD and Social Work Research Unit, National Maternity Hospital.

FRASER, D. (1984) *The Evolution of the British Welfare State: A History of Social Policy Since the Industrial Revolution*, 2nd Edn, London: Macmillan.

GARDINER, F. (1992) 'Political interest and participation of Irish women 1922–1992: the unfinished revolution', *The Canadian Journal of Irish Studies*, 18, 1, pp. 15–40.

GARDINER, F. (1993) 'Political interest and participation of Irish women 1922–1992: the unfinished revolution', in Smyth, A (Ed.), *Irish Women's Studies Reader*, pp. 45–78, Dublin: Attic Press.

GIRVAN, B. (1984) 'Industrialisation and the Irish working class since 1922', *Saothar*, No. 10.

GLENDINNING, C. and McLAUGHLIN, E. (1993) *Paying for Care: Lessons from Europe*, London: HMSO.

HARDEY, M. and CROW, G. (Eds) (1991) *Single Parenthood: Coping with Constraints and Making Opportunities*, London: Harvester Wheatsheaf.

HEALEY, G. (not dated) *Women and Enterprise Network: An Evaluation Report*, Dublin: Parents Alone Resource Centre.

HEARNE, D. (1992) 'The Irish citizen 1914–1916: nationalism, feminism, and militarism', *The Canadian Journal of Irish Studies*, **18**, 1, pp. 1–15.

KEE, R. (1976) *The Most Distressful Country*, London: Quartet.

KENNEDY, L. (1989) *The Modern Industrialisation of Ireland, 1940–1988*, Dublin: Economic and Social History Society of Ireland.

KOVEN, S. and MICHEL, S. (Eds) (1993) *Mothers of A New World?*, London: Routledge.

LANGAN, M. and OSTNER, I. (1991) 'Gender and welfare: towards a comparative framework', in Room, G. (Ed.) *Toward A European Welfare State*, Bristol: School of Advanced Urban Studies.

LEWIS, J. (1992) 'Gender and the development of welfare regimes', *Journal of European Social Policy*, **2**, 3, pp. 159–73.

LEWIS, J. and OSTNER, I. (1994) *Gender and the Evolution of European Social Policies*, Working Paper 4/94, Bremen: Centre for Social Policy Research.

LYNCH, K. and McLAUGHLIN, E. (1995) 'Caring labour and love labour', in Clancy, P., Drudy, S., Lynch, K. and O'Dowd, L. (Eds) *Irish Society: Sociological Perspectives*, pp. 250–92, Dublin: Institute of Public Administration.

MAGEE, C. (1994) *Teenage Parents: Issues of Policy and Practice*, Dublin: Combat Poverty Agency.

MAHON, E. (1995) 'From democracy to femocracy: the women's movement in the Republic of Ireland', in Clancy, P., Drudy, S., Lynch, K. and O'Dowd, L. (Eds) *Irish Society: Sociological Perspectives*, pp. 675–708, Dublin: Institute of Public Administration.

McCASHIN, A. (1993) *Single Parents in the Republic of Ireland: Enumeration, Description and Implications for Social Security*, Dublin: Economic and Social Research Institute.

McCASHIN, A. (1995) *Single Mothers in Ireland: A Local Study*, Dublin: Combat Poverty Agency.

McDEVITT, D. (1987) 'Marriage, maintenance and property', in Curtin, C., Jackson, P., and O'Connor, B. (Eds) *Gender in Irish Society*, Galway: Galway University Press.

McLAUGHLIN, E. (1993) 'Ireland: Catholic Corporatism', in Cochrane, A. and Clarke, J. (Eds) *Comparing Welfare States: Britain in International Context*, London: Sage and The Open University.

McWILLIAMS, M. (1993) 'The church, the state and the women's movement in Northern Ireland', in Smyth, A. (Eds.) *Irish Women' Studies Reader*, pp. 79–99, Dublin: Attic Press.

MEANEY, G. (1991) *Sex and Nation: Women in Irish Culture and Politics*, Dublin: Attic Press LAP Pamphlet.

MEANEY, G. (1993) 'Sex and the nation: women in Irish culture and politics', in Smyth, A. (Ed.) *Irish Women's Studies Reader*, pp. 230–44, Dublin: Attic Press.

MILLAR, J., LEEPER, S., AND DAVIES, C. (1992) *Single Parents, Poverty and Public Policy in Ireland: A Comparative Study*, Dublin: Combat Poverty Agency.

NCOPF (National Council for One Parent Families) (1995) *Key Facts*, Dublin: NCOPF.

NOLAN, B. and FARRELL, B. (1990) *Child Poverty in Ireland*, Dublin: Combat Poverty Agency.

O'HARE, A. (1983) *Mothers Alone: A Study of Women who Gave Birth Outside Marriage*, Dublin: Federation of Services for Unmarried Parents and their Children.

O'NEILL, C. (1992) *Telling it Like It Is*, Dublin: Combat Poverty Agency.

OWENS, R. (1983) 'Votes for ladies, votes for women: organised labour and the suffragette movement, 1876–1922', *Saothar*, **9**, pp. 32–47.

PEILLON, M. (1982) *Contemporary Irish Society*, Dublin: Gill & Macmillan.

PYLE, J. (1990) 'Export-led development and the under-employment of women: the impact of discriminatory development policy in the Republic of Ireland', in Ward, K. (Ed.) *Women Workers and Global Restructuring*, New York: Cornell University, ILR Press.

QUATAERT, J. (1993) 'Woman's work and the early welfare state in Germany: legislators, bureaucrats, and clients before the First World War', in Koven, S. and Michel, S. (Eds) *Mothers of a New World*, pp. 159–187, London: Routledge.

RICHARDSON, V. (1992) 'The family life styles of some single parents in Ireland', in Kiely, G. (Ed.) *In and Out of Marriage: Irish and European Experiences*, Dublin: Family Studies Centre.

ROLL, J. (1992) *Single Parent Families in the European Community*, Brussels: European Commission, European Family and Social Policy Unit.

SACHBE, C. (1993) 'Social-mothers: the bourgeois women's movement and German welfare state formation, 1820–1929', in Koven, S. and Michel, S. (Eds) *Mothers of a New World*, pp. 136–158, London: Routledge.

SAWYER, R. (1993) *We Are But Women: Women in Ireland's History*, London: Routledge.

SMYTH, A. (1992) 'A great day for the women of Ireland: the meaning of Mary Robinson's presidency for Irish women', *The Canadian Journal of Irish Studies*, **18**, 1, pp. 61–76.

SMYTH, A. (1993) 'The women's movement in the Republic of Ireland 1970–1990', in Smyth, A. (Ed.) *Irish Women's Studies Reader*, Dublin: Attic Press.

SMYTH, A. (1994) 'Paying our disrespects to the bloody states we're in: women, violence, culture and the state', in Griffin, G., Hester, M., Rai, S. and Roseneil, S. (Eds), *Stirring It: Challenges of Feminism*, pp. 13–39, London: Taylor & Francis.

WARD, M. (1983) *Unmanageable Revolutionaries*, London: Pluto Press.

WARD, M. (1993) 'Suffrage first – above all else!: an account of the Irish suffrage movement', in Smyth, A. (Ed.) *Irish Women's Studies Reader*, pp. 20–44, Dublin: Attic Press.

WRC SOCIAL AND ECONOMIC CONSULTANTS LTD. (1992) *Parenting Alone in West Tallaght*, Dublin: Parents Alone Tallaght.

YEATES, N., with STOLTZ, P., (1995) *Unequal Status, Unequal Treatment: The Gender Restructuring of Welfare – Ireland*, Working Paper of the Gender and European Welfare Regimes project, Human Capital Mobility Programme of the EC, Dublin: Women's Education, Research and Resource Centre, University College Dublin.

Chapter 3

Single Mothers in Britain: Unsupported Workers or Mothers?

Simon Duncan and Rosalind Edwards

1. Introduction

In British academic policy research, the term single mothers is most often used to denote mothers who have had children outside of marriage and without a cohabiting male partner. Lone mothers, as a description, tends to be a generic term, referring to a whole range of mothers bringing up children without a male partner in their household: divorced, separated, and widowed, as well as single (never-married) mothers. Throughout this chapter we use the general term 'lone mother' and retain 'single mother' to refer to never-married lone mothers. The route that mothers may take into lone motherhood is seen as important. While marital breakdown is the predominant factor creating lone-mother families in Britain, political consternation has largely focused around the increasing proportion of single mothers.

The increase which has occurred throughout Western Europe in lone mothers caring for dependent children is particularly marked in Britain. Moreover – contrary to the situation in many other West European countries – British lone-mother families are increasingly characterized by poverty and dependence on state benefits. The levels of such benefits in Britain mean that those who wholly or partially rely on them tend to exist on very low incomes. In fact, the uptake of paid work by British lone mothers has actually been decreasing, and few are in the full-time work that is more likely to provide a household wage. In contrast, the uptake of paid work by married or partnered mothers has increased substantially, including full-time employment, so that their employment rate has overtaken that for lone mothers. Again, this picture is in contrast to most other West European countries where, as other contributors show, more lone mothers are in paid work, especially full time, than married or cohabiting mothers (see Roll, 1992).

Lone motherhood in Britain also has a political significance wider than the policy issues directly raised. It has become a symbol, and a means of political mobilization, for alternative discourses about the nature of 'the family' and the welfare state (Bortolaia-Silva, 1996). This socio-political debate is becoming increasingly polarized between two major interpretations of lone motherhood. In one, lone mothers are seen as a threat to society, morally as well as financially, perversely enabled by overly supportive welfare state benefits and provisions. In the other, lone mothers are seen as a social problem who are prevented from undertaking paid work by the constraining structure and nature of the welfare state. We will discuss these discourses and their policy implications below, along with other, alternative, discourses which are less influential at the level of state policy in Britain.

Despite the oppositions between these dominant 'social threat' and 'social problem' discourses, both are essentially based on the simple stimulus–response model of social action critiqued in our introductory chapter to this volume. Within these discourses it is assumed that if state welfare provisions are changed (such as welfare benefits or child care) lone mothers will respond appropriately (by taking up paid work).[1] Lone mothers' own understandings of their role as mothers vis-à-vis paid work, and of what course of action is best for them and their children, are shut out. These understandings will be developed within a variety of social settings, including those provided by neighbourhoods and local labour markets, which will further influence the way lone mothers assess their situation.

The current debate in Britain downplays the basic issues of why, and how, lone mothers do or do not take up paid work. As Bradshaw and Millar note (1991: 33), there is actually little coherent empirical knowledge on this issue. In this chapter, following the theme of the book as a whole, we will focus more on the social processes through which lone mothers take up, or do not take up, paid work, as these develop within social settings at a variety of scales. Following section 2, which provides background information on lone motherhood in Britain, section 3 examines the nature of the discourses around lone motherhood in Britain. This is followed by an analysis of how the British welfare state regime and its policies position lone mothers (section 4). However, as we have argued, nation-states are not the only major context for social behaviour. Thus sections 5 and 6 go on to assess the influence of labour markets and neighbourhoods on lone mothers' assessments of their situation visa-à-vis paid work, which enable and/or constrain their desired courses of action.

2. Lone Motherhood in Britain

Numbers, prevalence and origins

Since 1971, the number of lone parent families in Britian – of which over 90 per cent are lone mother families – has more than doubled (see Table 3.1). Lonemother families now account for 19 per cent of all families with dependent children, compared with just 7 per cent in 1971 (Table 3.2). Between 1.8 to 2 million children are estimated to live in lone-parent families. Given current

Family type	1971		1986		1992*		% change 1971–92
	000s	%	000s	%	000s	%	
Single mothers	90	15.8	230	22.8	490	35.0	444
Separated and divorced mothers	290	50.8	600	59.4	730	52.1	152
Widowed mothers	120	21.0	80	7.9	60	4.3	−50
Lone fathers	70	12.3	90	9.9	120	8.6	71
All lone parents	570	100	1010	100	1400	100	146

Note *provisional
Source Haskey (1994)
Table 3.1 Estimated number and proportion of lone-parent families: Britain 1971–92

trends, therefore, increasingly large numbers of British mothers and children will experience life in a lone-motherhood household at least once during the course of their lives (Burghes, 1993).

From the late 1980s, just over half of new lone-parent families resulted from marital divorce or separation where the child/ren remained living with the mother, while nearly a third resulted from births to single mothers; over one-tenth are families headed by lone fathers and just 6 per cent resulted from widowhood. These figures are part of a continuing trend by which single mothers have increased steadily as a proportion of all lone parents (Table 3.1). However, the numbers of divorced and separated lone mothers are also increasing, alongside a decrease of half in the number of widows since 1971. Although the number of lone fathers has almost doubled over the same period, they also account for a smaller proportion of lone-parent families than formerly, and around a third are widowers.

It is important to note that the category 'single mother' is in itself quite diverse. Commentators, particularly those working from the 'social threat' discourse, tend to assume that single mothers are young women who have an

Family type	1971 %	1981 %	1986 %	1991 %
Married/ cohabiting couples	92	87	86	80
Lone mothers:	7	11	13	19
single	1	2	3	6
separated and divorced	4	7	9	11
widowed	2	2	1	1
Lone fathers	1	2	1	1
All lone parents	8	12	14	20

Source adapted from Burghes (1993)
Table 3.2 Families with dependent children by type: Britain 1971–92

unplanned pregnancy and/or who have chosen to have a child on their own. However, in the national statistics, it is impossible to distinguish these groups from ex-cohabitees, who are also counted as 'single' lone mothers. In these families, children were conceived, born and/or brought up in a couple relationship, where the partners separated later. In fact, 54 per cent of single mothers in 1990–92 were over 25 years old, and only 8.6 per cent were teenagers. The ex-cohabiting group is undoubtedly the larger, and will share many of the characteristics of divorced and separated mothers (Bradshaw and Millar, 1991). Indeed, over the last twenty years teenage women have accounted for a declining proportion of all out-of-marriage births, and the average age at which women first give birth continues to rise.

It is the case that the number of teenage births to unmarried (but mostly partnered) teenagers has risen fairly consistently since the 1970s, but this is because of a decline in 'shotgun' weddings (these are marriages taking place after conception but before the baby is born) and a corresponding rise in the number of cohabiting unmarried couples. Similarly, while breakdown rates for cohabitees are higher than for married couples as a whole, the evidence shows that marital breakdown is particularly likely for 'shotgun' weddings (Burghes and Brown, 1995). Statistically, the breakdown of a shotgun wedding produces a separated or divorced lone mother, while a breakdown in a cohabiting relationship produces a single mother. All that may be happening, therefore, is a net statistical shift between categories, with little change in the behaviour or characteristics of the people involved. Certainly, there is little evidence of any major increase in births to unattached young women, nor that most women who become lone mothers have done so without attempting or hoping to establish a cohabiting relationship with the father (ibid.). Similarly, the average duration for lone motherhood is only four years, before remarriage or repartnership, and if anything single mothers repartner even earlier (Burghes, 1993). However, as we shall see in section 3, facts like these count for little in the face of sensationalist discourses emphasizing moral and cultural break-down.

Families and households

The role of cohabitation in mediating changes in the British family form is also reflected in statistics on family characteristics, as Table 3.3 shows. The families of 'other' lone mothers (i.e., divorced, separated and widowed) are similar in size and age to those of married couples, except that these lone mothers and their children are a little older and there is a slight likelihood of more children. Single mothers are much more likely to be younger, with just one child under five. However, cohabiting couples occupy a middle position between married and single mothers, again reinforcing the view that the rise in single motherhood reflects the rise in cohabitation for younger adults. While in 1971, 55 per cent of extra-marital births were registered by the mother alone, by 1993

Family type	Parent under 25 years old (%)	With one child (%)	With youngest child under 5 (%)	With youngest child over 10 (%)
Never-married lone mothers	46.0	70.1	71.3	7.7
Cohabiting couples	24.2	52.8	61.8	18.7
Divorced/separated lone mothers	4.7	41.1	31.7	39.5
Married couples	4.7	37.6	41.8	33.9

Note children defined as dependent children under 19
Source Burghes and Brown (1995) from General Household Survey
Table 3.3 Family characteristics by type of family: Britain 1990–92

	Single lone mothers (%)	Other lone mothers (%)	Cohabiting couples (%)	Married couples (%)
Living alone	75.9	90.8	95.1	95.8
With parents	20.9	6.1	1.6	3.1
With others	3.3	3.1	3.3	1.1
All	100	100	100	100

Source Burghes and Brown (1995), from General Household Survey
Table 3.4 Proportion of families living alone or with others: Britain 1990–92

three-quarters were registered by parents living at the same address (whom we can presume were mostly cohabiting), with most of the change being accounted for by births to women under 25 years old.

Where single mothers do stand out as rather different, though, is in the proportion living with their parents (the child's maternal grandparents) – see Table 3.4. Even so, only around one in five single mothers are in this intergenerational household form, with 76 per cent living alone with their children. Given the very small proportion of cohabiting mothers who live with their parents or with others (e.g. the father's parents), this implies that most of the single mothers who do live with their parents have not cohabited. Only 6 per cent of other lone mothers live with their parents, and this means that altogether almost 90 per cent of lone mothers in Britain live alone with their children. Lone motherhood must be considered an autonomous household type which, therefore, requires independent resourcing and income. How this is to be achieved, of course, is at the root of much of the debate in Britain.

Employment and income

On average, in 1993, British lone parents received 63 per cent of their income from state benefits, as Table 3.5 shows (according to the 1993 DSS/PSI survey,

Ford et al., 1995). The major source was Income Support, the main social assistance benefit, with smaller proportions provided by the universal Child Benefit (including one-parent benefit), and Family Credit which is available to low-income earners with dependent children. (The benefits available to lone mothers are discussed in section 4.) Only 24 per cent of average income was provided by earnings from paid work. Levels of maintenance paid by the absent partner (usually the father) have generally been low and unreliable, and provided just 9 per cent of average income in 1993. These figures aggregate across all lone mothers, and in this sense are statistical fiction. Put another way, over half of lone mothers relied on Income Support for the bulk of their income, with only 23 per cent gaining most income from earnings (ibid.).

	Income Support %	Family Credit %	Child Benefit %	Net earnings %	Maintenance %	All five sources %
Single mother	54	4	16	17	5	96
Divorced mother	35	6	16	26	13	96
Separated mother	33	6	16	29	12	96
Lone father	24	2	15	49	1	91
Working over 24 hrs	–	9	8	74	8	99
Working 16–23 hrs	4	24	10	49	12	99
Working 1–15 hrs	50	1	15	23	8	97
No paid work	64	–	20	–	9	93
All	42	5	16	24	9	96

Source adapted from Ford et al. (1993)

Table 3.5   Mean proportion of lone parents' income by source: Britain 1993

The levels and adequacy of state benefits, chiefly Income Support, is therefore of some concern. Calculations have repeatedly shown that Income Support rates are insufficient for even the bare necessities for families with children, especially for those with young school-age children (Burghes, 1993). In short, reliance on state benefits for the bulk of income normally means poverty.

Paid work is the major means for lone mothers to escape poverty and state dependency – where the income of those lone mothers in work was double those without in 1993. Despite this, in Britain the uptake of paid work by lone mothers has decreased over recent decades. Around half of lone mothers held employment in the mid 1970s, with about a quarter in full-time jobs. By 1990 this had fallen to 38 per cent, with only 19 per cent in full-time work. As Table 3.6 shows, the employment position of lone mothers is much weaker than for other household types, and by 1990 over 60 per cent of lone mothers had incomes less than half the national average.

	Lone mothers %	Couple mothers* %	Lone fathers %	All men 16–64 %
In employment:[†]	37.7	58.1	63.4	74.9
full-time	19.2	21.0	53.2	64.7
part-time	18.5	37.1	10.2	10.2
Without employment	62.3	41.9	36.6	25.1
	100	100	100	100

Notes *married and cohabiting
†full-time includes self-employed with employees, part-time self-employed without employees
Source 1991 Sample of Anonymised Records (SARs), authors' calculations
Table 3.6 Economic activity by household type: Britain 1991

Much part-time work undertaken by women in Britain is both 'short' in hours of work and badly paid (Lonsdale, 1992). As a result, therefore, few part-time jobs will provide enough income to support a family. However, over half of lone mothers who were in employment in 1991 worked less than 30 hours a week. As many as 31 per cent worked less than 21 hours. Not surprisingly, average earnings for the minority of lone-mother households who were in paid work in 1990–92 were less than half those for couples (see Table 3.7). Consequently, many lone mothers in paid work continue to depend on state benefits (see Table 3.5). As Table 3.7 also shows, it is only single mothers in work who earn significantly less than other employed women (largely because over a third work less than 16 hours a week). Rather, it is the male partner's income that makes most difference to couple income. Exit from lone-mother status itself, through repartnership, will therefore also usually mean increased household income – although the evidence suggests that this extra income will not necessarily accrue to the mother or her children (Graham, 1987; Pahl, 1989).

While the debate is often couched in terms of 'getting lone mothers back to work', it is clear that it is access to well-paid, full-time or 'long' part-time jobs that is in issue, and that this applies to women as a whole as much as to lone mothers. Despite this, current policy development is focused on part-time work (see section 4). This is likely to put lone mothers in a more stressful position as they try to combine several insecure and inadequate sources of income.

	Mothers alone (£)	Couples (£)
Single lone mothers	87.4	–
Other lone mothers	102.0	–
Cohabiting couples	105.2	266.3
Married couples	100.1	320.8

Source Burghes and Brown (1995), from General Household Survey
Table 3.7 Average net weekly earnings of employed persons by household type: Britain 1990–92

Housing

Lone mothers are less likely than their partnered counterparts to be in owner-occupied housing, and more likely to be tenants, or even in temporary accommodation (Table 3.8). In Britain, public rented housing, particularly local authority (council) housing, has become increasingly residualized both economically and socially, and by 1993 the majority of tenants had no paid work and were dependent on benefits. Even within this sector, lone parents have tended to get the worst housing, especially those who could be classified as 'undeserving' such as young, single mothers (Crow and Hardey, 1991). They often received 'older rather than newer; flats rather than houses; higher floors rather than lower' (Harrison, 1983: 225). Table 3.8 also shows how the various routes into lone motherhood structure current access, and this will also be important in terms of the strategies lone mothers can employ for the future (cf. Crow and Hardey, 1991). Single lone mothers are the most likely to be in rented accommodation. However, the largest proportion of lone mothers are in public housing, compared with married mothers, rather than owner-occupied housing. This indicates that material disadvantage and downward social mobility is consequent on divorce and separation. Again, cohabiting mothers hold a position midway between married and single mothers.

Housing tenure	Single lone mothers (%)	Other lone mothers (%)	Cohabiting Mothers (%)	Married mothers (%)
Owner occupation	19.4	43.0	48.0	78.5
Public renting*	72.6	50.8	42.2	16.2
Private renting	7.9	6.2	9.8	5.3
All	100	100	100	100

Note *local authority or housing association
Source adapted from Burghes and Brown (1995)
Table 3.8 Housing tenure by family type Britain 1990–92

As Table 3.4 shows, single mothers are also more likely to be sharing with parents and friends, although the evidence suggests this is often involuntary (Holme, 1985). While sharing can be advantageous, it may mean overcrowding, frequent moves and a high risk of homelessness. In addition, many divorced and separated lone mothers have to find new accommodation on partnership breakdown; Bradshaw and Millar (1991) found that 58 per cent of such lone mother families had moved home. The PSI studies found that a sixth of lone mothers in their samples had had to stay in temporary bed and breakfast accommodation at some period, a quarter of these for more than a year (Ford et al., 1995). While around a third of lone mothers are in owner-occupied housing, we should not assume this necessarily means housing advantage – certainly around a fifth are in mortgage arrears and/or experience problems paying for repairs (Bradshaw and Millar, 1991; see also Leeming et al., 1994). Lone mothers are also more likely to live in inner-city areas, and in both a tenurial and a geographical sense are therefore concentrated in the poorer parts of the urban system (Crow and Hardey, 1991).

Quality of life

Surveys regularly show that lone mothers are strikingly worse off than other low-income families in Britain, and that this is almost entirely a consequence of their exclusion from paid work and the lack of an alternative income such as maintenance (Marsh and McKay, 1993). This situation is in stark contrast, for example, with the combination of state-advanced maintenance and high levels of paid work in Sweden (Björnberg, chapter 9). Not surprisingly then, lone-mother households are twice as likely as couples to suffer material hardship, and they are generally in poorer health.

In comparable surveys carried out in 1991 and 1993 (McKay and Marsh, 1993; Ford et al., 1995), 25 per cent of lone mothers were in 'severe hardship' at any one time (using an index based on levels of debt, inability to afford food and other necessities, and financial worry). As many as 40 per cent had been in severe hardship at some time over the three years. Similarly, almost half were in debt (including rent and mortgage arrears), while three-quarters had experienced debt over the period. A relatively high incidence of housing stress was also found, measured in terms of dampness, poor repair etc. Another survey showed that poorer lone mothers in London had a limited nutrient base in their diets – although the mothers attempted to protect their children from the worst nutritional effects of poverty (Dowler and Calvert, 1995 – and see also Graham, 1993). A large proportion of lone mothers smoke, where – as Marsh and McKay (1994) have argued – smoking is the easiest, locally approved and legal anodyne to deal with discouraging circumstances.

Hardship, poor diet and smoking can be expected to combine with the stresses of parenting alone, and possible relationship breakdown, to produce high levels of poor health. Over a fifth of lone mothers report limiting, long-standing illness in surveys carried out over the last decade (Popay and Jones, 1990; McKay and Marsh, 1993), and about a third suffer illness over the long term – figures around 50 per cent higher than for partnered mothers. As many as 10 per cent state that illness prevents them obtaining a job.

Nonetheless, both surveys and in-depth studies also show that most lone mothers report a considerable advantage in lone motherhood – independence and increased control of their lives within the household – even where they are living on inadequate state benefits (Graham, 1987; Bradshaw and Millar, 1991; Shaw, 1991; Dean and Taylor-Gooby, 1992). Thus a sense of independence may compensate for the material hardships involved. We also should not assume that lone motherhood means passivity or inevitable poverty. In working within a mix of both constraints and opportunities (even if, in Britain, the constraints are often more severe than elsewhere in Western Europe) lone mothers are often able to provide a good quality of life for themselves and their children: it is just that circumstances often mean it is harder for them to do so.

Lone motherhood – diversity and variability

Lone mothers are often presented as a 'categorical' group, where it is assumed that, because the family type is distinguished by mothers caring for their children with the father living elsewhere, then lone mothers must necessarily share all other characteristics and behaviour. This incorrect assumption is particularly convenient for the sweeping generalizations often made in discourses on lone motherhood (see section 3). In the discussion up to now we have pointed to the differences between single and other lone mothers (mostly divorced and separated). The position of cohabiting mothers, often more like single mothers than ex-married and married mothers, also counteracts this simplistic 'categorical' view. There are also other dimensions of diversity, distinguished by overlapping patterns of constraints and resources and – although strangely neglected in the literature – class, ethnicity and geographical location.

We can briefly illustrate this point in terms of the major means by which lone mothers can escape poverty and state dependency – the uptake of paid work, especially full-time work. In 1991 only 20 per cent of lone mothers with three or more children, who were more constrained in terms of child care, had a job, and just 8 per cent were in full-time work. In constrast, these figures were 42 per cent and 20 per cent respectively for those with only one child. Similarly, where the youngest child was aged 0–4 years, only 21 per cent held a job, just 10 per cent full time, with corresponding figures of 59 and 37 per cent for those where the youngest child was over 12. In terms of personal resources, 81 per cent of lone mothers with higher education were employed, as many as 55 per cent full-time, and while 61 per cent of owner-occupiers were in work (33 per cent full time) only 24 per cent of public housing tenants were (just 9.5 per cent full time). These variations by individual characteristics of lone mothers overlap with variations by local labour market and neighbourhood (see sections 5 and 6). In some areas as many as 70 per cent of lone mothers were in paid work in 1991, with 30 per cent or so in full-time jobs, while in other areas these rates sank to single figures (Duncan and Edwards, 1996).

There are also substantial ethnic contrasts in the uptake of paid work, as Table 3.9 shows. Black minority groups in Britain show a particularly high rate of lone motherhood, with around half of mothers in this status in 1991, compared with just 14 per cent of White mothers. This has been taken to support some racialized versions of the underclass discourse (see section 3). However, Black lone mothers are also far more likely to be in paid work, especially full-time jobs. Indeed, the most constrained and least resourced in terms of number and age of children, tenure and age, show uptake levels as

Ethnicity	In paid work (%)	(of which full-time)[†][*] (%)	No paid work (%)
White	37.7	(18.5)	62.3
African-Caribbean/ Black	57.1	(30.2)	44.9
African	55.9	(32.3)	45.1
Indian and Pakistani	23.7	(15.1)	74.3

Notes *ethnicity defined as in 1991 Census; 'Black' = 'Black British'
†including self-employed with employees
Source 1991 SARs, authors' calculations
Table 3.9 Lone mothers' uptake of paid work by ethnicity*: Britain 1991

high as the most resourced and least constrained White lone mothers. Similarly, the most resourced and least constrained Black lone mothers show employment patterns nearer to the male norm of majority full-time work (see Duncan and Edwards, 1997). Black lone mothers are also better educated than White lone mothers and their children are far less likely to be deprived (Moore, 1996). Even those Black lone mothers who are poor smoke less and eat better food than their White counterparts (Dowler and Calvert, 1995).

These variations show that it is wrong to see lone mothers as one homogeneous group, and incorrect to assume that they hold similar views or behave in the same way. Unfortunately, this is how lone mothers are portrayed in much of the debate. As soon as we recognize this variety of experience, and stop treating lone mothers as a categorical group, then a focus on the social processes and relations by which lone mothers do, or do not, take up paid work becomes important. This is the task of succeeding sections of this chapter.

3. Discourses Around Lone Motherhood in Britain

As discussed in our introductory chapter to this volume, political rhetoric, based on particular ideological stances about the welfare state and 'the family', both influences legislation and affects public perceptions of lone motherhood. Such discourses thus provide another layer of the social processes lone mothers must negotiate. Four major discourses about lone motherhood have currency in Britain, each competing for legitimacy but having different potencies within the national context (as well as in the neighbourhood context we discuss later). These discourses are: lone motherhood as a social threat; as a social problem; as part of lifestyle change; and as an escape from patriarchy. We deal with each of them in turn.

Lone motherhood as a social threat

This discourse links into the underclass debate, which has developed in the USA in particular (see de Acosta, chapter 4), but has been imported into

Britain (Morris, 1993). The underclass theory posits that, in spatially segregated areas, there is a developing class that has no stake in the social order, is alienated from it and hostile to it, and thus is the source of crime, deviancy and social breakdown. In turn, this links into a New Right political view of the state in society, where the welfare state is viewed as encouraging state dependency, leading to the collapse of both the work ethic and the traditional family.

Lone mothers are seen as active agents in the creation of this underclass. Until recently, in Britain, young single mothers have been pointed to as the central culprits, but – as has long been the case in the USA (see de Acosta, chapter 4) – elements of a racialized discourse are now emerging (see below). These lone mothers are said to choose to have children to gain benefits and then, supported by the state, they choose not to work. Their sons, assumed to be without male authority or roles, thus are said to drift into delinquency, crime and the drug culture, while their daughters learn to repeat the cycle of promiscuity and dependency. The fathers of these children – without the 'civilizing' influence of the family – supposedly lapse into inherent aggressive selfishness (Morgan, 1995).

Academic versions of the social threat discourse tone down the emotive signifiers somewhat (see, e.g., Segalman and Marsland, 1989; Murray, 1990; Morgan, 1995). Popularizing versions use emotional symbolism more fully (see Mann and Roseneil, 1996 for review) – and are sometimes written by academic authors. The American academic Charles Murray, in particular, has been given a platform in the British broadsheet newspaper, *The Sunday Times*. There are regular 'wedded to welfare' and 'babies on benefits' stories in the media, displaying raw prejudices. For example:

> It is becoming increasingly clear to all but the most blinkered of social scientists that the disintegration of the nuclear family is the principal source of so much unrest and misery. . . . It is not just a question of a few families without fathers; it is a matter of whole communities with barely a single worthwhile role model.
> (*The Sunday Times*, quoted in *Search*, 16 June 1993)

And specifically relating to Black families, under the banner headline 'The ethnic timebomb', the tabloid newspaper *The Sunday Express* claimed:

> Almost six in 10 black mothers are bringing up children on their own, urged on by our benefit system.

(See Song and Edwards, 1996, for a review of discourses on Black lone motherhood in Britain.)

The underclass social threat discourse has been taken up by sections of the Conservative Party – in government at the time of writing – with stress placed on the role of the welfare state's provision of housing and benefits in encouraging single motherhood especially. For example, Stephen Green, Chairman of the Conservative Family Campaign has stated: 'Putting girls into council flats and providing taxpayer funded child care is a policy from hell' (quoted in *The Observer*, 14 November 1993). Socialists and feminists are targeted as supporting social breakdown, and the scapegoating of lone mothers as self-created threats avoids (at least temporarily) having to make the choice of seeing mothers as workers or home-makers (see section 4).

Those who promulgate a view of lone motherhood as a threat to society campaign for policies that do not encourage or reward such 'self-damaging conduct'. There are proposals to reduce or remove the benefits paid to lone mothers, such as the extra allowances available to lone parents on both the universal Child Benefit payment and targeted income-related benefits; restricting payments for lone mothers who have more children while receiving benefit (now a practice in the USA – see de Acosta, chapter 4); and making grandparents responsible for both lone parent and grandchildren (as is theoretically the case in Germany – see Klett-Davies, chapter 7). There are suggestions that young single mothers on benefit should be placed in hostels where their sexual relations and children's upbringing can be supervised, so as to enforce 'good behaviour' (see Zulauf, 1997). Encouragement and reward for traditional male-breadwinner/female-home-maker married couples is also stressed, with proposals to tighten up the divorce laws, so that fewer lone-mother families are created in the first place, and to place 'moral' family education on the school curriculum.

In contrast to this view of lone motherhood as a threat to the social order, the next discourse sees lone mothers as victims who need help.

Lone motherhood as a social problem

The view of lone mothers as victims of society posits that they should get more help, not less. Here, it is social circumstances that are seen as placing both lone mothers and their children in economically and socially disadvantaged positions. Stress is laid on the 'facts', whereby the majority of lone mothers are 'mature' divorced, separated or widowed women, rather than young single mothers (see Tables 3.1 and 3.3). Within the social problem discourse, there is no underclass in the sense of a self-reproducing distinct part of society who stand outside cultural, political and economic norms. Rather, there are growing numbers of people in poverty, where the economic and social causes are beyond the control of those they affect, and where shrinking the welfare state only makes the problems worse. Lone mothers are just one group affected by these processes (see e.g., Morris, 1993); they do the best they can in unfavourable circumstances.

According to the social problem discourse, lone mothers want jobs, but they are simply prevented from taking them by the costs of child care and the poverty trap. Indeed recent surveys show that as many as 90 per cent of lone mothers who are not in paid work say they would like a job, over half of them saying they would take a job immediately if child care were available (Bradshaw and Millar, 1991; McKay and Marsh, 1994). However, widows (seen as the most 'deserving' in the social threat discourse) are less likely to want employment, while young single mothers (seen as least 'deserving') are keenest. Overall, lone mothers' estimates of the wages they would accept were extremely modest, so it is not such expectations that keep them out of the labour market (McKay and Marsh, 1994).

In order to create more favourable circumstances for lone-mother families, proponents of the social problem view of lone motherhood argue for changes in the benefit and child-care systems. Lone mothers will then be enabled to get paid work and escape both poverty and state dependence. For example, at a minimum, child-care costs should be taken into account when calculating Income Support (the 'safety net' benefit payable to lone mothers and others who are not in paid work) and Family Credit payments (a benefit payable to parents with dependent children who have low paid jobs). In 1993, an earnings disregard for formal child-care costs was made available to all parents claiming Family Credit, but at a level that would not even cover full-time care of one child. Nevertheless, the measure does suggest that the social problem approach retains a foothold in British policy-making circles, despite the growing prevalence of the social threat discourse.

Other policy suggestions under this discourse include increases in lone-parent top-up on benefits, measures to encourage lone mothers to pursue training and higher education, and the establishment of a public child-care system that matches other West European levels. Not only would lone mothers (and other mothers) be able to take full-time jobs, but the system would soon pay for itself in terms of lower benefit outlay and higher tax income (see, e.g. Cohen and Fraser, 1991; Holtermann, 1992).[2]

The social problem view is dominant in much of the social policy academic discipline and among practitioners (such as a social workers, health visitors and so on) – reflecting a Fabian political inheritance of enlightened state intervention. Figures in the liberal establishment, such as church leaders, often also take this line. Unsurprisingly, this becomes the perfect foil for those on the New Right in lambasting the excesses of the 'permissive leftists' of the 1960s. Perhaps because of this outdated intellectual and political inheritance, however, in Britain the social problem discourse is fragmenting. The lines upon which this break up is occurring take us deeper into debates on the causes of social disadvantage.

That British lone mothers and their children are socially disadvantaged is not in dispute – most of these families are poor. Analyses of the National Child Development Study data (a major survey that follows the lives of all babies born in one week in 1946 and 1958) reveal that the children of the lone mothers in these samples were more likely to be unemployed, less well-qualified, suffer illness, and die earlier (e.g. Elliott and Richards, 1991; Kiernan, 1992). However, there are no inevitable associations between lone mothering and poor outcomes for children (Burghes, 1994). What is in dispute here, however, is the causal explanation of these associations between lone motherhood, poverty and disadvantage – the issue around which the social problem discourse is fragmenting.

One explanation is associated with the distinguished British sociologists A. H. Halsey and Norman Dennis (erstwhile supporters of the Labour Governments in the 1960s, but now writing for the right-wing think tank, the Institute for Economic Affairs). They argue that it is because lone-parent families do not follow the 'norms of the traditional family' that children suffer (e.g. Halsey, *The Financial Times*, 12 August 1991; Halsey, 1993). The absence of fathers not only causes social disadvantage, but also results in social deviancy, crime and hooliganism (Dennis, 1993; Dennis and Erdos, 1993). Thus, within this strand of the discourse, social policy changes seeking to bring lone mothers into the labour market will not have much effect on the fundamental cause of disadvantage: the lack of fathers. Rather, policies are required that reinforce traditional families.

While this emphasis on the absence of fathers and a desire to reinforce traditional families clearly links in with the New Right espousal of lone mothers as a social threat – as in Halsey's linkage between the break up of the traditional family structure and destruction of the modern state (quoted in *Daily Mail* 16 October 1995) – it does not totally collapse into it. This is because, in this view, marketization has been extended to the social world of partnerships, families and child rearing, replacing non-monetary moral codes. Halsey views Margaret Thatcher (the radical 'free market' Conservative prime minister during the 1980s) as 'a major architect of the demolition of the traditional family' (Halsey 1993: 129). Now, according to Dennis, market values have been extended even to sexual relations, with a high priority being given to 'sexual excitation' and the encouragement of a 'please myself sexual conduct' (Dennis, 1991a and b). One might detect an undercurrent of older, socially more powerful men seeking to regulate the private lives of economically weaker, younger women: freedom in markets normally leaves older White men in control, but freedom in sexuality does not. For Halsey, Dennis and others like them, the ideal is a return of the political left to 'ethical socialism', with its historic mission 'to spread the values of the family throughout all the relationships of society' (*The Observer*, 14 November 1993). Such views ignore the point raised by the 'lone motherhood as escaping patriarchy discourse', outlined later, that the 'traditional' father was often markedly uninvolved with his children (McKee and O'Brien, 1992), and that some fathers are violent or abusive, so that their absence is surely a bonus. Indeed, conflict between parents has been shown to affect children's educational and social ajustment prior to separation or divorce (Elliott and Richards, 1991; Burghes, 1994). Additionally, some 'absent' fathers keep in close contact with their children.

The other view of the cause of disadvantage in lone-mother families prioritizes poverty rather than family. As we note above, it is argued that most lone-mother families are created by divorce or separation, rather than the single mothers who are central to the 'fatherless' version. Moreover, even Dennis accepts that any statistical associations between 'fatherlessness' and crime and delinquency have to be seen in the context of time and place. In the 1940s, and 1950s (as in the National Child Development Study database), single mothers were a much smaller group who already tended to come from the most disadvantaged sections of society. They were mostly young White women from the poorest working-class families, often with poor social networks and education. So, controlling for class, income and housing, Ferri (1976) shows that children from lone-parent families in the 1958 sample did no worse than other children in educational performance, for example. Lone motherhood as such does not cause disadvantage, but poverty does (see also analysis by Lambert and Streather, 1980).

Nevertheless, if poverty is part and parcel of lone motherhood, as we have said, within Western Europe it is a particularly British phenomenon. The dominant academic view argues that this is the result of poor social policy making. As one leading British academic social policy researcher put it:

> The family form is changing very rapidly. Social policy has failed to recognise the change and the least useful thing to do now is to start stigmatising the victims of these changes.
>
> (Prof. Jonathan Bradshaw, *The Guardian*, 13 October 1993)

However, the very notion of 'the family form' would be challenged by those who believe there is not, and should not be, one family form. This brings us on to the third discourse on lone mothers.

Lone motherhood as lifestyle change

Both the social threat and the social problem discourses portray lone motherhood in a basically negative way: the former views lone mothers as actively choosing to be anti-social, while the latter places lone mothers as passive victims. The lifestyle change discourse puts lone mothers into a more positive position.

In this view, long-term changes are taking place in family patterns and gender relations, resulting from people's choices about how they live their lives, within a context of overarching economic, cultural and social change. At worst, these changes should be accepted; at best, they should be welcomed. Either way, they are certainly not to be feared. Proponents of such a view point to historical research showing that the assumed 'traditional family' never was that standard, normal or successful; it was created in particular historical circumstances (Gittins, 1985; Lewis, 1989a, 1992a). Overall, historically, changes to family forms are very much an ongoing process. Current trends are not some epoch-shattering development, there was no golden age of family life, and there is little chance that government policy can reverse such deeply embedded processes. As the Deputy Director of the left-wing think tank. The Institute for Public Policy Research put it, '1990s women are not going to give up on the right to earn a living and 1990s men and women are not going to give up on the right to divorce' (*The Guardian*, 13 October 1993). Indeed, in Britain, popular embeddedness of a lifestyle discourse are signalled by the launch of magazines such as *Singled Out* and *Solo*, aimed at the lone-parent market and covering all aspects of their lives, from holidays and cookery to financial and legal matters.

To some extent, elements of the lifestyle discourse overlap with the social problem view. Lifestyle changes are seen as inevitably creating specific social problems, particularly as social institutions take some time to adapt. Marriage and taxation laws, for instance, will be outmoded, and social welfare legislation generally will address past problems. Thus policy recommendations are similar to those put forward in the 'poverty as causal' version of the social problem discourse; with social policy being developed so as to allow lone mothers to take up paid work and escape poverty, and child-care provision also seen as decisive.

However, the element that differentiates it from the social problem discourse is a 'postmodern' emphasis on 'family' as a fluid and everchanging concept (Cheal, 1991; Giddens, 1991). The spotlight is taken off lone mothers because they are simply one part of wider diversities in family forms and gender relations. Some proponents of this view counterpose current trends with a stable, traditional, and stultifying, family past – as opposed to their forming a continuation of historically fluid family forms. The influential sociologist Anthony Giddens, for example, presents an argument that may seem rather romanticized from the point of view of many British lone mothers:

> in experiencing the unravelling of traditional family patterns . . . individuals are actively pioneering new social territory and construct-ing innovative forms of familial relations. . . . Individuals are actively restructuring new forms of gender and kinship relations out of the detritus of pre-established forms of family life. Such restructurings are not merely local and they are certainly not trivial.
>
> (1991: 176–7)

In this view, then, policies should aim to create better conditions for all families in the context of changing circumstances.

The lifestyle discourse and its policy recommendations, however, impli-citly mean facing up more squarely to changes in gender relations and the power of women vis-à-vis men. But it is precisely this issue of treating women as equal citizens with independent economic and sexual power, with its threat to established relations, that helps fuel the social threat discourse! It is also this issue that fuels the fourth, and final, discourse.

Lone mothers as women escaping patriarchy

One of the reasons for the changes in family forms, as central to the lifestyle discourse described above, is the change in gender relations, or even a 'gender revolution', as highlighted by feminist research. Increasingly, women are said to be no longer willing to accept control over their lives by individual men. Other social changes, such as access to paid work, contraception, divorce, and so on, give the means to affect this. Some feminists argue that private patriarchy – control by husbands or fathers – is merely replaced by public patriarchy – subordination to men in paid work and politics (e.g. Walby, 1990). Nevertheless, whatever judgement is taken on the contemporary nature of patriarchy, there is the implication of another discourse on lone mother-hood, as women escaping private patriarchy.

Describing such changes as a 'gender revolution' also embodies ideas that while women have changed – or at least their expectations have – men have not (Hochschild, 1989). Cohabitation and marriage are increasingly likely to lead to break-up and divorce, therefore, where both partners have different ideas of what a heterosexual relationship involves. There is evidence that whilst women very rarely 'choose' lone motherhood, once in this situation they do find advantages in it. They value their independence, making their own decisions about their lives, even if they do so in relative poverty (Graham, 1987; Bradshaw and Millar, 1991; Shaw, 1991; Dean and Taylor-Gooby, 1992). Similarly, while many continue, ideally, to see life with a male partner as preferable, the trouble is that the right sort of man, sharing their expectations about gender roles and relations, is not available. Indeed, past experience can be with inadequate, abusive or violent men (Bradshaw and Millar, 1991). Lone motherhood thus can be seen as representing one way by which women are attempting to escape the immediate patriarchy of the domestic situation.

This view has become apparent in some of the campaigning against the Child Support Act 1991 (e.g. Campaign Against the Child Support Act, 1993; Wages for Housework, 1993). (Although some feminists appear to see the Act as favourable to women – Toynbee, 1994). As one of its aims, this Act attempts to ensure that absent parents – overwhelmingly fathers – take financial responsibility for their children, and financially penalizes lone mothers who do not name the father/s of their child/ren. Within the escaping patriarchy discourse, the Act can be regarded as representing an attempt to enforce a relationship with a male 'head of household' (the absent father) even where he is not physically in situ. The patriarchal political establishment, acting through the state, is threatened by the growing independence of women; especially by lone mothers, who have shown that women and children can live their lives without men (for further discussion of the Child Support Act, see section 4).

This discourse finds inspiration in radical feminism, where the family and sexuality are identified as major sites of women's oppression (e.g. Delphy and Leonard, 1992). It can also share some of radical feminism's policy prescriptions, such as more support for women to leave violent men and set up separate households, and wages for housework (although the latter proposal is contentious even amongst feminists).

In one sense, the lone motherhood as escaping patriarchy discourse returns us to the social threat view with which we started this discussion of discourses on lone motherhood. Yes, the traditional family is breaking up, but it is not young women who are the threat and who are to be blamed – rather, it is men who are the problem.

The potency of the discourses

In Britain, lone motherhood serves to highlight social expectations about gender roles and relations because of its social 'deviancy' from assumed or idealized norms. Discourses about lone motherhood, therefore, play a particularly powerful role. Currently, the social threat discourse is increasingly influential nationally, although still strongly challenged by the social problem view. The contradictions of a liberal state regime and a New Right government, exacerbated by the change from private to public patriarchy in terms of female power vis-à-vis men, give the social threat view particular resonance. The lifestyle change and women escaping patriarchy discourses have little national influence. However, as we discuss later in this chapter, these latter two discourses may hold sway amongst particular groups of lone mothers living in particular neighbourhoods, affecting their views of themselves and their integration into society.

Dominant discourses on lone motherhood, as we explained in our introductory chapter, can have very practical consequences in the form of policies (as well as vice versa). Hence there are also material consequences in the form of the provision of resources and supports to lone mothers. We now turn to the British welfare regime and policies that provide one of the contexts for lone mothers' abilities to take up paid work.

4. The British Welfare State Regime and Lone Motherhood

Esping-Andersen (1990) locates Britain within the Liberal welfare state regime, where social policy is used to uphold the market and traditional work-ethic norms, with modest and means-tested benefits aimed at a residualized and stigmatized group of welfare recipients. Esping-Andersen's classification, and the theory behind it, has been criticized for being gender blind. However, most of the resulting alternatives retain and build on Esping-Andersen's insights (see Sainsbury, 1994; Duncan, 1995). As Hobson puts it, 'both women and men are more or less poor in certain welfare states because of the fact that their welfare regimes are systems of stratification' (1994: 175). While no one country represents a pure case of any regime (e.g. in Britain, aspects of the Social Democratic welfare regime, have been historically important where the state is used to compensate for market failure and advances welfare to all at equally high standards), there seems little doubt that lone mothers in Britain fit into this classic definition of the Liberal welfare state regime.

Supporting lone mothers: the balance between pubic and private responsibilities

There are basically three sources of support potentially available to lone mothers: public support from the state, private support through lone mothers' own earnings, and private support from men. The beginning of the 1990s, in Britain, saw a major shift in the prevailing balance of these sources, away from the state and towards the fathers of children and lone mothers undertaking paid work. Prior to this, British Governments had treated lone mothers less as workers and more as non-working mothers supported by the state, albeit experiencing dilemmas over this (Bradshaw, 1989; Lewis, 1989b; Millar, 1989). Lone mothers received a 'top-up' to the universal Child Benefit – 'One-parent Benefit', in recognition of their additional needs – a recognition that drew on the social problem discourse of lone motherhood (due to be removed for new lone mother claimants from April 1998). Maintenance from fathers was seen as a matter for the courts and for parents themselves.

The 1991 Child Support Act, however, required the biological fathers of lone mothers' children – termed 'absent' parents – to support them according to a fixed formula. The amount payable under the formula is a proportion of the biological father's assessable income (Eekelaar, 1991). Maintenance is enforced by the state through the Child Support Agency. The Agency formula does not take account of a man's need to support any non-biological children he may live with in a second family, presuming they are supported by their own 'absent' father. Subsequent biological children are included in Agency calculations. Thus biological, rather than social, parenthood is posited as the relevant factor.

The Act itself and the Agency formula demonstrate the underlying policy–response notion we have discussed previously – getting lone mothers and 'absent' fathers to change their behaviour – as well as the influence of the social threat/underclass discourse on policy developments. The idea that men should father only as many children as they can afford to support financially is implicit. Men will thus be deterred from feckless sexual behaviour or they will have to accept responsibility for their actions. They will be attached to families (financially) by the state, even if they choose to remove themselves physically. The mothers of their children are thus rendered privately dependent on men in their rightful breadwinning role, even if 'absent', rather than publicly on the state as breadwinner. Thus traditional familial and gendered divisions of labour are reproduced, rather than there being adaptation to the changes of the lifestyle discourse (Millar, 1994). This is in some contrast to the Swedish 'advanced maintenance system' (see Björnberg, chapter 9).

The CSA also shifts support for lone mothers onto their own private efforts as breadwinners, at least in a part-time way. As noted, the previous UK benefit system was predicated on non-working mothers, where motherhood and paid work were seen as incompatible. Coupled mothers, however, have more and more taken up employment, and part-time work is now considered compatible with motherhood (although it is still seen as a personal choice not a government responsibility, and so does not need policy support through public child care, extended parental leave, etc.).

The CSA seeks to manipulate financial incentives so that paid work, especially part-time, is attractive for lone mothers. The Act extended eligibility for Family Credit – a cash benefit with some associated provisions, that may be claimed by lone mothers and other parents with dependent children who work but whose net family income falls below a specified level – to those who work 16 hours or more per week (the previous threshold being 24 hours). Moreover, the first £15 of maintenance being paid by the 'absent' father is disregarded in calculating a lone mother's entitlement to Family Credit (plus other in-work benefits) and, if the mother pays for professional child care for her children aged under 11 years, she can offset a proportion of the costs against her earnings. Employed lone mothers who do not claim in-work benefits can keep all of any maintenance from 'absent' fathers (and CSA involvement is voluntary in their case). Lone mothers who do not move into, or continue, employment and are living on Income Support – the state 'safety net' benefit for those with no other source of income – gain nothing from the child support paid by the father. Indeed, lone mothers claiming state benefits who do not reveal the name and, if known, the whereabouts of the 'absent' father can suffer financial penalties to their already minimal benefit payments unless they can demonstrate 'good cause' to withhold this information. In addition, lone mothers on Income Support receive slightly less in One-parent Benefit than do working lone mothers. In an effort to further lure lone mothers on Income Support into the labour market, the British Government put forward plans to have a deferred £5 per week credit against their Child Support which lone mothers can claim as a lump sum if they subsequently take up 16 hours or more employment.

Again it is assumed that changes to policy will mean corresponding changes in lone mothers' behaviour, and again the influence of the social threat discourse can be seen. In a White Paper issued prior to the introduction of the CSA, the government argued that getting lone mothers off benefit and into employment would mean that they were providing their children with appropriate role models, teaching them 'a more positive attitude to work and independence' (DSS, 1990: 41). Both dependence on state benefits and transmission of the attitude that this is acceptable to the next generation are supposed features of underclass behaviour. However, as Millar (1994) points out, there is some ambivalence underlying this for underclass theorists, as they also often see mothers who are workers, rather than home-makers, as creating the delinquents of the future. The British Government also currently proposes freezing One-parent Benefit, so that it will eventually disappear, signalling yet another move away from the influence of the social problem discourse towards that of social threat.

The CSA has been the subject of much criticism, with calls either for changes or its abolition. Arguments include the following:

> that it is driven by a desire to save state expenditure rather than a concern with children, pushing women into low-paid, insecure jobs and reducing their entitlement to support for bringing up children (Wages for Housework, 1993);
>
> that the interaction of the CSA, Family Credit and other benefits is complex and insecure (Millar, 1994);
>
> that the child-care offset meets only minimal costs, excludes those who use informal child care (the source for the majority of working mothers, including lone mothers – Popay and Jones, 1990; Bradshaw and Millar, 1991) and does not address the actual lack of provision itself (with Britain amongst the lowest public child-care providers in Europe – Moss 1990);
>
> that enforced financial dependency means that lone mothers are enmeshed in patterns of control by their former partners (Clarke et al., 1993);
>
> and that changes in family structure and employment make the idea of a 'family wage' obsolete, so increasing numbers of men cannot support even one family on their own (Millar, 1994).

The gendered regime

Paradoxically, the shift from public to private responsibility for supporting lone mothers in Britain is, in fact, underlaid by considerable state intervention. Overall, the situation of lone mothers points up the British welfare regime's lack of clarity over whether women generally are basically integrated into society as workers in the labour market (as in Sweden – see Björnberg, chapter 9) or as mothers and housewives in families (as in Germany and Ireland – see Klett-Davies, chapter 7, and McLoughlin and Rodgers, chapter 2). On the one hand, if the state provides sufficient support to lone mothers to enable them to become paid workers (e.g., by providing high levels of affordable public child care), then the government is implicitly stating that all mothers are primarily workers. It would hardly be politically feasible to deny partnered mothers access to public child-care provision, and the category of 'lone mother' is not an empirically sustainable child-care rationing device (see Edwards, 1993). On the other hand, treating lone mothers as primarily mothers and home-makers makes heavy demands on Treasury expenditure, even at minimum levels – a cost the British Government is currently baulking at. This strategy also flies in the face of demands from all angles of the political spectrum that women should be both economically and socially independent. Both policy courses, therefore, are fraught with political implications vis-à-vis the relations between men and women, and the nature of 'the family'. This situation helps explain why lone motherhood in Britain is often seen as such a threat to the social order.

As Hobson (1994) points out, lone mothers are the 'residuum' in the gendering of policy, so that they can be taken as a 'litmus test', or indicator, of gendered social rights in different welfare regimes. If this is the case, then where Sweden is 'women-friendly' (Hernes, 1988), Britain must be 'women-hostile'. However, even were the British state to provide adequate child care and proper benefit packages that allowed lone mothers to take employment and hence escape poverty, jobs have to be available for them. This brings us on to the next context for considering lone mothers' uptake of paid work.

5. Local Labour Markets in Britain

National labour market

In Britain, John Ermisch (1991) has shown that lone mothers' employment rate falls in recessions, reflecting the fact that job availability is a factor in lone mothers' ability to take up paid work (see also Bartholomew et al., 1992). Moreover, because of the process of horizontal and vertical occupational sex segregation (whereby women are concentrated in particular occupations and at lower status levels) the jobs available to women are generally the least well paid and less secure (Millar and Glendinning, 1989; Crompton and Sanderson, 1990; MacEwen Scott, 1994). Black women are doubly disadvantaged in the labour market because of the cross-cutting of this process with racism (Bhavnani, 1995).

Indeed, Britain is notorious in the European Union for the development of a particularly low-paid and insecure part-time workforce that is predominantly female (OECD, 1994) – and the government has been assiduous in blocking European Union reforms that might give this female workforce greater rights and pay, such as the Social Chapter or the extension of maternity/paternity leave. Many 'women's jobs', therefore, do not pay a wage sufficient alone to maintain a household adequately, and in addition threaten a severe poverty trap, with benefits cut at a faster rate than wages increase. It is for these reasons that, for mothers in particular, participation in the labour force is often part of a dual-earner strategy (alongside their male partners), with women also doing the 'double shift' of domestic labour (Brannen and Moss, 1991). Clearly, lone mothers by definition cannot take part in a dual-earner strategy, and yet benefits and maintenance are not usually adequate to replace the missing male partner's wage. Even if jobs are available in a quantitative sense, therefore, the sort of jobs on offer to lone mothers in Britain may not pay them enough to allow them to run an independent household or escape the poverty trap (and that is not even taking the cost of child care into account).

Spatial variation in local labour markets

The supply of different sorts of jobs, crucially, is spatially structured through local labour markets. This was particularly marked in Britain during the 1980s, with the concentration on new 'high-tech' and production service jobs in the so-called 'western crescent' stretching around London from Cambridge, through Berkshire, to Southampton. At the same time, the older industrial areas and cities recorded substantial job losses (Townsend, 1993). In addition, different areas, reflecting different gendered spatial divisions of labour, will supply different amounts and types of 'women's jobs' (Massey, 1984; Walby, 1986). Furthermore, women – and mothers especially – have particularly limited job search areas because their time is constrained by their domestic responsibilities, transport difficulties and because of sexual harassment (Pickup, 1988). These constraints are likely to be even more severe for lone mothers who in addition, are concentrated in economically declining areas (Winchester, 1990; Hardey and Crow, 1991). Thus the decline on lone mothers' paid work during the 1980s was particularly marked in inner-city areas; elsewhere it was more stable, fluctuating with the economic cycle (Bartholomew et al., 1992).

In 1991, in different labour markets within Britain, the rate of employment as a whole for lone mothers varied between 25 per cent and 70 per cent, and for full-time work between 6 per cent and 29 per cent (using District Councils as measuring units) (Duncan and Edwards, forthcoming). However, the spatial variation of lone mothers' employment across local labour markets is very similar to the geography of female employment as a whole.

Areas with high employment rates for lone mothers (over 45 per cent in employment and 20 per cent full time) include the Lancashire cotton towns and Staffordshire 'potteries' (both in the north west of England), some east Midland labour markets (around Northampton and Leicester), west London, and parts of southern Scotland and the aforementioned 'western crescent' (Duncan and Edwards, ibid.). These areas have a general tradition of women's full-time work and women's jobs in textiles, clothing manufacture or services – areas where women are seen as paid workers as much as home-makers (see McDowell and Massey, 1984; Walby, 1986; Lewis, 1989a).

Low employment areas for lone mothers (below 30 per cent in employment and 15 per cent full time) include Merseyside (also in the north west of England), most of Wales and the northeast, South Yorkshire, much of the south west, and parts of East Anglia. These are areas with less tradition of women as paid workers. They are also often declining labour markets; for example, the dock work of Merseyside or the coalmining and heavy industry of the north east, South Wales and South Yorkshire.

This association with local economic structure and history is not the whole picture, however. Many of the areas most favourable for women's full-time employment, in fact, are also areas of industrial decline. For example, women's participation in the cotton textile and woollen mills (Lancashire and south Scotland), and the potteries (Staffordshire) may have been very high, but these industries now scarcely exist. Other areas of favourable economic growth, such as light industrial and service jobs in East Anglia, do not show a similar development of women's status as paid workers – the proportion of women taking on full-time paid work remains relatively low. (See Martin and Rowthorne, 1986; Townsend, 1993, for regional economic change in Britain.) This suggests that historical and cultural definition of gender divisions of labour play an important role in explaining women's (and thus lone mothers') propensity to take up paid work in different regions.

Historical and cultural regional gender divisions of labour

Traditional regional divisions of labour are not merely a function of local economic structures; they are reflections of the way that women in a particular local area are socially integrated into society, either through the labour market or through 'home and family' (domestic work and child care). On the one hand, for example, in the Fenlands and East Anglia women have always been exploited as a casual, ill-paid and unskilled labour force, and have remained in similar status jobs even once completely new service and manufacturing jobs were introduced from the 1960s (McDowell and Massey, 1984). Social institutions and gender relations in family farming areas combine to minimize women's independent role (Whatmore, 1991). On the other hand, for example, in industrial Lancashire, not only was there a tradition of women's full-time paid work, women also gained greater power within the private sphere of households and the public sphere of politics (Mark-Lawson et al., 1985; Mark-Lawson, 1988). Such regional cultural traditions seem to be enduring, although immigration and the concentrated residence of different ethnic groupings may bring different traditions to particular localities.

Thus a crucial context for lone mothers' abilities to take up paid work or not are the sets of social expectations (within the variety of British labour markets) about whether women are primarily seen locally as paid workers or as home-makers. The issue is not related to lone mothers only but to gendered divisions of labour generally in various localities. Even within a particular local labour market though, there can be significant variations in lone mothers' paid employment. It is to the social and material processes operating at this level, and which also affect lone mothers' decisions about taking up paid work, that we now turn.

6. Lone Mothers in Neighbourhoods

Empirical research on British lone mothers' uptake of paid work has tended to focus on either the characteristics of social policies or the characteristics of lone mothers, such as route into lone motherhood, age and number of children, educational and vocational qualifications, receipt and level of maintenance, and so on (e.g. Marsh and McKay, 1993; McKay and Marsh, 1994; Ford et al., 1995). As argued in our Introduction to this book, while these national and individual characteristics are undoubtedly influential, they can fail to capture the more subtle, informal neighbourhood-based contexts in which lone mothers negotiate their identities as mothers and/or as workers. Indeed, there are considerable variations in lone mothers' uptake of paid work between neighbourhoods. For example, in the contiguous urban towns of Brighton and Hove on the south coast of England, uptake rates varied between neighbourhoods (using electoral districts as measurement units) from 6 per cent to 25 per cent for full-time work, and 20 per cent to 58 per cent for employment rates as a whole (Duncan and Edwards, forthcoming).

Moreover, as an outcome of the British Government's stance that central and local government have little part to play in providing day-care resources, there is enormous local variation and a diversity of sectoral child-care provision in Britain (Moss, 1991). This patchwork of child care varies in its use to working mothers and in cost and quality. Furthermore, access to much day-care provision has been found to be more difficult for lower socio-economic and minority ethnic groups than it is for those with greater resources (Cohen and Fraser, 1991). Child care often proves too expensive for lone mothers who wish to work full or part time as there is only one wage coming into the household (McKay and Marsh, 1994).

For the most part, British lone – and other – mothers rely on family and other support networks for child care. Some aspects of this may be decreasingly available to lone mothers. In 1990, 88 per cent of lone mothers lived in households on their own, and grandmothers were more likely to be in paid employment themselves. This is in contrast to the situation in 1974, when a higher percentage of lone mothers (then a smaller overall proportion of families as a whole) had paid work. Then, 45 per cent of lone mothers with a child under five were living with other adults in the household, and 90 per cent of lone mothers with a child under five who had paid work lived in multi-unit households, usually their own parents' home (Land, 1994). Indeed, while the majority of today's working lone mothers still rely on their own mothers or other relatives for child care, half of all lone mothers do not use any form of child care at all (Bradshaw and Millar, 1990; Popay and Jones, 1990).

In general, mothers' local networks can also be significant for shared social identities (Bell and Ribbens, 1994). The prevalent discourses about lone motherhood, and the relationship between motherhood and paid work within social networks and neighbourhoods, can play a role in lone mothers' decisions to take paid employment, quite apart from benefit, labour market and child-care structures, and thus contributing to the variations of lone mothers' uptake of paid work at the neighbourhood level. Data from an empirical research project we are currently conducting on lone mothers' uptake of paid work illustrate the influence of socially held conceptions of motherhood vis-à-vis paid work (see also Edwards and Duncan, 1997; and Duncan and Edwards, forthcoming for full results).[3]

Identity and neighbourhood process in the uptake of paid work

Mothering identity

As part of our research into the contexts for lone mothers' uptake of paid work, 65 lone mothers were interviewed, living either in the inner London boroughs of Lambeth and Southwark (containing the highest percentage of lone mothers in Great Britain), or in the contiguous south coast towns of Brighton and Hove (containing near average proportions of lone mothers). The lone mothers came from different neighbourhoods and seven particular social groups. In Lambeth/Southwark we interviewed two groups of African-Caribbean lone mothers (9 younger and 10 older women), and a group of African lone mothers (10 women), all three groups living in neighbourhoods of public housing; and a group of White lone mothers with 'alternative' and feminist views, also mainly living in public housing. In Brighton/Hove, the lone mothers we interviewed were all White: another group with 'alternative' views, living in a gentrified owner-occupied neighbourhood (10 women); a group living on a peripheral public housing estate (10 women); and a group living in a suburban owner-occupied neighbourhood (6 women). (See Edwards and Duncan, 1997 for the rationale underlying the choice of groups and access to them.)

Our interview data reveal that the groups of lone mothers held particular understandings about their identity as mothers, and as lone mothers in particular, in relation to paid work (which elsewhere we have termed 'gendered moral rationalities' – Duncan and Edwards, 1997; Edwards and Duncan, 1996). From the interviews with lone mothers themselves, we have identified three main 'ideal forms' of this overall type of understanding:

(i) *Primarily mother* In this form, lone mothers give primacy to the moral benefits of physically caring for their children themselves over and above any financial benefits of undertaking paid work. The sorts of statements that the lone mothers interviewed for our research made that fall within this view include: 'If you have children you should be with them, not leave them with someone else'; 'Bringing up children is a job in itself'; and 'If you work you miss out on your children growing up'.

(ii) *Mother/worker integral*   Here, lone mothers may see financial provision through employment as part of their moral responsibilities towards their children. The sorts of views in this vein expressed by lone mothers include: 'You need to earn money to take care of your children'; 'Working means that I can provide for my child and give him a better life'; and 'Working sets a good example to my children, so they'll want to get on in life themselves'.

(iii) *Primarily worker*   Within this form, lone mothers give primacy to paid work for themselves separate to their identity as mothers. In this vein, the lone mothers interviewed said things like: 'I think of myself as a career person rather than a mother'; 'Staying at home and just looking after children feels like a trap'; and 'Working gives me status and self-respect'.

In terms of the seven social groups of lone mothers taking part in our research, the White lone mothers living on a peripheral council estate in Brighton, all working-class, were much more likely to give primacy to caring for their children themselves, over and above paid work (as Jordan et al., 1992, also found for White working-class lone mothers living on a deprived Exeter council estate). The White, mainly middle-class, lone mothers living in a suburban are of Brighton/Hove, tended to combine this primacy with some elements of a separate, even contradictory, identity as workers. Few in these two groups expressed any views that saw paid work and motherhood as integral, especially amongst the 'suburban' lone mothers.

The older group of African-Caribbean lone mothers, mainly living in smaller pockets of council housing in Southwark, also expressed views giving primacy to motherhood, but had more elements of both a separate identity as workers, and of motherhood and paid work as integral. The younger group of African-Caribbean lone mothers and the African (mainly West African) lone mothers, mainly living on larger council estates in Lambeth/Southwark, tended to give equal weight to motherhood and paid work as integral, and to having a separate work identity for themselves.

Both groups of White 'alternative' lone mothers, living in Southwark/ Lambeth and in a gentrified area of Brighton, were much more likely to have identities as workers for themselves, separate to motherhood.

Thus, on an overall level, the White lone mothers we interviewed largely saw motherhood and employment as dichotomous, incompatible or separate activities, demanding different identities (primarily mother – primarily worker). Generally, however, the Black lone mothers, to varying extents, were more able to integrate the two within their views.

Neighbourhood supports

The lone mothers' views about the compatibility of motherhood and employment were often socially sustained by norms held in common with others in their local social networks. Transgressing local norms can result in any available familial or friendship support, including child care, being withdrawn (see Jordan et al., 1992). For example, in our research, Sylvia, one of the lone mothers who lived on the peripheral Brighton council estate, said she would love to have paid work as she thought she would be better off than living on benefits. She was very aware of the social threat view of lone mothers as scroungers on the state. Her own mother, who lived nearby, was not in employment and offered Sylvia child care and other support when she needed it. However, her mother would not look after Sylvia's children to enable her to work because her mother believed that mothers should stay at home and look after their children. Thus if Sylvia took up paid work it would cause problems in her relationship with her mother, and would go against her own views of what is 'right', morally if not financially.

In contrast, Kim, one of the younger African-Caribbean lone mothers living on a council estate in Lambeth, was in paid work (and was also conscious of social threat views of lone motherhood). She said she was better off financially working than being on benefits, that she was not the sort of person who could stay at home with her children all the time, and that working allowed her to better herself and her children, including her children learning that education was important so they could eventually find good jobs. Kim's family and friends were supportive of her working, and child care was provided by Kim's ex-partner, with whom she maintained a supportive relationship, with back up support from her sisters.

Indeed, there is evidence that, in holding social norms about mother-hood and paid work as integral (as we noted in section 2), Black lone mothers are much more likely to be economically active and to work full time than their White counterparts (Bartholomew et al., 1992; Duncan and Edwards, 1997). In our research it is noticeable that those neighbourhoods in Brighton/Hove with the lowest lone-mother employment rates include the large public housing estates, mainly housing a White working-class popu-lation (Duncan and Edwards, 1996). Thus, overall, lone mothers holding socially sustained views of motherhood that fall outside those dominant in British society – 'mother/worker integral' and 'primarily worker' – are more able to combine these with paid work. In contrast, those subscribing to, and supported in, traditional dominant notions of mothering – 'primarily mother' – are less able to combine this view of themselves with one of being paid workers.

In this way, different social groups of lone mothers, living in different neighbourhoods, and with different social network supports, respond differ-ently to the local and national structures within which they live. These responses are not organized around their position as lone mothers per se, but are more to do with their views about the general compatibility of motherhood and paid work. Thus, again, the issue is infused largely with gendered ideas about whether women should be home-makers or paid workers.

7. Conclusion

The debate – or rather moral panic – surrounding lone motherhood in Britain is not about lone mothers' situation in itself. Rather, it is about the relations between men and women; about their roles and situations in relation to one another and their integration into society.

In Britain, lone mothers are seen as a separate category from other families, not least by the state, where different types of behaviour are deemed appropriate, or expected, for women in two-parent and lone-mother families, and where policies are influenced by particular discourses around lone motherhood. Currently British policies, strongly influenced by the social threat discourse, are moving away from the state financially supporting lone mothers towards a combination of reimposing or imposing the (ex) male breadwinner and lone mothers' own earnings. This latter aim is not supported by publicly provided child care, as maternal employment generally (posed as coupled rather than lone mothers) is regarded by the state as a 'private' and individual choice.

The issue of lone mothers' uptake of paid work is significantly shaped by expectations and beliefs about women's, especially mothers', roles – about gendered divisions of labour – at other levels as well as policy. Lone mothers' job opportunities and their propensity to take up paid work are locally differentiated. This occurs at the level of local labour markets, where both particular jobs (especially socially defined women's jobs) and conceptions as to whether women are mothers or workers are differently distributed. It also occurs at the levels of neighbourhoods and social networks, with different social groups of lone mothers having access to varying resources in terms of child-care support and in terms of socially held conceptions of the meaning of motherhood and its compatibility with paid work.

These various contextual levels, providing opportunities and constraints for lone mothers' uptake of paid work, interact in a number of ways. The overall existence and, crucially, the importance of social networks and support at a neighbourhood level, for example, may well be related to the British welfare state regime, whereby policies generally do not support maternal employment or child-care provision. Lone mothers are left especially reliant on opportunities and constraints provided by informal kin and friendship support networks in terms of their conceptions of themselves as mothers who should, or should not, take up paid work.

Notes

1 In turn, this is based on the assumption of 'rational economic man'. Lone mothers as individual economic agents, maximize their personal welfare on cost–benefit calculations (see Duncan and Edwards, forthcoming; Edwards and Duncan, 1996).

2 The policy debate over child care in Britain is most often expressed in terms of

mothers' access to the labour market, rather than the social and educational benefits for children (Edwards, 1993).

3   This research is funded by the Economic and Social Research Council under grant number R000234960. For full results from the study see Duncan and Edwards, forthcoming. Vignettes of, and quotes from, lone mothers in the text are based on data from interviews carried out during the summer of 1994.

References

BARTHOLOMEW, R., HIBBETT, A. and SIDAWAY, J. (1992) 'Lone parents and the labour market: evidence from the LFS', *Employment Gazette*, November, pp. 559–77.

BELL, L. and RIBBENS, J. (1994) 'Isolated housewives and complex maternal worlds: the significance of social contacts between women with young children in industrial societies', *Sociological Review* **42**, 4, pp. 227–62.

BHAVNANI, R. (1995) *Black Women and the Labour Market: A Research Review*, Manchester: Equal Opportunities Commission.

BORTOLAIA-SILVA, E. (Ed.) (1996) *Good Enough Mothering? Feminist Perspectives on Lone Motherhood*, London: Routledge.

BRADSHAW, J. (1989) *Lone Parents: Policy in the Doldrums*, London: Family Policy Studies Centre.

BRADSHAW, J. and MILLAR, J. (1991) *Lone Parent Families in the U.K.*, London: HMSO.

BRANNEN, J. and MOSS, P. (1991) *Managing Mothers: Dual Earner Households After Maternity Leave*, London: Unwin Hyman.

BURGHES, L. (1993) *One Parent families: Policy Options for the 1990s*, York: Joseph Rowntree Foundation.

BURGHES, L. (1994) *Lone Parenthood and Family Disruption: The Outcomes for Children*, London: Family Policy Studies Centre.

BURGHES, L. and BROWN, M. (1995) *Single Lone Mothers: Problems, Prospects and Policies*, London: Family Policy Studies Centre.

CAMPAIGN AGAINST THE CHILD SUPPORT ACT (1993) *Dossier of DSS Illegalities*, London: CACSA.

CHEAL, D. (1991) *The Family and the State of Theory*, London: Harvester/Wheatsheaf.

CLARKE, K., CRAIG, G. and GLENDINNING, C. (1993) *Children Come First? The Child Support Act and Lone Parent Families*, London: Barnardos/Children's Society/ NCH/NSPCC/SCF.

COHEN, B. and FRASER, N. (1991) *Childcare in a Modern Welfare State*, London: Institute of Public Policy Research.

CROMPTON, R. and SANDERSON, K. (1990) *Gendered Jobs and Social Change*, London: Unwin Hyman.

CROW, G. and HARDEY, M. (1991) 'The housing strategies of lone parents', in Hardey, M. and Crow, G. (Eds).

DEAN, H. and TAYLOR-GOOBY, P. (1992) *Dependency Culture: The Explosion of the Myth*, Hemel Hempstead: Harvester/Wheatsheaf.

DELPHY, C. and LEONARD, D. (1992) *Familiar Exploitation: A New Analysis of Marriage in Contemporary Western Society*, Cambridge: Polity Press.

DENNIS, N. (1991a) 'Common sense, social science knowledge and social change in the late 1960s', paper presented at Institute of Economic Affairs Consensus Conference, London, July.

DENNIS, N. (1991b) 'What's "left" and "right" in sex, childrearing and face to face mutual aid', paper presented at Institute of Economic Affairs Consensus Conference, London, July.

DENNIS, N. (1993) *Rising Crime and the Dismembered Family*, London: Institute for Economic Affairs.

DENNIS, N. and ERDOS, G. (1993) *Families Without Fatherhood*, London: Institute for Economic Affairs.

DEPARTMENT OF SOCIAL SECURITY (1990) *Children Come First*, London: HMSO.

DOWLER, E. and CALVERT, C. (1995) *Nutrition and Diet in Lone Parent Families in London*, London: Family Policy Studies Centre.

DUNCAN, S. S. (1995) 'Theorising European gender systems', *Journal of European Social Policy*, **5**, 4, pp. 263–84.

DUNCAN, S. and EDWARDS, R. (1996) 'Lone mothers and paid work: neighbourhoods, local labour markets and welfare state regimes', *Social Politics*, **3**, 4 pp. 195–222.

DUNCAN, S. and EDWARDS, R. (1997) 'Lone mothers and paid work: rational or economic man or gendered moral rationalities', *Feminist Economics*, **3**, 2.

DUNCAN, S. and EDWARDS, R. (forthcoming) *Lone Mothers and Paid Work: Context, Discourse and Action*, London: Macmillan.

EDWARDS, R. (1993) 'Taking the initiative: the government, lone mothers and day care provision', *Critical Social Policy* **39**, pp. 36–50.

EDWARDS, R. and DUNCAN, S. (1996) 'Rational economic man or lone mothers in context? The uptake of paid work and social policy', in Bortolaia-Silva, E. (Ed.).

EDWARDS, R. and DUNCAN, S. (1997) 'Supporting the family: lone mothers, paid work and the underclass debate', *Critical Social Policy*, **5**, 2.

EEKELAAR, J. (1991) *Regulating Divorce*, Oxford: Clarendon.

ELLIOTT, J. and RICHARDS, M. (1991) 'Parental divorce and the life chances of children', *Family Law*, November, pp. 481–4.

ERMISCH, J. (1991) *Lone Parents: An Economic Analysis*, Cambridge: Polity Press.

ESPING-ANDERSEN, G. (1990) *Three Worlds of Welfare Capitalism*, Cambridge: Polity Press.

FERRI, E. (1976) *Growing Up In A One Parent Family*, London: National Children's Bureau.

FORD, R., MARSH, A. and McKAY, J. (1995) *Changes in Lone Parenthood*, Department of Social Security Research Report 40, London: HMSO.

GIDDENS, A. (1991) *Modernity and Self-Identity: Self and Society in the Late Modern Age*, Cambridge: Polity Press.

GITTINS, D. (1985) *The Family in Question*, Basingstoke: Macmillan.

GRAHAM, H. (1987) 'Being poor: perceptions and coping strategies of lone mothers', in Brannen, J. and Wilson, G. (Eds) *Give and Take in Families*, London: Allen & Unwin.

GRAHAM, H. (1993) *Hardship and Health in Women's Lives*, Hemel Hempstead: Harvester/Wheatsheaf.

HALSEY, A. H. (1993) 'Changes in the family', *Children and Society*, **7**, 2, pp. 125–36.

HARDEY, M. and CROW, G. (Eds) (1991) *Lone Parenthood: Coping With Constraints and Making Opportunities*, London: Harvester.

HARRISON, P. (1983) *Inside the Inner City: Life Under the Cutting Edge*, Harmondsworth: Penguin.

HASKEY, J. (1994) 'Estimated numbers of one parent families and their prevalence in Great Britain 1991', *Population Trends*, 78, London: HMSO.

HERNES, M. (1988) 'The welfare state citizenship of Scandinavian women', in Jones, K. and Jonasdottir, A. (Eds) *The Political Interests of Gender*, London: Sage.

HOBSON, B. (1994) 'Solo mothers, social policy regimes and the logics of gender', in Sainsbury D. (Ed.).

HOCHSCHILD, A. (1989) *The Second Shift: Working Parents and the Revolution at Home*, London: Piatkus.

HOLME, A. (1985) *Housing and Young Families in East London*, London: Routledge & Kegan Paul.

HOLTERMANN, S. (1992) *Investing in Young Children: Costing an Education and Daycare Service*, London: National Children's Bureau.

JORDAN, B., SIMON, B., KAY, H. and REDLEY, M. (1992) *Trapped in Poverty?*, London: Routledge.

KIERNAN, K. E. (1992) 'The impact of family disruption in childhood on transitions in young adulthood', *Population Studies*, **46**, pp. 213–21.

LAMBERT, L. and STREATHER, J. (1980) *Children in Changing Families*, London: Macmillan.

LAND, H. (1994) 'The demise of the male breadwinner in practice but not in theory: a challenge for social security systems', in Baldwin, S. and Falkingham, J. (Eds) *Social Security and Social Change*, London: Simon & Schuster.

LEEMING, A., UNELL, J. and WALKER, R. (1994) *Lone Mothers: Coping With the Consequences of Separation*, Department of Social Security Research Report No. 30, London: HMSO.

LEWIS, J. (1989a) *Labour and Love: Women at Work and Home 1850–1939*, Oxford: Blackwell.

LEWIS, J. (1989b) 'Lone parent families: politics and economics', *Journal of Social Policy*, **18**, 4, pp. 595–600.

LEWIS, J. (1992a) *Women in England Since 1945*, Oxford: Blackwell.

LEWIS, J. (1992b) 'Gender and the development of welfare regimes', *Journal of European Social Policy*, **2** 3, pp. 159–73.

LONSDALE, S. (1992) 'Patterns of paid work', in Glendinning, C. and Millar, J. (Eds) *Women and Poverty in Britain*, Hemel Hempstead: Harvester/Wheatsheaf.

McDOWELL, L. and MASSEY, D. (1984) 'A woman's place?', in Massey, D. and Aldlen, J. (Eds) *Geography Matters*, Milton Keynes: Open University.

MacEWEN SCOTT, A. (Ed.) (1994) *Gender Segregation and Social Change*, Oxford: Oxford University Press.

McKAY, S. and MARSH, A. (1994) *Lone Parents and Work*, Department of Social Security Research Report 25, London: HMSO.

McKEE, L. and O'BRIEN, M. (1992) *The Father Figure*, London: Tavistock.

MANN, K. and ROSENEIL, S. (1996) 'Lone mothers, the underclass and the backlash', in Bortolaia-Silva, E. (Ed.).

MARK-LAWSON, J. (1988) 'Occupational segregation and women's politics', in Walby, S. (Ed.) *Gender Segregation at Work*, Milton Keynes: Open University.

MARK-LAWSON, J., SAVAGE, M. and WARD, A. (1985) 'Gender and local politics: struggles over welfare policies 1918–39', in Murgatroyd L., Savage, M., Shapiro, D., Urry, J., Walby, S. and WARKE, A. (Eds) *Locality, Class and Gender*, London: Dion.

MARSH, A. and McKAY, S. (1993) *Families, Work and Benefits*, London: Policy Studies Centre.

MARSH, A. AND McKAY, S. (1994) *Poor Smokers*, London: Policy Studies Centre.

MARTIN, R. and ROWTHORNE, B. (1986) *The Geography of Deindustrialisation*, London: Macmillan.

MASSEY, D. (1984) *Spatial Divisions of Labour*, (2nd Edn, 1995) London: Macmillan.

MILLAR, J. (1989) *Poverty and the Lone Parent Family: The Challenge to Social Policy*, London: Avebury.

MILLAR, J. (1994) 'Poor mothers and absent fathers: support for lone parents in comparative perspective', paper presented at the Social Policy Association Annual Conference, University of Liverpool, July.

MILLAR, J. and GLENDINNING, C. (1989) 'Gender and poverty', *journal of Social Policy*, **18**, 3, pp. 363–82.

MOORE, R. (1996) 'Deprivation and the ethnic minority child', paper presented at the British Sociological Association annual conference, University of Reading, April.

MORGAN, P. (1995) *Farewell to the Family: Public Policy and Family Breakdown in Britain and USA*, London: Institute of Economic Affairs.

MORRIS, L. (1993) *Dangerous Classes: The Underclass and Social Citizenship*, London: Routledge.

MOSS, P. (1990) *Childcare in the European Community 1985–1990*, Brussels: EU Commission.

MOSS, P. (1991) 'Daycare policy and provision in Britain', in Moss, P. and Melhuish, E. (Eds) *Current Issues in Day Care for Young Children*, London: HMSO.

MURRAY, C. (1990) *The Emerging British Underclass*, London: Institute of Economic Affairs.

OECD (1994) *Women and Structural Change: New Perspectives*, Paris: Organisation for Economic Co-operation and Development.

PICKUP, L. (1988) 'Hard to get around: a study of women's travel mobility', in Little, J., Peake, L. and Richardson, P. (Eds) *Women in Cities*, London: Macmillan.

PAHL, J. (1989) *Money and Marriage*, London: Macmillan.

POPAY, J. and JONES, G. (1990) 'Patterns of health and illness amongst lone parents', *Journal of Social Policy*, **19**, 4, pp. 499–534.

ROLL, J. (1992) *Lone Parent Families in the E.C.*, Brussels: EC Commission.

SAINSBURY, D. (Ed.) (1994) *Gendering Welfare States*, London: Sage.

SEGALMAN, R. AND MARSLAND, D. (1989) *Cradle to Grave*, London: Macmillan.

SHAW, S. (1991) 'The conflicting experiences of lone parenthood', in Hardey, M. and Crow, G. (eds).

SONG, M. and EDWARDS, R. (1996) 'Comment: raising questions about perspectives on black lone motherhood', *Journal of Social Policy*, pp. 377–97.

TOWNSEND, A. (1993) *Uneven Regional Change in Britain*, Cambridge: Cambridge University Press.

TOYNBEE, P. (1994) 'Family fortunes', *The Guardian*, 2 February.

WAGES FOR HOUSEWORK AND PAYDAY MEN'S NETWORK (1993) 'Against redistributing poverty', *Centrepiece* 8, London: Wages for Housework Campaign.

WALBY, S. (1986) *Patriarchy At Work: Patriarchal and Capitalist Relations in Employment*, Cambridge: Polity Press.

WALBY, S. (1990) *Theorising Patriarchy*, Oxford: Blackwell.

WHATMORE, S. (1991) *Farming Women: Gender, Work and Family Enterprises*, London: Macmillan.

WINCHESTER, H. (1990) 'Women and children last: the poverty and marginalisation of one-parent families', *Transactions, Institute of British Geographers*, **15**, 1, pp. 70–86.

ZULAUF, M. (1997) 'Mother and baby homes: a viable solution for young single mothers?', unpublished paper, London School of Economics.

Chapter 4

Single Mothers in the USA: Unsupported Workers and Mothers

Martha de Acosta

1. Introduction

This chapter brings together data on single mothers'[1] participation in the labour force in the USA, with an analysis of how a small group of low-income single mothers living in Cleveland, Ohio decided whether or not to take paid work. The chapter focuses on the factors that single mothers take into account when making this choice, and relates information from three different spatial levels – national, local labour market, and neighbourhood.

Local service providers in one low-income city district of Cleveland furnished the research staff with lists of single mothers who were potential interviewees for this project. A small opportunistic sample of 14, mainly young, single mothers resulted. Although not statistically representative of single mothers in the Near West Side of Cleveland, it gives us 'a point of entry, the locus of an experiencing subject or subjects, into a larger social and economic process' (Smith, 1987: 157). Interviews of one to one-and-a-half hours were conducted with each of the women. During the course of the interviews, the single mothers gave accounts that began to reveal how they decided on courses of action to secure resources, and how they made sense of their circumstances. This snapshot interaction could capture only a partial picture of the ways these mothers made sense of the constraints and opportunities in their immediate lives, of the different courses of action they considered, and of those they embarked upon. Nonetheless, important insights were gained. Moreover, while we did not expect the women to talk about the larger social conditions that shaped their everyday lives, the analysis of their practices and the lines of action they embark upon show their situated interpretation of macro-structural factors and social and material conditions (Smith, 1987; Bourdieu and Wacquant, 1992).

2. Single Motherhood in the USA

The growth of female-headed families

Increases in the number of families headed by single mothers, and changes in the distribution of these families in terms of race, ethnicity, marital status, and age of the mother are at the centre of current debates about the state of families. Single mothers caring for their children comprise an increasingly large percentage of families in the USA. Married-couple families have decreased from 70.5 per cent of all families in 1976, to 56 per cent in 1990 (Current Population Reports, 1991). Between 1976 and 1991, the number of families maintained by single parents increased more than twofold – from 3.8 million to 10.1 million, and of those, the overwhelming majority (86 per cent) were maintained by mothers. While the proportion of families headed by women rose from 11 per cent to 13 per cent between 1970 and 1988 and reached 25 per cent in 1994, the proportion of families headed by Black women rose from 28 per cent to 43 per cent (Garwood, 1991). Divorced mothers were the largest category of single mothers (31.9 per cent) among one-parent families maintained by mothers, followed by never-married mothers (30.7 per cent) in 1991, but their prevalence varied according to race and ethnicity. While divorced mothers were the largest category among Whites (39.2%), those never-married were the most numerous among Blacks (54.2%). Among Hispanics the situation was somewhat different. Both separated (29.5 per cent) – legally separated or otherwise absent from spouse but not legally divorced – and never-married (29.2 per cent) single mothers were most prevalent, while divorced mothers were less numerous (21.7 per cent). Single-mother situations were more prevalent among Blacks whose children were more likely to be living with the mother only (54 per cent), than Hispanic (28 per cent) or White children (17 per cent) (Current Population Reports, 1993).

Single-mother households with children under 18 years of age represented slightly more than half of all families who were poor in 1990 – up from one-third of the families in poverty in 1970 (Current Population Reports, 1991). Moreover, about four in ten depended on welfare at one time during the year (Moffit, 1992). This has diverted attention from middle-class mother-only families, which have shown the faster increase. Consequently, families headed by mothers with children under 18 years of age who are poor comprised only 16 per cent of all families headed by single mothers with children under 18 years of age.

The growth in the number of families headed by single mothers who are poor has multiple causes. First, to a large extend it is due to a minimum wage that has remained unchanged and to changes in the labour market. During much of the 1980s the minimum wage was not raised, and by the end of that decade nearly half of all poor families had one employed member; only 16 per cent had a full-time worker (Economic Report to the President, 1991 cited in Gaffikin and Morrissey, 1994). Moreover, a reduction in the number of full-time jobs declined and the number of temporary part-time ones increased.

The median income of single mothers caring for children under 18 years ($16,443) is far lower than that of families with children under 18 years who live with both parents ($44,053). Even subtracting working wives' contribution to two-earner families with children, calculated at 31 per cent of family income, this indicates a wide gap which separates the median income of families with children from the median income of single mothers.

A second cause of impoverishment for many families headed by single mothers is inadequate alimony (divorce settlement) and child support (maintenance). Notwithstanding the passage of The Family Support Act of 1988, aimed at improving child-support systems, more than half of children eligible for child support do not receive it (Current Population Reports, 1991). Furthermore, child-support awards are low. In 1982, alimony and child support accounted for less than 10 per cent of White mothers' income and about 3 per cent of that of Black mothers (Garfinkel and McLanahan, 1986).

A third cause of the growth of poor families headed by single mothers is inadequate public assistance. In the USA a stratified welfare system gives more support to those considered 'deserving' of it; widows receive a higher level of assistance than never-married, divorced or separated mothers. About one-third of the families headed by widows are poor, compared to approximately half of all families headed by single women (Garfinkel and McLanahan, 1986).

A little-acknowledged trend in mother-only families is that the number of births to teenage mothers *declined* by 25 per cent between 1972 and 1986. The social conditions in which early child bearing occurs, and its negative outcomes, have focused media attention on teenage motherhood and fuelled social and public policy. Seven out of 10 teenage mothers are unmarried, and the majority raise their children without the father's support, shifting much of the financial support to the state. Mothers who give birth before completing their education do not achieve an education comparable to that of those who give birth when they are older. Furthermore, in recent times, income loss to young women who drop out of high school or become single mothers at an early age has increased (Duncan and Hoffman, 1991). Many public and non-profit agencies that target their services to teenage mothers have contributed to improving the social conditions in which these mothers raise their children. Nevertheless, teenage single mothers and their children are considered to be at risk of negative health and social outcomes. For example, teenage mothers make less use of prenatal care and have a higher incidence of low-birth-weight babies (Hardy and Zabin, 1991).

Labour force participation of single mothers

Working mothers' participation in the labour force has increased rapidly and substantially. Sixteen million workers were employed in March of 1980, 23 million in March of 1992 (US Department of Labor, 1993). In accounting for the growth of mothers' labour-force participation, four factors stand out: first, the decline in real income of families with children, which made two-earner families the norm; second, increases in the divorce rate which pushed divorced single mothers with children under 18 years of age to the highest level of employment (80 per cent) among single mothers in March of 1992; third, among never-married mothers with children under age 18 a higher percentage worked (73.2 per cent) than among married mothers with children in that age range (67.8 per cent) (US Labor Department, 1993) (Tables 4.1 and 4.2); fourth, dominant societal views which became more favourable to working mothers, even mothers of young children, with a trend for mothers to go to work when their children are younger.

In 1992, over half of married mothers with children under three years of age, whose husbands were absent or who were widowed or divorced, participated in the labour force, and four out of ten never-married mothers did so (Table 4.3).

The unequal distribution of educational achievement among mothers according to marital status, race and ethnicity is one of the factors that accounts for their differential labour-force participation. Divorced mothers in the labour force were more likely to have at least a high school education than were widowed and never-married mothers. More White single mothers have completed high school than Black single mothers, with Hispanic mothers lagging behind (Current Population Reports, 1993).

Single mothers' participation in the labour force and positioning in the labour market has been affected by structural changes in the US economy and

Marital and labour force status	Women with children under 18 years	With youngest child			
		14 to 17	6 to 13	3 to 5	Under 3
All women 16 years and over					
Labour-force participation rate (%)	58.1	65.8	65.3	56.1	44.3
Unemployment rate (%)	8.0	5.1	7.4	8.4	11.7
Married, husband present					
Labour-force participation rate (%)	55.7	63.3	62.1	54.8	43.7
Unemployment rate (%)	6.5	4.2	5.9	6.7	9.4
Single Mothers					
Never married					
Labour-force participation rate (%)	52.3	(*)	64.9	54.7	41.0
Unemployment rate (%)	26.8	(*)	22.2	26.3	33.8
Married, husband absent					
Labour-force participation rate (%)	61.7	70.1	69.9	53.9	48.7
Unemployment rate (%)	16.4	8.6	16.7	17.5	22.6
Widowed					
Labour-force participation rate (%)	60.3	64.7	61.3	(*)	(*)
Unemployment rate (%)	10.2	9.8	10.5	(*)	(*)
Divorced					
Labour-force participation rate (%)	78.1	81.2	84.3	69.9	58.1
Unemployment rate (%)	7.9	5.5	7.8	8.0	14.7

Note *rate not shown where base is less than 75,000
Due to rounding, sums of individual items may not equal totals
Source US Department of Labor, Bureau of Labor Statistics
Table 4.1 Labour-force status of women 16 years and over, by marital status and presence and age of youngest child: USA, March 1981

Marital and labour force status	Women with children under 18 years	With youngest child			
		14 to 17	6 to 13	3 to 5	Under 3
All women 16 years and over					
Labour-force participation rate (%)	66.6	76.4	73.6	64.4	54.5
Unemployment rate (%)	7.0	4.2	5.8	7.8	10.1
Married, husband present					
Labour-force participation rate (%)	66.8	75.7	72.8	64.7	56.8
Unemployment rate (%)	5.3	3.4	4.5	6.3	7.1
Single Mothers					
Never married					
Labour-force participation rate (%)	53.6	70.5	63.5	59.3	43.9
Unemployment rate (%)	17.9	8.0	11.3	17.9	24.6
Married, husband absent					
Labour-force participation rate (%)	63.8	77.0	74.0	55.0	49.8
Unemployment rate (%)	12.9	10.2	10.8	9.9	22.3
Widowed					
Labour-force participation rate (%)	59.1	58.4	62.2	65.3	38.2
Unemployment rate (%)	9.8	6.2	11.5	14.2	7.5
Divorced					
Labour-force participation rate (%)	80.2	85.9	84.0	75.4	58.7
Unemployment rate (%)	7.3	4.9	7.2	7.3	14.6

Note Due to rounding, sums of individual items may not equal total
Source US Department of Labor, Bureau of Labor Statistics
Table 4.2 Labour-force status of women 16 years and over, by marital status and presence and age of youngest child: USA, March 1991

by labour market segmentation. The largest job increase in the labour market has been in the secondary market where jobs are low paid, and have little stability or continuity. The gender and racial compositions of jobs influence the organization of the labour process, the kind of control workers have over their work, and the level of their earnings (Tomaskovic-Devey, 1993).

While single mothers' distribution across occupations resembles that of other women workers, they are more highly concentrated in blue-collar jobs (15.1 per cent) and in service jobs (21.6 per cent) than other women workers (Amott, 1988). For Black and Hispanic mothers, labour-force participation is even more concentrated in service occupations in the secondary labour market, while for Whites, participation is more concentrated in professional and white-collar[2] jobs where there is a higher return for education and better defined career paths. Moreover, in each of these labour markets, women earn less than men do.

Although labour participation rates have increased for both minority and non-minority women, persistent differences in participation and unequal returns for schooling prevail (Smith and Tienda, 1987). The decline in manufacturing jobs has pushed Blacks and Hispanics with low skills out of the labour force. In particular, joblessness has increased disproportionately among women of colour with less than a high school education (Tienda, Donato and Cordero-Guzman, 1992).

Marital status and age of children	(% in labour-force)			
	1970	1980	1990	1992
Married, husband present	40.9	50.1	58.2	59.3
Children under 6	30.5	45.1	58.9	59.9
Children under 3	25.9	41.3	55.5	57.5
Single Mothers				
Never married	(1)	61.5	66.4	64.7
Children under 6	(1)	44.1	48.7	45.8
Children under 3	(1)	41.7	41.9	41.0
Married, husband absent	55.9	59.4	63.6	61.8
Children under 6	45.4	52.2	59.3	55.7
Children under 3	42.5	42.4	51.6	48.8
Widowed	27.3	22.5	19.5	18.8
Children under 6	36.8	44.7	50.1	56.3
Children under 3	(2)	(2)	(2)	(2)
Divorced	73.0	74.5	75.5	74.0
Children under 6	63.3	68.3	69.8	65.9
Children under 3	52.1	56.8	57.6	55.6

Source US Department of Labor, Bureau of Labor Statistics, 'Number of Working Mothers Now at Record Levels', press release, July 26, 1984, and Current Population Survey, March 1990 and 1992

Table 4.3 Labour-force participation rates of mothers with pre-school children, marital status, selected years: USA, March 1970–92

3. Discourses Around Single Motherhood in the USA

Discourses on single mothers pivot around ideal notions of gender roles and relations, and are structured by notions of race and class. These discourses shape single mothers' construction of their identities and the direction of their lines of action. Discourses on single mothers also cast the terms of policies that create constraints and possibilities for single mothers. Edwards and Duncan (1997) have identified four competing discourses on single motherhood: single mothers as lifestyle change, single mothers as women escaping patriarchy, single mothers as social problem, and single mothers as social threat (see chapter 3, this volume).

The discourse on single mothers as lifestyle change has been put forward by feminists and social scientists. Changes in gender roles and in attitudes towards sexuality have removed much of the stigma of being a single mother (Stannard, 1977). Emphasis on individual rights and self-fulfilment, changes in gender roles, and more permissive attitudes toward sexuality have increased the number of women opting for single motherhood (Stannard, 1977; Garfinkel and McLanahan, 1986). Changes in lifestyle appear even more pronounced because single-parent families are compared to fictionalized, two-parent families of TV shows in the 1950s and early 1960s, rather than to more realistic images (Coontz, 1992).

Growing economic independence of women allowed them to support themselves outside marriage, to become more selective in their decision to marry, or to leave a bad marriage (McLanahan, 1994). Public recognition that a large number of married mothers had joined the workforce reduced support for single mothers to stay at home on public assistance. By 1988, women on public assistance with children over age three were required either to take paid work or participate in 20 weekly hours of training.

The discourse of single mothers as escaping patriarchy has welcomed the breakdown of the family as freeing women from an identity defined in relationship to a man (wife of —), of having a husband 'to have both a sex life and respectability' (Stannard, 1977: 337). Some women of colour, who see their families 'as sites of shared resistance to racism' (Blum, 1993: 293) and viewing power differentials within the families as an outcome of racist relations, have criticized this interpretation of family distintegration.

The social problem discourse explains the behaviour of single mothers in terms of social and economic forces that affect their lives, but are beyond their control. Post-industrial capitalism has had a destructive effect on the traditional family. Fewer men are earning a family wage and fewer women have access to a man's earnings. Such economic dislocation puts women in a position of being 'torn by increasingly incompatible work and family demands' (Blum, 1993: 294).

The social problem discourse has been used extensively by social scientists and policy analysts to understand teenage pregnancy. Based on extensive ethnographic studies of urban youth, Anderson (1991) concluded that the teenagers most likely to give birth out of wedlock were those who saw no way out for them. Duncan and Hoffman (1991) found that while raising government benefits to single mothers increased their chances of giving birth to children out of wedlock, labour market and marital opportunities had a much stronger effect in the opposite direction.

Strong at the beginning of the century, incorporated into federal legislation passed in the 1930s, and part of programmes to eradicate long-term poverty in the 1960s, the view of single mothers as a social problem has recently been in retreat. The War on Poverty programmes of the President Lyndon Johnson era saw the poor as victims, as individuals wanting to get jobs, but prevented from doing so because of social and economic factors beyond their control, such as race, limited skills, or lack of child care. The poor were deserving of state support.

According to this view the persistence of poverty among single mothers is due to the fragmentary and discriminatory nature of the welfare state. First, services are provided by a patchwork of institutions and programmes. Second, the welfare state in the USA has been less comprehensive than in many European countries, and has historically separated those deserving help from those who do not deserve it (Peterson, 1991).

The mid-1970s saw the beginnings of the social threat discourse, articulated by a rising new political right, whose project has been characterized as the reassertion of patriarchy and the rearticulation of racial ideology (Omi and

Winant, 1986). The defining characteristics of this project are the formulation of social questions as issues of individual guilt and responsibility and a strong anti-statism. Economic dislocations in the 1970s marked the end of the American Dream, and an awareness that the economy would not continue to grow evenly and continuously. Social scientists and political thinkers became interested in those who remained in poverty for long periods of time; the concept of 'underclass' gained wide currency. The concept refers to those who are seen as having no productive role in society, characterized by long-term joblessness, weak attachment to the labour force, and increased isolation. Conservatives, liberals, and radicals, in their quest to understand why poverty persisted despite programmes to eliminate it, were drawn to the concept of the underclass (Peterson, 1991).

The authoritarian populism articulated by the New Right blamed the welfare state for the breakdown of the work ethic and the nuclear family (feminists and other social movements were also blamed for the breakdown of traditional values). Government benefits had perverse effects: increasing the percentage of unemployed males, thus destroying 'the father's key role and authority' (Gilder, 1981: 114) and increasing the percentage of children born out of wedlock. Articulated as the social threat discourse, these arguments are being used to increase the surveillance over single mothers and institute workfare policies. Entitlements have ceased to be citizens' rights, instead they 'have become a code word for undeserving benefits' (Gordon, 1994: 288).

Central to this discourse is the image of an underclass characterized by social pathologies and 'behavioral deficiencies' (Auletta, 1981; Murray, 1980, cited in Ricketts, 1992). According to Murray, federal government benefits have created a sector of the poor who are irresponsible, 'characteristically take jobs sporadically if at all, do not share the social burdens of the neighborhoods in which they live, shirk the responsibility of fatherhood and are indifferent or often simply incompetent mothers' (Murray, 1980, cited in Ricketts, 1992: 48).

A different perspective on the underclass had been put forth by those who consider it a product of socio-structural phenomena resulting from the spatial and industrial restructuring of capitalism in the USA. Wilson (1987) argues that the increase in female-headed households among Blacks is due to the increasing difficulty women have in finding a mate with stable employment. Along the same lines, Reed (1992) concludes that economic alienation on the one hand and crime and contact with the criminal justice system on the other are the major reasons for the unavailability of marriageable men. Articulated as part of the social problem discourse, these arguments have been used to advocate policies that will result in a full-employment economy and universal rather than means-tested federal policies.

Discourses on single mothers that characterize them as a social threat integrate classist and racist themes that shape policies that affect women – particularly welfare legislation and child-care policies (Quadagno, 1994), which I turn to next.

4. The USA State Welfare Regime

Social welfare policies

The USA is generally regarded as the type case of a 'liberal welfare state regime', where social policy is used to uphold the market and traditional work-ethic norms, and modest means-tested benefits are aimed at a residualized and stigmatized group of welfare recipients. Such a regime places single mothers in a particular position of disadvantage. In the USA, single mothers are not only poor, but are also regarded as 'a trope for dependency or family breakdown' (Hobson, 1995: 176). However, at times the USA has also deviated from the 'liberal' ideal type, as with the more 'social democratic' policies of Lyndon Johnson's 'great society' of the 1960s.

The Social Security Act of 1935 shaped the basic parameters of the liberal model. This Act set up a stratified system in which social insurance programmes provided better payments, and were better regarded, than public assistance programmes (Gordon, 1994). From the start, government provision excluded some groups, particularly Blacks and single mothers. Blacks were deliberately excluded by a Congress controlled by Southern Democrats who wanted to be ensured of cheap labour. Single mothers were marginalized by government provision that labelled them undeserving.

Between 1911 and 1920, 40 states provided pensions to poor widowed mothers caring for dependent children. Local, state, and national women's groups argued that, just like disabled veteran soldiers, widowed mothers should be adequately and honourably supported by government when bread-winner husbands were not available (Skocpol, 1995). Notwithstanding lofty aims, spotty implementation, limited funding, and surveillance of mothers through 'proper home' investigations undermined mothers' pensions. When the programme was federalized as Aid to Dependent Children (ADC) under the Social Security Act of 1935, those problems persisted. In 1939, surviving dependents of contributing workers were removed from ADC and placed under social security's old age and survivors' insurance, thus marginalizing the programme. Skocpol analyses the transition in this way:

> Benefits remained low and their distribution geographically uneven. And traditions of surveillance established by social workers became even more intrusive once southerners, blacks, and unmarried mothers began to represent a significant number of clients. Directly contradicting the original sponsors' intentions, mothers' pensions, ADC-AFDC, evolved into the core program of what is today pejoratively known as 'welfare'.
>
> (1995: 417)

Not only does the government provision separate people into two groups, it deepens their inequality. Gordon finds this to be true in extreme form in the Aid to Families With Dependent Children (AFDC) where,

The stigmas of 'welfare' and of single motherhood intersect; hostility to the poor and hostility to deviant family forms reinforce each other. The resentment undercuts political support for the program, and benefits fall farther and farther behind inflation.

(1994: 6)

Cuts to welfare programmes such as food stamps, low-income housing, and AFDC are shaped by our ideas of the 'good society'. Priority spending in the federal budget benefits corporate sectors and high-income groups, and cuts aid to single mothers (Gordon, 1994). In 1992 the national average of AFDC and food stamps income for a mother without any other source of income was $7,479 (Committee on Ways and Means, US House of Representatives, 1993 *Green Book*, cited in Gans, 1995). Unable to live on this amount, they at times supplement their welfare benefits with informal work. Mothers avoid better paid official labour because they fear losing welfare and health-care benefits (Hobson, 1995).

Child-care policies

In a climate where traditional two-headed families with husbands as providers and wives as home-makers were highly valued, non-maternal child care was frowned upon until not too long ago. Moreover, in the USA, child rearing is considered a private matter because children are not seen as a social good. Unlike the situation in many European countries (see, e.g., the chapters on France and Sweden, this volume), no national maternity leave or child-care provisions support mothers' paid work.

Historically, in the USA, independent sectors took the initiative. A patchwork system evolved, characterized by a variety of purposes. Beginning in the 1850s, social service agencies began to provide child care to poor families, while charitable organizations and the settlement house movements, assisting in the assimilation of immigrant families to the USA, expanded the availability of child-care services. The child-care services provided by these agencies were meant to be custodial in nature, building character and preventing future problems. Later, educators put forward the educational function of child care and pushed for schools as child-care sites (Klein, 1992).

In the 1960s, when the federal government intervened in child care, the social service and educational sectors tried to maintain their turf. The resulting legislation reflected compromises among professional interests and was coloured by the ideological debate about the role of government vis-à-vis family functions.

Given the fragmentary nature of child care in the USA compared to that of other industrialized countries, it is perplexing to many that the women's movement did not play a vocal role in shaping progressive child-care policies. The women's movement's initial lack of interest in the problems of combining motherhood and work was due in part to its focus on establishing legal equality between women and men, breaking down legal and economic barriers to employment and education, eliminating discrimination against women, and advocating reproductive freedom. Composed mainly of White middle-class women, this movement did not press for working mothers' rights in its early stages. This was because those rights were perceived as requiring special treatment for women, and therefore undermining their equal treatment under the law (Hewlett, 1986). Only when more middle-class mothers have been affected by the scarcity, inaccessibility and indifferent quality of child care has the issue been given attention by women's groups (Klein, 1992).

Labour shortages during the Second World War produced changes in gender roles that, in turn, spurred federal allocation of funding to the states to provide child care. During the War, the Lanham Act of 1941 provided federally funded child-care centres for women working in the war industries. These centres closed at the end of the war, when notions of traditional gender roles were re-established. Federal involvement in child care did not recur until the 1960s; in 1962, the Public Welfare Amendment to the Social Security Act was passed, shaped by workfare advocates and those who saw poor families as a social problem (Klein, 1992).

A later amendment to the Social Security Act in 1967 allocated child-care funding for participants in the Work Incentive Program (WIN), and for recipients of Aid for Dependent Children (AFDC), and also had a workfare/training target (Norgren, 1981, cited in Klein, 1992). In the early 1970s, Congress passed the Comprehensive Child Development Act, aimed at providing federal support for day care for all children, but it was vetoed by President Richard Nixon.

In a message to the Senate, explaining his reasons for vetoing the 1971 Bill, Nixon pointed to its 'family weakening implications' as a flaw (Nixon, 1971, cited in Klein, 1992). He argued that the response to the challenge of child care should be that it 'be consciously designed to cement the family in its rightful position as the keystone of our civilization' (Nixon, 1971, cited in Klein, 1992). When the child-care debate was renewed in 1975, conservative groups attacked federal intervention in child care as the 'sovietization' of American children (Steiner, 1976, cited in Klein, 1992).

As early as the 1960s, a coalition of fiscal conservatives, intent on rolling back the welfare state, and religious conservatives, working to restore traditional family values, began to emerge. Public policy during the 1970s and 1980s was geared to sending mothers on public assistance back to work – privileging their role as workers. On the other hand, working mothers not on public assistance were denied adequate child-care support, thus privileging their roles as mothers (Quadagno, 1994).

Although child-care programmes for low-income families comprise all but one of the child-care programmes currently funded by the federal government, they still fall short of meeting the needs of these families. Funding for child-care programmes for low-income families was negatively affected by budget cuts in the early 1980s. Moreover, the different objectives, target populations, and programme requirements of federal child-care programmes make it difficult for the states to create seamless systems and have resulted in large gaps in child-care subsidies (US General Accounting Office, 1994).

The only programme not restricted to low-income families is the dependent care tax credit, which allows families to deduct part of their child-care expenses from their income taxes. Dependent care tax credit grew from one-third of federal expenditures for child care in the early 1980s to two-thirds by the end of the decade, making it the main form of federal support for child care (Hayes, Palmer and Zaslow, 1990).

The absence of comprehensive child-care policies forces most working mothers to put together their own ensemble of child-care arrangements. They choose and combine from the most common forms of child care in the USA, which are:

- at home, cared for either by a relative or a home child-care provider;
- at the home of relatives or the home of a child-care provider;
- in a pre-school programme; and
- at school, either in kindergarten (a class for children 4–6 years old) or in elementary school.

The kind of child-care families choose varies with the children's ages and the income and education of the parents. Relatives and home child-care providers (childminders) are usually chosen for infants and toddlers, while day-care settings are used for children between the ages of three and six. Parents with children in that age group and with higher income and educational levels prefer pre-school programmes (Friedman, 1986). Single working mothers of pre-schoolers tend to use care in the caretaker's home (37.6 per cent) slightly more than care in the mother's own home (31.7 per cent), and only 24.5 per cent use organized child-care facilities. To a large extent, single working mothers are more likely than married working mothers to rely on relatives to provide child care at home or at a home away from home (O'Connell, 1993). Single mothers of children who are of kindergarten and elementary school age use school as their preferred child-care arrangement. Care by relatives, including grandparents, both at home and in another home, represents a second but much less likely form of child-care arrangement for single mothers of children in that age group (O'Connell, 1993).

The hourly cost of day care in the USA in 1988 was estimated to range from $1.00 to $1.30/hour for family home child-care providers, and from $1.35 to $2.50 for centre care (Hofferth, 1989; Kisker et al., 1989). Not unexpectedly, the lower the income, the higher the burden of paying for child care. In 1989, low-income families who used market services were estimated to spend 20–25 per cent of their income on child care; high-income families were estimated to spend under 5 per cent (Hofferth, 1989).

Aware that affordable, accessible, good-quality child care is still a scarce commodity for middle- and low-income working mothers, policy makers have devised plans to expand child-care assistance to encourage single mothers to find employment and enhance their employability through education and job training (Bowen, Desimone and McKay, 1995). Bowen and Neenan (1992) found that subsidized child care was an economic incentive for poor working parents of pre-school children who: (i) had already found an interim form of child care, and (ii) were on a waiting list for subsidized care. They note, however, that although subsidized child care may be a necessary condition for the employment of low-income parents, it may not be sufficient. The presence of other barriers these parents may face, such as low levels of education and training, little work experience, and limited availability of jobs, is likely to mediate the impact of subsidized child care as an incentive to employment. However, as I discuss later, there may be other intervening variables, in terms of mothers' values on the suitability of combining motherhood with paid work.

5. Lone Mothers in One Local Labour Market: The Cleveland Case

Urban geographers have noted that the growth of capitalist industrialization produces geographically uneven development. Neighbourhoods, cities and regions have found that their economic fortunes are volatile; cities and states compete to attract new businesses in a new economic and political climate. Changes in technology and the organization of labour and increased global competition create new growth centres with their peripheries, produce disinvestment in some areas, and spur radical restructuring of others (Storper and Walker, 1989; Sayer and Walker, 1992). Storper and Walker (1989) have used Cleveland as a counter-example to refute the spatial division of labour theorists who have argued that city systems reflect a particular spatial division based on hierarchies of labour skill and the command structure of large corporations. Cleveland serves as a counter-example because during the 1970s and 1980s Cleveland lost half its population while remaining one of the top ten headquarter cities in the USA.

Closing of manufacturing plants hit cities such as Cleveland harder than others because the area remains dependent on industries that are declining in terms of employment (Bingham and Austrian, 1994, cited in Hill, 1995). Furthermore, plant closings have had more impact on racial minorities than on Whites, and on women more than men. Non-White and racial minorities are concentrated in industries that have undergone the largest plant closings – automobile, rubber, and steel, in particular (Bluestone and Harrison, 1982). Nearly a quarter of blue-collar jobs were lost during this period; only a small part of that loss was made up by growth in professional white-collar jobs (12 per cent). Blue-collar jobs still represent the single largest occupation for Cleveland residents, followed by 'other professional' jobs (Bingham and Kalich, 1995).

Touted as a come-back city because of revitalization initiatives, Cleveland still ranks only 76th among the nation's 77 major cities by median income, 15th by unemployment rate, 4th by percentage of the population below poverty level[3] (29.7 per cent), and 3rd by percentage of public assistance households (McQueen, 1995).

Labour-force participation in the city remains low. In 1990, 6 out of 10 males and 5 out of 10 females were in the labour force, and the rate of unemployment stood at 15.1 per cent for men and 12.8 per cent for women. The situation was even less promising for single mothers of children aged 18 and under, only 46.5 per cent of whom were in the labour force and 16.4 per cent of whom were unemployed (Current Population Reports, 1990).

This low level of participation of Cleveland city residents in the labour force is largely due to a widening gap between the skills they possess and those demanded for technical and professional positions that have been created. Between 1970 and 1980, jobs requiring less than a high school degree dropped by 48.2 per cent and those requiring only high school education decreased by 14 per cent. At the same time, jobs requiring some college education increased by 53.5 per cent and those requiring a college degree increased by 31 per cent (Kasarda, 1989). While only 13 per cent of Cleveland residents working in the city had college degrees, and 70 per cent of Cleveland workers held low-paying jobs, 29 per cent of suburbanites working in Cleveland had either completed four years of college or had advanced degrees, and close to half held jobs that paid over $40,000. Most of the high-paying jobs created in Cleveland have gone to suburbanites (Bingham and Kalich, 1995).

These shifts in the labour market have diminished Cleveland residents' opportunities to be employed full-time, year round. In 1990, just over half (55 per cent) of city males were employed full time compared to 62 per cent of suburbanite males. While only 5 out of 10 Cleveland women were employed full-time for 40 weeks or more, 9 out of 10 suburban Cleveland women worked full-time year round (Current Population Reports, 1990).

In Cleveland almost half of all single mothers with children under 18 years of age were gainfully employed in 1990 – a figure that was higher in the suburbs where almost 6 out of 10 single mothers had paid work (US Census of Population and Housing, 1990). About two out of four working single mothers with children under 18 years of age were in 'other' professional and service occupations (US Census of Population and Housing, 1990; Current Population Reports, 1993). Not surprisingly, given their position in the labour market, the income level of single mothers in Cleveland was extremely low in 1990. Seven in 10 mothers had incomes of less than $10,000, and less than 2 in 10 had incomes between $10,000 and $20,000. Incomes above $20,000 were extremely rare. These income levels placed a large proportion of single mothers below the poverty level. The income of single mothers in the suburbs was slightly better. Almost 6 in 10 (59.8 per cent) earned less than $10,000, and slightly more than 2 out of 10 earned between $10,000 and $20,000. Sixteen per cent earned more than $20,000 (US Census of Population and Housing, 1990).

Low levels of education limited single mothers' access to well-paid jobs. Seven out of 10 single mothers in Cleveland had a high school education or less, and almost 4 in 10 had less than a high school education. Less than 3 in 10 had completed college or had some college education. In the suburbs, the level of education was higher, almost 4 in 10 had either had some college education or had completed four years of college (US Census of Population and Housing, 1990).

The loss of manufacturing jobs also restricted single mothers' participation in the labour force. During the early 1980s, the inner city lost 27 per cent of its manufacturing jobs, while the suburbs lost a mere 4 per cent (Garofalo and Park, 1988). Furthermore, Cleveland's transportation system, as that of many older American cities, was designed for jobs in central areas, not in distant suburbs (Hughes, 1989). Consequently, the predominantly Black single mothers in the inner cities find access to the newly created jobs extremely difficult.

Cleveland's history of racial segregation aggravates the effects of the economic shift on minority populations. In 1980, continuing a long history of segregation indices, Douglas Massey rated 60 of the largest cities in the USA on a scale of 0 to 100, with 0 being totally integrated and 100 being totally segregated. Cleveland scored 87.5 on the segregation scale (Brazaitis, 1988). Although much progress has been made in race relations in the last 25 years in terms of education and housing, the marks of segregation still persist. In the 1980s, a court order began the desegregation of the Cleveland schools. Ninety per cent of Cleveland's Blacks lived on the east side of the city in 1970. Since that time, housing has opened up in other parts of the city and many Blacks have moved to the eastern suburbs.

In the 1970s, as the economic base of urban areas declined and poor minority students became the predominant majority in urban schools, inequalities between urban and suburban districts became more pronounced. Public school funding in the USA is based on property taxes; consequently wealthier districts have better funded schools. The declining tax base in the city of Cleveland has resulted in a financial crisis in the school district. Furthermore, inner-city children face a host of problems that negatively affect their readiness to learn and the schools have not addressed these problems adequately. As a result, many city students perform well below national norms in reading and maths, and have poor attendance; less than half of the students who enter the ninth grade graduate with a high school diploma. Sub-standard public education has pushed many residents with school-age children to the suburbs, and many of those who remain in the city, and can afford it, send their children to private or parochial schools.

Another constraint on single mothers' ability to take paid work is inadequate child care. The supply of child-care facilities for working mothers in Cleveland does not meet the demand. While 56.8 per cent of mothers with children under six years of age in Cuyahoga County (the largest county in the state of Ohio, of which Cleveland is the largest city) are in the labour force, and child care in the county averages $80 a week – 5.3% higher than in 1991 – only 12 per cent of children from working poor families are receiving child-care assistance (Children's Defense Fund, 1995). Most of the unmet demand is predominantly from single mothers (Ellison, 1990).

Constraints and opportunities on Cleveland's Near West Side

The area in Cleveland designated as the Near West Side comprises the three neighbourhoods closest to the Cuyahoga River, a geographic feature which divides the city into two distinct areas: the East Side and the West Side. These neighbourhoods have been hard hit by the economic restructuring and downsizing that shook Cleveland. Coulton, Chow and Finn (1990) and Chow and Coulton (1990) have assessed the differential effect of the shrinking manufacturing job-base on the poverty level of Cleveland neighbourhoods. They found that one of the three Near West Side neighbourhoods comprises a traditional poverty area – an area that has had a proportionately larger number of residents who have been out of the labour force for quite some time. The other two Near West Side neighbourhoods are emerging poverty areas; that is to say, they had a large contingent of workers in the manufacturing industries in the late 1970s, but as labour market shifts began, these neighbourhoods began to fall into poverty. Finally, starting in the 1970s, a small sector of one of the Near West Side neighbourhoods has attracted gentrifying young professionals who want a city environment and wish to renovate old houses.

Poverty has powerful effects on its residents. For one thing, the likelihood that poor persons in Cleveland will encounter non-poor persons has declined considerably, while their chance to interact with other poor persons has increased (Chow and Coulton, 1994). The number of AFDC cases per 1,000 residents in the Near West Side area increased by 31 per cent between 1979 and 1988 (Coulton, Chow and Finn, 1990).

Adverse social conditions and low quality of life are corollaries of concentrated poverty. On the Near West Side, a 13 per cent population loss (a decrease from 44,223 residents in 1980 to 38,543 in 1990), resulted in an 82 per cent occupancy rate in 1990. About half of those who live on the Near West Side are tenants. In 1990, the median value of housing units was $22,500 – close to half that of the city as a whole – and a median rent of $275 was 15 per cent lower than the median rent in the rest of the city (Current Population Reports, 1990).

An increase in crime has been another corollary of poverty. The rate of type I crimes (which include aggravated assault, assault, auto theft, burglary, homicide, larceny, rape, and robbery) as well as other crime violations against property and person, was three times higher on the Near West Side than the average for the city (Cleveland Area Network for Data and Organizing, 1994).

Despite those negative conditions associated with poverty, the Near West Side makes available a number of resources to single mothers. Coulton and her collaborators have calculated the amount of adult supervision available for children in the community, which they label 'child-care burden' (Coulton et al., 1993). In calculating the resources available to mothers in caring for their children, the index includes the ratio of children to adults, the ratio of males to females, and the percentage of the population that is elderly. The Near West Side has slightly more favourable child/adult and male/female ratios than average for the city, but in the population above 65 years of age it stands just below the city's average, in contrast to some inner-city neighbourhoods where very few elderly persons live. Compared to other Cleveland neighbourhoods, the Near West Side fares relatively well regarding its child-care burden.

A considerable number and variety of social service agencies serve the neighbourhood. Non-profit organizations, churches, and public agencies offer job training, assistance and job searches, education, and health and social services. This network of support adds to the social capital available to single mothers and has improved a few selected quality-of-life indicators. For example, between 1980 and 1990 the number of deaths per 1,000 live births, although still higher than the national average of 9.2, dropped from 16 to 11 (US Bureau of the Census, 1994). Day-care supply has also improved; day and after-care programmes increased from 7 to 12, and capacity grew 58 per cent to a total of 715 available spaces (Ellison, 1990). Still, however, the available spaces were capable of serving only 16 per cent of the population under six years of age.

The labour-force participation of single mothers on Cleveland's Near West Side

The low level of educational attainment of Near West Side residents, as compared to that of Clevelanders in other neighbourhoods, restrict access to job opportunities and puts them at a disadvantage in competing with suburbanites (US Census of Population and Housing, 1990). Thirty per cent of Near West Side residents had 9 to 12 years of education, but only 25 per cent were high school graduates, and a mere 4 per cent had a college a degree.

In 1990, 6 in 10 men and 4 in 10 women on the Near West Side participated in the labour force – a significant drop since 1980 when 80.7 per cent of the men and 47.6 per cent of the women were in the labour force (Chow and Coulton, 1990). Forty-eight per cent of the male residents and 33 per cent of the female residents of the Near West Side were employed in 1990; however only 30 per cent of the men and 49 per cent of the employed males worked 35 or more hours a week year-round. These figures are even lower for female residents of the Near West Side, only 18 per cent of whom worked year-round; of those employed, a mere 42 per cent worked 35 or more hours a week year-round. The two top job opportunities for residents of the Near West Side were as labourers – close to one-third of employed persons over 16 years of age – and sales, technical, administrative and clerical support – almost one-quarter of employed persons over 16 years of age.

Having children under the age of 6 reduces the likelihood that single mothers will be employed. Single mothers of children below the age of 6 (26 per cent) and single mothers who had children both under the age of 6 and between the ages of 6 and 17 (22 per cent) had a lower employment rate than single mothers of children between the ages of 6 and 17 (US Census of Population and Housing, 1990).

6. Lone Mothers in a Case Study Neighbourhood: Mothering and Work on the Near West Side

In this section I will analyse the accounts of 14 single mothers on Cleveland's Near West Side – to elaborate on how they made decisions regarding taking paid work, and the lines of action they were willing to pursue regarding work. These lines of action were shaped, but not determined, by the structural and practical conditions the mothers encountered. Faced with specific circumstances, the mothers' belief and what they had learned from previous experiences were brought to bear on the choices they made.

We interviewed 14 women, ten of whom were White and four of whom classified themselves as Puerto Rican or of Puerto Rican descent – officially classified as Hispanic in the USA. The average age of the mothers was 21, four of whom had become mothers before they turned 17; the oldest mother interviewed was 40 years old. Nine mothers had never married, four had divorced or separated, and one had terminated cohabitation. A large majority had been single mothers for less than five years, with four having acquired this status less than one year before; three had been single mothers for more than 16 years. Most of the women had only one child, one of them had three. The children's ages ranged from two months to 20 years, but all mothers had at least one child under 14. More than half of the mothers lived alone with their children, one took care of a younger brother as well, and four lived with their families. One mother had completed elementary school only, nine had some high school experience, three had completed high school, and one mother was attending a two-year college. The distribution of educational attainment among these mothers paralleled national trends; those who had never married had less education than separated mothers.

The criterion these single mothers used for considering themselves as such was that they were raising the children by themselves. The children's fathers either did not help or helped little with money, mostly by buying diapers (nappies), clothes, or milk. The mothers talked about not being able to count on the children's fathers and of fathers doing little or nothing to help:

> It means raising my daughter on my own, just myself. Me providing for her and just stuff like that. Just me doing it on my own.

'On my own', 'me providing for her', 'just me' – in a short statement, this single mother restates her independence, emphasizing that the whole responsibility for her daughter lies with her.

Views of single motherhood at the national and local level as perceived by single mothers in the case study

The mothers in this case study had beliefs about mothering which set tasks and responsibilities for them and provided practical and moral reasons for the ways they balanced child rearing and study, child rearing and work, and mothering and social life. Overall, these women saw single motherhood as a viable option for themselves. In their view, they were part of a larger group of single mothers who shared similar life situations: taking care of their children without a father's support and holding a job. One young mother compared herself to other teenage mothers when she observed that, as many of her peers, she had dropped out of school when she became a single mother. Indeed, dropping out of school is part of a national trend for teenagers who get pregnant while in high school.

Some women felt that responses to single mothers had become more favourable:

It's getting to be more and more normal, I think, and more accepted as a part of society because there are more and more single mothers,

one mother noted. Another said that society considers them 'important' because they perform a vital social function, that is 'they take care of their kids'.

While the climate towards single mothers has improved in the last decades, and expressions such as 'broken home' are heard only sporadically, the women we talked to perceived the contempt felt for mothers who received government subsidies. Several mothers who were on public assistance sensed that they were 'put down'; some described the societal view of single mothers as 'a problem to society'. These women were aware of the increasingly common belief that mothers should not have children unless they are able to support them. One of those who thought single mothers were seen as a 'problem to society', thought that women were victims of irresponsible men:

Most people would rather have them be with the fathers and everything but I mean, they can't always be . . . because half of 'em are dirt! Too lazy or they don't want to be with the mother because they found she was pregnant and they dumped her . . . because they don't want to. Yeah, single mothers are a problem to society, yeh . . . some . . . like the teen mothers.

Taken by itself, this mother's account might be used to provide support to advocates of the social threat discourse, who have pointed to irresponsible fatherhood as typical of the underclass, and who have recommended restrictions to federal assistance to young unwed mothers. Other young mothers were aware of the disdain for young unmarried women who are seen as throwing away their future to have babies and having become dependent on public assistance. One mother described the consequences of the social threat discourse on single mothers:

> They're trying to down us because we all had the kids and stuff like that. They think we shouldn't have kids and we should go to school . . . like we are trying to go to school. Now they're trying to talk about cutting off welfare and cut this and cut this. Now they passed this bill, they're gonna make us go to work and get paid $2.35 an hour just because we're on welfare. I don't think that's gonna be all right for the people that are on welfare. If they're gonna give them a job . . . they're gonna make us work for $2.35. Maybe we won't get no food stamps, only get $350 a month and cut your food stamps back . . . that means some people would get more money but less food stamps, you probably still won't be able to make it.

This mother uncovered some of the contradictions in what single mothers are hearing. She understands that education is important, but while she is studying – as she thinks she is expected to – she is worrying about new measures that will have her work at below the minimum wage and will cut down on her food stamps.

While this group of single mothers was aware of public censure at the national level for single mothers, especially those who are teenaged, they largely ignored the views of their neighbours or considered those views irrelevant. They contended that they did not know what neighbours thought – or said that those opinions did not matter because neighbours were of divided opinions. A few young mothers noted that older neighbours 'condemn' teenage mothers, but were able to minimize this disapproval by interpreting it as a manifestation of the critics' age. The young mothers we interviewed did not indicate that they felt stigmatized by the older neighbours' moral condemnation.

While mothers claimed that they were affected by neighbours' views, they sensed their neighbours' disdain, as well as that of the nation, for welfare assistance. While mindful of this disdain, the women we talked to seemed to feel better about themselves than mothers on public assistance who were part of an ethnographic study that found they felt both stigmatized and depressed (Coles, n.d., cited in Garfinkel and McLanahan, 1986).

When the rewards of being a single mother were considered, many put the accent on *mother*: 'it's a joy to see them growing up'; 'being there to see the kid's first steps'. Others put the accent on *single* – a status that positioned them so that their children's exclusive attention came to them: 'all her attention just comes to me', a mother said about the relationship with her daughter. Being a *single* mother also brought independence, and 'not having to put up with men'. Women who valued being single mothers for these reasons lend support to the escaping patriarchy discourse; the mothers celebrated freedom from a husband, being the adult in charge, making decisions, and rejoiced in their accomplishments.

Not having a partner had its drawbacks, including limited resources, reduced opportunities for sharing responsibilities and earning a satisfactory income. One mother related:

> Yeah, money's always a problem and, you know, sometimes just extra help and things like that. You get stressed out real easy.

Only one mother talked about having to explain the absence of a father to her child, a situation she was particularly sensible to because of her child's mixed race:

> I have to explain to my daughter why her father's not always around and explain to people why . . . 'cause she is mixed, she's half black and half white . . . so explain to her why people cut her down sometimes. When she goes on, I'm the one that's gonna have to deal with all that . . . when she gets older.

Having crossed two boundaries – giving birth to a biracial child, and raising her in a mother-only family – this single mother found herself having to address processes that remained invisible for the most part to the rest of the mothers.

Conditions for single motherhood on the Near West Side

The single mothers in this case study made choices that made practical and moral sense to them – choices that took into account the favourable conditions, as well as the constraints that the neighbourhood presented. In choosing a place to live, social connections guided their choice: four of the women had grown up on the Near West Side and another four came back to the neighbourhood because their mother, father or friends lived there. Five women chose the neighbourhood because of economic considerations; they appreciated the nice, inexpensive housing available.

One mother said this was the fifth time she had come into this neighbourhood from Puerto Rico – a pattern characteristic of the shuttle between the island and the mainland in which many Puerto Rican residents of this neighbourhood engage. They come to Cleveland looking for jobs; if prospects look bad, they lose their jobs, or if family emergencies arise either in

Cleveland or in Puerto Rico, they return to their homeland. After a while, they return to Cleveland looking for job opportunities once again. In the 1950s Puerto Ricans settled in this area because of its closeness to the steel mills. Although many of those jobs are gone, Puerto Ricans continue to live and come to the Near West Side where relatives and friends live.

While friends and family and inexpensive housing had drawn the women to the neighbourhood, the availability of jobs or day care had not been a consideration. Given that it is well known that few jobs are available in town for those with the limited job skills of the mothers in our study, it is not surprising that they had not inquired about jobs before moving. The mothers knew that the few jobs that were available in the area were in the fast-food places and drug stores, paid minimum wages, or were part-time. Most thought that the best way to obtain these available jobs was to put in applications at the stores or to search the newspapers for classified advertisements. (Most fast-food places post ads on their windows when they are looking for help and some of the larger stores place them in local newspapers.) Those in our sample who were working, however, got their jobs through personal connections.

Another choice made by some of the mothers was to live on their own with their children. Most of the younger women in our study indicated that they had come to be on their own with children by moving out of their parents' home. These young mothers described how having a child had prompted them to move out of their parents' home. Sometimes they did not get along with their parents: 'both my parents were drinking and I just don't like it'; others felt that if they stayed they would be a burden on their family. Whatever the motivation, having children had changed the way they related to family members and had triggered the move. Other women described how a change in their relationship with the children's father had led to being on their own with the children – the children's fathers were divorced or separated from the women or had never cohabitated with them.

While the children's fathers offered little support, brothers, sisters, mothers, and fathers who lived close to the mothers, exchanged favours and services, such as advice, day care, driving, and financial assistance. The majority of single mothers reported that those who were closest to them and who they saw often were female family members: mothers, sisters, daughters, and grandmothers. Fathers, brothers and grandfathers were mentioned as male family members who helped in a variety of ways as well. One grandfather drove the single mother to school and the child to day care every day. Given the limited job opportunities these women had, family support and government services were their main sources of support.

Neighbourhood qualities of the Near West Side offered additional support for these single women in their mothering role. Not only were relatives close by, but neighbours were friendly, and older people as well as young people lived in the district. The mothers in our study credited the presence of elderly people for contributing to the quiet and the feeling of safety in raising children in the neighbourhood. The layout of the Near West Side offered another advantage to most of the women in our study who did not own a car: closeness to stores, a park and a hospital.

In a few ways the Near West Side is not a good place to raise children according to the mothers. It is a centrally located district with busy streets and fast drivers and shows signs of deterioration associated with the area's increasing impoverishment; the parks and other public spaces have become unsafe due to drugs and drinking.

The jobs the women were able to secure before having children and the work experience they had gained in those jobs were factors that shaped their thinking about taking paid work afterwards. Before having the children, these women had held a variety of service jobs, such as cleaning, waitressing, clerking in fast-food restaurants, and acting as custodians. Three of the women had been too young to work before they had children, and they had been supported by their parents with whom they lived.

Combining motherhood and work

At the time of the interview two mothers were working, another had been working until recently, a fourth was looking for a job, one was unemployed and took care of a sick son full-time, and the rest of the mothers were in school. The high number of single mothers in school in our case studies resulted from the method of accessing them. During the time in question, the job market had not changed much, nor had the women's skills. As a result, the kind of jobs the single mothers had held since having the children were not very different from the ones they had held before: factory work, bank cashiering, babysitting, house and office cleaning, and beauty products sales.

The mothers who chose to work were motivated by financial, emotional, and moral reasons. One mother simply mentioned financial reasons: 'I decided to work because of financial reasons'; another captured a complex set of reasons when she said she had gone to work 'to get out of welfare'. This response encompasses her ability to provide for herself and her children and to exclude herself from being seen as a problem to society. 'Getting out of welfare' denotes financial as well as psychological and moral reasons for choosing work. Other mothers also touched on emotional and moral reasons from a succinct, 'I feel better about working', to an acknowledgement of assuming the role of the child's provider. One mother said:

> You're bringing home the food, you know, you're taking care of your baby and I think that makes you feel better about yourself.

Work also provided women with a stage where they could show their skills. One mother felt proud about possessing the knowledge to do the job: 'I have to work with computers, every day on a computer. You have to know how to work with computers, everything, to get the job'.

Finding a job, being able to work, and bringing home enough money to support themselves was not easy. One mother, who had talked to her social worker about going to work, found she could not because she would lose the medical benefits she needed for her sick son. She was the only mother in our study who thought that it was better to receive government benefits than to work.

These single mothers' preference for work appears to contradict the argument of proponents of the social threat discourse that welfare dependency breeds a weak attachment to the labour market. In this neighbourhood, the mothers' choice not to work was strongly shaped by the scarcity of jobs to which women with low-level skills could apply. One mother pointed to low wages as another disincentive to work: when asked what she would do after she completed her studies she said she wanted to work, but in her words, 'I wouldn't work for just two bucks an hour'.

The low-paying jobs, especially if part-time with no benefits, did not pay the bills. These single mothers, as many other workers in the secondary labour market, have become part of a large contingent of workers earning a minimum wage, with no benefits and no career ladder. One of the mothers worked 48 hours a week – over the norm for full-time workers – but made only $4.25 an hour, not enough to put her above the poverty threshold.

As already noted, the mothers' decisions about what to do were sustained by their interpretation of prevailing societal views. In particular, feelings and beliefs about mothering shaped decisions regarding work and study. The majority of the mothers felt that when the children were young they should stay at home. One mother said that she could go back to work full-time when her child was two, and another when the child was one year of age. Many preferred part-time work to be able to spend more time with their children – a choice characteristic of single mothers across the USA, who work fewer hours than married mothers. One mother, who was receiving welfare benefits that she deemed insufficient, preferred to stay at home with her small child, but recognized the need to work:

> When you really have to go out there and get some money coming in 'cause if there's no money coming in you cannot stay home with the kids, it doesn't matter how old is the baby, nothing like that, you have to be out there. I think part-time would be better so I could spend more time with the baby.

The mothers thought that neighbours' opinion on whether mothers should stay at home or go to work fell on both sides:

> Some people are really against it, they think that it's just horrible if the mother goes out and works while her kids are at a babysitter, at day care, and then some people think that it's the best thing to do.

As a result, neighbours' views did not figure prominently in framing mothers' choices – except for one mother who used the neighbours' opinion – that she should find a boyfriend to support her – to distance herself from their views and express her own position: she felt she was young and still had the opportunity to 'fire her oats' ('live it up'). She chose independence from a man and the freedom that gave her to express her sexuality rather than financial security – a view consistent with the discourse that portrays single mothers as escaping patriarchy.

These single mothers found balancing work and mothering difficult. Echoing discourses that mothers should be at home with their children, these women felt that work robbed them of time with their children and they were afraid that it might affect their relationship with the children. One mother related:

> The time you lose that you don't spend with the baby, that's difficult. They are always doing stuff and I don't want to miss anything. Now he's learning to talk and I have to watch what I say 'cause he will repeat it. It is a beautiful experience.

While she felt robbed of the experience of watching her child grow, being away from him was made easier by the knowledge that he has been well cared for by relatives. The same mother continued:

> The people around me make it easier, the people that help out. I can go to work knowing that my baby is safe 'cause I know that the people that take care of him love him, they wouldn't let nothing happen to him.

The younger mothers we interviewed were studying for a General Equivalency Diploma (GED), a course of study to obtain a diploma equivalent to graduating from high school. Although, on the average, women who become single mothers at a young age have a higher risk of dependency on public assistance and low income, these young mothers were on public assistance but were optimistic about the course of action they had taken and the future. They talked about the courses they wanted to take, which included, among others, cosmetology, vocational training, and nursing, and the jobs they would seek, mostly secretarial and nursing.

In our study we found variations in the mothers' confidence and feeling that they could overcome their circumstances. Among the younger mothers we found several whose confidence was supported by the resources and views they found in the community. Those mothers who felt that combining coursework with raising children was easy referred to the advantage of having a child-care site where they were taking the GED courses and the help they got from their families. Those for whom studying was difficult were weighed down not only by practical matters but by a sense that it was not good to put the child through so much for the mothers to get an education. They complained about the daily routine of taking their small children from home to a day-care provider or to the school. One mother wished somebody would come to her home to watch her child so that she wouldn't have to 'drag my son out every day'. Another mother indicated that her daughter's health took precedence over her studies; if the daughter was sick or had to go to the doctor, the mother had to miss class and make it up at another time, 'but I'd rather miss out on schooling than I would . . . , my daughter's important, you know'.

Two other, somewhat older mothers were taking clerical training for a two-year associate degree. One of these women, a mother of older children, talked about the difficulty of combining her schoolwork with helping her children with their homework. Time was a precious commodity both for the mothers who worked and those who studied.

In brief, the mothers who worked and who studied felt the need to work or to prepare for work through education, but they felt pulled to be at home in so far as their views of mothering required them to spend more time with their children. Overall, available support through relatives or accessible and trustworthy day care made their decision to work easier.

As with other working mothers across the nation, these single mothers orchestrated complex child-care arrangements to be able to go to work or to become employable through coursework. Aside from child care at the place where many of these women were taking their GED classes, mothers relied on family and friends to look after their children when they went to work, to the store, or out with friends. One mother who had applied for a job and was expecting a response shortly was concerned that she would not find child care for the evening hours she would be working. If relatives were not looking after the children, the mother's main criteria for selecting a child-care facility were convenience or closeness to home and being able to trust the child-care provider. In a child-care market that is unlicensed to a large extent, mothers are forced to be extremely careful in inspecting the care their children receive.

Having someone to talk to about how to get jobs, where to work, and about career plans was a resource the mothers in our study had. The younger women discussed whether to work and what work they might get with their mothers. A 23-year-old, unemployed mother of two small children talked about work with her father:

> I discuss it with my dad a lot. We talk about it quite a bit. He always looks in the papers for me and tries to find me jobs and he knows that I want to go back to school and be a medical secretary.

By regularly reading the classified ads and talking with her about work, this father supported his daughter's ambition to get back to work.

Most mothers, hopeful about their future, described it in terms of the education and work they sought: those in school looked forward to finishing school, working part- or full-time, and several wanted to go to college. Other mothers wanted better jobs; one dreamed of making a lot of money and being able to send her son to a private school – 'no public school for him' she concluded, anticipating that a good education would give him better opportunities. Only one mother described her future exclusively in terms of her mothering by indicating that she would like to have another child.

Given these mothers' participation in the workforce, advocates of the social threat discourse might label these single mothers as disengaged from work and posing a threat to society. Granted only a few of the mothers who talked to us were employed, several were receiving public assistance, and all were poor; but they were emotionally and morally attached to work, which they preferred over public assistance. Even the younger mothers, those most punished by new welfare policies, showed that engagement by taking classes to prepare themselves for work.

At the same time, these single mothers found combining motherhood and work difficult, despite the neighbourhood's resources, accessible child care, and the support of family and friends which most of them could access. They were responding to contradictory messages that prescribed work and self-sufficiency for poor mothers and their views about good mothering.

7. Conclusion

In this chapter I examined the conditions that structured and created opportunities to take paid work for a group of single mothers on the Near West Side of Cleveland in the context of the local labour market, national discourses around single motherhood, and welfare policies. Attention was given to the multiple, inter-dependent factors these single mothers attended to in negotiating their identities as mothers and as workers. Unique to this analysis has been the inclusion of national, regional and local data and the consideration of neighbourhood resources available to the mothers and the role of dominant discourses on these single mothers' practices.

The ability of the mothers in our study, who at best had a high school education, to take paid work was determined by national and regional economic restructuring and declining labour market conditions. The mothers found that most of the jobs being created in the local labour market for women with less than a college education were low paid and dead end; many jobs were part time with no benefits, and would not raise them above the poverty level.

At the neighbourhood level, convenient, safe child care enabled some mothers to take paid work, and others to take classes to prepare for work, while maintaining a sense that they remained good mothers. Social networks also supported mothers in their work and in their studies. Friends and relatives looked after the children, helped with chores, and offered other forms of assistance. Family's and friends' moral support was as important as the material support offered to mothers in enabling them to be workers now and to become workers in the future.

Mothers felt a tension between the notion that good mothers stay at home with their children and the notion that single mothers should be self-sufficient.

Although these mothers claimed that societal and local views about poor single mothers did not affect them, their preference for work and preparing for work was fuelled in part by the negative attitude toward single mothers on public assistance. These women's views on mothering also strongly affected their decisions about whether to take work and the number of hours they could stay away from home.

A group of young women who had become single mothers when they were teenagers, were taking GED classes – an alternative route to graduating from high school – at the time of the study. Several of them planned to go to college after that. Those choices appeared sound to them because hardly any jobs are available to those who have not completed high school and only minimum wage jobs for those without some post-secondary education. The day-care facilities at the GED site made their course of action easier than it is for most single mothers in the area, and enabled them to prepare for work while feeling they were good mothers.

The mothers who had jobs found themselves at the margins of the secondary labour market, making minimum wage in dead-end jobs. In spite of this, their dignity was boosted by providing for their children and by the skills they possessed.

Dominant discourses about single mothers have been used to interpret the social circumstances and the behaviour of single mothers. The social problem discourse, for instance, has been used to understand the economic and social circumstances that make becoming a teenage mother desirable, and shapes much of the practice of social service agencies serving young women. In examining the increasingly difficult circumstances that the single mothers in our study faced, we are confronted by the consequences of policies inspired by the social threat discourse. The mothers' preference for work and their motivation to lift themselves off welfare shows single mothers who share the beliefs of mainstream society and do not fit the image of isolated disaffected individuals. Those mothers who cherished the independence that being single brought, who were proud of their accomplishments, echoed themes of the women escaping patriarchy discourse. None of these discourses, however, captures the ways the mothers in our study, in conditions that they took for granted and without elaborating much on why they chose certain courses of action, actively construed an identity for themselves as mothers and/or workers.

This chapter has shown the central role that these women's interpretation of mothering played in their decisions to take work and how long they worked. All the mothers faced the same tight local labour market, although we found differences in the extent to which they had access to good, convenient child care and had support from friends, neighbours and relatives. This local support also played an important role in these women's choice of courses of action, in so far as it allowed them to work or prepare for work while they continued to be good mothers.

While all the mothers in our study experienced tension between the roles of mother and worker, and they all faced a declining labour market, their reading of cultural frameworks, their access to good, convenient child care, the support they got from friends, neighbours, and relatives interacted in dynamic ways to shape their courses of action regarding mothering and work.

Notes

1 In this chapter the term 'single mothers' is used to designate never-married and what the US Bureau of the Census calls other-married mothers (separated, divorced and widowed).
2 'Professional white collar' is one of five occupational categories that combine the 13 major occupational categories, excluding military occupations, used by the Census Bureau (Bingham and Kalich, 1995):
  (i) Professional white collar: managers, professional speciality occupations (executives, engineers, architects, scientists, teachers, social scientists, urban planners, lawyers, judges, social and religious workers, writers, artists, entertainers, and athletes) supervisors and proprietors in sales.
  (ii) Other professionals: technicians, retail sales and administrative supports, personal services.
  (iii) Blue collar: precision craft and repair, transportation and moving, operators, fabricators, and labourers.
  (iv) Service: private household occupations, protective services, personal and health services.
  (v) Other: forestry, farming, and fishing.
3 The federal cash income poverty threshold was set at $12,590 for a family of three and $15,150 for a family of four in 1995 (Council for Economic Opportunities in Great Cleveland, 1994)

References

AMOTT, T. (1988) 'Working for less: single mothers in the workplace', in Mulroy, E. A. (Ed.) *Women as Single Parents: Confronting Institutional Barriers in the Courts, the Workplace, and the Housing Market*, pp. 99–122, Dover, MA: Auburn House Publishing Co.

ANDERSON, E. (1991) 'Neighbourhood effects on teenage pregnancy', in Jencks, C., Christopher, W., and Peterson, P. E. (Eds) *The Urban Underclass*, pp. 375–94, Washington D.C.: The Brookings Institute.

AULETTA, K. (1981) *The Underclass*, Random House.

BIER, T., WELD, E., HOFFMAN, M. and MARIC, I. (1988) *Housing Supply and Demand: Cleveland Metropolitan Area, 1950–2005*, Cleveland, OH: Cleveland State University.

BINGHAM, R. D. and KALICH, V. Z. (1995) 'Blest be the tie that binds: suburbs and the dependence hypothesis', presentation at Urban Affairs Association Annual Conference, Portland, OR, 3–7 May, 1995.

BLUESTONE, B. and HARRISON, B. (1982) *The Deindustrialization of America*, New York: Basic Books, Inc.

BLUM, L. M. (1993) 'Mothers, babies, and breastfeeding in late capitalist America: the shifting context of feminist theory', *Feminist Studies*, **19**, pp. 291–311.

BOURDIEU, P. and WACQUANT, L. J. D. (1992) *An Invitation to Reflexive Sociology*, Chicago, IL: The University of Chicago Press.

BOWEN, G. L., DESIMONE, L. M. and MCKAY, J. K. (1995) 'Poverty and the single mother family: a macroeconomic perspective', *Marriage and Family Review*, **20**, pp. 115–42.

BOWEN, G. L. and NEENAN, P. A. (1992) 'Child care as an economic incentive for the working poor', *Families in Society*, **73**, pp. 295–303.

BOWEN, G. L. and NEENAN, P. A. (1993) 'Child day care and the employment of AFDC recipients with preschool children', *Journal of Family and Economic Issues*, **14**, pp. 49–68.

BRAZAITIS, T. J. (1988) 'Study ranks Cleveland among most segregated', *The Cleveland Plain Dealer*, 23 June, p. 9-A.

CHILDREN'S DEFENSE FUND (1995) *Helping Families Work: A 1995/1996 Factbook*, Columbus, OH: Children's Defense Fund-Ohio.

CHOW, J. and COULTON, C. J. (1990) *Labor Force Profiles in Cleveland's Low-income Neighborhoods*, Cleveland, OH: Center for Urban Poverty and Social Change, Mandel School of Applied Social Sciences, Case Western Reserve University.

CHOW, J. and COULTON, C. (1992) *Was There a Social Transformation of Urban Neighborhoods in the 80s? A Decade of Changing Structure in Cleveland, Ohio*, Cleveland, OH: Center for Urban Poverty and Social Change, Mandel School of Applied Social Sciences, Case Western Reserve University.

CLEVELAND AREA NETWORK FOR DATA AND ORGANIZING (CAN DO) (VERSION 1.0) [Electronic Database System] (1994) Cleveland, OH: Center for Urban Poverty and Social Change, Mandel School of Applied Social Sciences, Case Western Reserve University.

COONTZ, S. (1992) *The Way We Never Were: American Families and the Nostalgia Trap*, New York: Basic Books.

COULTON, C. J., CHOW, J. and FINN, C. M. (1990) *Social Conditions Affecting People in Cleveland's Low-income Neighborhoods*, Cleveland, OH: Center for Urban Poverty and Social Change, Mandel School of Applied Social Sciences, Case Western Reserve University.

COULTON, C., KORBIN, J., SU, M. and CHOW, J. (1993) *Community Level Factors and Child Maltreatment Rates*, Cleveland, OH: Center for Urban Poverty and Social Change, Mandel School of Applied Social Sciences, Case Western Reserve University.

CURRENT POPULATION REPORTS (1990) Series P-20, no. 447, *Household and Family Characteristics: March 1990 and 1989*, Washington, DC: Government Printing Office.

CURRENT POPULATION REPORTS (1991) Series P-20, no. 458, *Household and Family Characteristics*: March. Washington, DC: Government Printing Office.

CURRENT POPULATION REPORTS (1993) Series P-20, no. 478, *Marital Status and Living Arrangements*: March. Washington, DC: Government Printing Office.

DUNCAN, G. T. and HOFFMAN, S. D. (1991) 'Teenage underclass behavior and subsequent poverty: have the rules changed?', in Jencks, C., Christopher, W. and Peterson, P. E. (Eds) *The Urban Underclass*, pp. 155–174, Washington DC: The Brookings Institute.

EDWARDS, R. and DUNCAN, S. (1997) 'Lone mothers and economic activity', in Williams, F. (Ed.), *Social Policy: A Critical Reader*, Cambridge: Polity Press.

ELLISON, C. (1990) *Profiles and Patterns: Cuyahoga County Child Care 1986–1989*, Child Day Care Planning Project, Cuyahoga County.

FISHMAN, R. (1987) *Bourgeois Utopias: The Rise and Fall of Suburbia*, New York: Basic Books.

FRIEDMAN, D. E. (1986) 'Painting the child care landscape: a palette of inadequacy and innovation', in Hewlett, S. A., Ilchman, A. S. and Sweeney, J. J. (Eds) *Family and Work: Bridging the Gap*, pp. 67–90, Cambridge, MA: Ballinger Publishing Co.

GAFFIKIN, F. and MORRISSEY, M. (1994) 'Poverty in the 1980s: a comparison of the United States and the United Kingdom', *Policy and Politics*, **22**, pp. 43–58.

GANS, H. J. (1995) *The War Against the Poor: The Underclass and Antipoverty Policy*, New York: Basic Books.

GARFINKEL, I. and McLANAHAN, S. (1986) *Single Mothers and Their Children: A New American Dilemma*, Washington DC: The Urban Institute Press.

GAROFALO, G. and PARK, C. (1988) 'The location of manufacturing in CALE', *REI Review*, Fall, pp. 14–23.

GARWOOD, A. N. (1991) *Black Americans: A Statistical Sourcebook*, Boulder, CO: Numbers and Concepts.

GILDER, G. (1981) *Wealth and Poverty*, New York: Basic Books.

GORDON, L. (1994) *Pitied but Not Entitled: Single Mothers and the History of Welfare 1890–1935*, New York: The Free Press.

HARDY, J. B. and ZABIN, L. S. (1991) *Adolescent Pregnancy in an Urban Environment: Issues, Programs, and Evaluation*, Washington, DC: The Urban Institute Press.

HAYES, C., PALMER, J. and ZASLOW, M. (1990) *Who Cares for America's Children: Child Care Policy for the 1990s*, Washington, DC: National Academy Press.

HEWLETT, S. A. (1986) *A Lesser Life: The Myth of Women's Liberation in America*, New York: William Morrow and Co., Inc.

HILL, E. W. (1995) 'The Cleveland economy: a case study of economic restructuring', in Keating, W. D., Krumholz, N. and Perry, D. C. (Eds) *Cleveland: A Metropolitan Reader*, pp. 53–86, Kent: The Kent State University Press.

HOBSON, B. (1995) 'Solo mothers, social policy regimes, and the logics of gender', in Sainsbury, D. (Ed) *Gendering Welfare States*, London: Sage.

HOFFERTH, S. (1989) *National Child Care Survey*, Washington, DC: Urban Institute, June.

HUGHES, M. (1989) 'Misspeaking truth to power: a geographical perspective on the "underclass" fallacy', *Journal of Policy Analysis and Management*, **8**, pp. 274–82.

KASARDA, J. D. (1989) 'Urban industrial transition and the underclass', *Annals of the American Academy of Political and Social Science*, **501**, pp. 26–47.

KISKER, E. E., MAYNARD, R., GORDON, A. and STRAIN, M. (1989) *The Child Care Challenge: What Parents Need and What is Available in Three Metropolitan Areas*, Washington, DC: US Department of Health and Human Services. [Prepared by Mathematica Policy Research, Inc. (Principal Investigator: R. Maynard and D. Polit)].

KLEIN, A. G. (1992) *The Debate over Child Care: 1979–1990*, Albany: State University of New York Press.

McLANAHAN, S. S. (1994) 'The consequences of single motherhood', *The American Prospect*, **18**, pp. 48–58.

McQueen, A. (1995) 'Cities keep their eyes on the prize: jobs', *The Cleveland Plain Dealer*, 24 September, p. 15-A.

Moffit, R. (1992) 'Incentive effects of the US welfare system: a review', *Journal of Economic Literature*, **30**, pp. 1–61.

Murray, C. 'Here's the bad news on the underclass', *Wall Street Journal*, 8 March, p. A14.

O'Connell, M. (1993) 'Where's papa! Fathers' role in child care', Population Reference Bureau, No. 20, in Table A-2, p. 19, *Primary Child Care Arrangement Used by Working Mothers for School-Age Children (Ages 5–14), 1985–1991*, Washington, DC: Bureau of the Census.

Omi, M. and Winant, H. (1986) *Racial Formation in the United States: From the 1960s to the 1980s*, New York: Routledge & Kegan Paul.

Open Housing Report (1986) 'US vs. Parma: the lessons learned', in *Cleveland, Past, Present, and Future*, Cleveland, OH: Cuyahoga Plan of Ohio.

Peterson, P. E. (1991) 'The urban underclass and the poverty paradox', in Jencks, C., Christopher, W. and Peterson, P. E. (Eds) *The Urban Underclass*, pp. 3–27, Washington DC: The Brookings Institute.

Quadagno, J. (1994) *The Color of Welfare: How Racism Undermined the War on Poverty*, New York: Oxford University Press.

Reed, W. L. (1992) 'Black men and their families: issues and options', *Challenge*, **3**, pp. 28–38.

Ricketts, E. (1992) 'The underclass: causes and responses', in Galster, G. C. and Hill, E. W. (Eds) *The Metropolis in Black and White*, pp. 216–35, New Brunswick, NJ: Center for Urban Policy Research.

Sayer, R. A. and Walker, R. (1992) *The New Social Economy: Reworking the Division of Labor*, Cambridge, MA: Blackwell Publishers.

Skocpol, T. (1995) *Social Policy in the United States: Future Possibilities in Historical Perspective*, Princeton: Princeton University Press.

Smith, D. E. (1987) *The Everyday World as Problematic: A Feminist Sociology*, Boston, MA: Northeastern University Press.

Smith, S. A. and Tienda, M. (1987) 'The doubly disadvantaged: women of color in the US labor force', in Stromberg, A. and Horkes, S. (Eds) *Working Women* 2nd Edn., pp. 61–80, Palo Alto, California: Mayfield.

Stannard, U. (1977) *Mrs. Man*, San Francisco: Germainbooks.

Staples, R. (1985) 'Changes in black family structure: the conflict between family ideology and structural considerations,' *Journal of Marriage and the Family*, **47**, pp. 1005–14.

Storper, M. and Walker, R. (1989) *The Capitalist Imperative: Territory, Technology, and Industrial Growth*, New York: Basil Blackwell.

Tienda, M., Donato, K. M. and Cordero-Guzman, H. (1992) 'Schooling, color, and the labor force activity of women,' *Social Forces*, **71**, pp. 365–95.

Tomaskovic-Devey, D. (1993) *Gender and Racial Inequality at Work: The Sources and Consequences of Job Segregation*, Ithaca, NY: ILR Press.

US Bureau of the Census (1991) *Statistical Abstract of the United States: 1991*, Washington, DC: Government Printing Office.

US Bureau of the Census (1994) *Statistical Abstract of the United States: 1994*, Washington, DC: Government Printing Office.

US Census of Population and Housing (1990) Public Use Microdata Samples US [machine-readable data files], Washington, DC: The Bureau of Census.

US Department of Labor (1993) *1993 Handbook on Women Workers: Trends and Issues*, Washington, DC: Government Printing Office.

US General Accounting Office (May 1994) *Child Care: Working Poor and Welfare Recipients Face Service Gaps*, Washington, DC: Government Printing Office.

Wilson, W. J. (1987) *The Truly Disadvantaged: The Inner City, the Underclass and Public Policy*, Chicago: University of Chicago.

Chapter 5

Single Mothers in Japan: Unsupported Mothers Who Work

Ito Peng

1. Introduction

Contrary to the common assumption about the traditional and enduring familialistic nature of Japanese society, lone-mother families have been on the increase in this country since the 1970s. In this chapter I use the term 'lone mother' to refer to all those households where mothers live without current partners, and 'single mother' to refer particularly to never-married lone mothers. Between 1973 and 1986 the estimated proportion of lone-mother families in Japan doubled, from about 4 per cent of all families with dependent children to about 8 per cent (Betania Homu, 1986). Reasons commonly given for this increase are: (i) women's greater independence; (ii) the greater emphasis placed on the importance of the 'modern' (Western) notion of conjugal marriage based on love and partnership; and (iii) women's greater choice whether to remain married or not.

However, there are also some important but less widely recognized reasons for this increase. First, lone motherhood has simply become more public in that it is no longer hidden as it was before. This may be partly due to an increased public acceptance of divorce as an alternative to a bad marriage, and to slightly more acceptance of marital break-up and lone parenthood compared with before. Secondly, since the mid-1960s there has been a noticeable change in the legal attitude to child custody on divorce. Prior to the mid-1960s, fathers were expected to have, and were therefore more often given, the exclusive custody of their children in accordance with the tradition of Japanese patrilineal household structure – the '*ie* system'. The *ie* system formed the legal basis of the Japanese family structure until its constitutional abolition after the Second World War. It was premised on the primogeniture system and the household economic structure in which the head of the household is charged with the power and the responsibility to maintain the primary objective of the system, namely the continuity of the family name. In most cases, however, the children were actually taken care of by female members of the father's family, such as grandmothers and aunts. Although, from the end of the Second World War, there was a gradual shift towards giving mothers the custody of their children, the proportion of children in their mother's custody only became equal to that in their father's in 1965. Since then custody favouring mothers has increased dramatically. By 1990, about three-quarters of child custody cases gave custody to the mothers as opposed to the fathers whereas the reverse was true only about 50 years ago (Japan, 1992b). The idea of joint custody, which is now increasingly the case in Western countries, has been introduced to Japan in recent years; however, this practice is very rarely adopted by the court. For example, in 1989, custody was given to the mother in 71.3 per cent of the cases, while in 22.6 per cent custody was granted to the father. In the remaining 6.1 per cent of cases custody was granted to others, most often to relatives other than the mother or the father (Japan, Ministry of Health and Welfare, 1991).

My examination of welfare policies directed towards lone-mother families in Japan shows that the welfare regime is characterized by a strong emphasis on social cohesion and social order, as opposed to individual social citizenship, and gender asymmetry. I situate lone mothers within the Japanese social context which structures the patterns of care and work and undertake both material and discourse analyses: the former based on examination of the current welfare system and labour market conditions; the latter based on my own in-depth interviews with lone mothers living in Tokyo.

This chapter is divided into five sections. First, I will outline the national trends concerning lone motherhood in Japan, including their prevalence and characteristics, economic status, and patterns of labour-market participation. In the second section I will examine the dominant and alternative political and popular discourses around lone motherhood in Japan. This section will discuss how the 'problems' of lone-mother families are defined, and how the notion of the family and mothers' paid work are perceived. The third section will analyse the welfare regime in Japan and how it positions lone mothers within a policy context. The fourth section will look at the varying constraints and opportunities presented by the local labour market and the employment conditions of women and lone mothers. Finally, the last section will deal with neighbourhood contexts for the support networks and informal support given to lone-mother families.

2. Lone Mothers in Japan

Trends in the prevalence of lone motherhood

Since the 1970s there has been a large increase in the number of lone mothers arising from divorce, and a steady decline in those due to widowhood (see Table 5.1). In comparison, the number of unmarried (i.e. single) lone mothers has been very low throughout the post-war period, remaining less than 6 per cent of the total, and now even declining. This is in considerable contrast to the USA, Britain and some countries where single lone motherhood is increasing.

	1973		1983		1991	
	000s	%	000s	%	000s	%
Single (unmarried)	15	2.4	38	5.3	30	3.6
Divorced	165	26.4	353	49.1	529	62.3
Widowed	387	61.9	259	36.1	252	29.7
No information	59	9.4	68	9.8	37	4.4
Total	626	100	718	100	848	100

Source Figures are based on National Surveys of Lone Mother Families, Ministry of Health and Welfare

Table 5.1 Civil status of lone mothers: Japan 1973, 1983, 1991

As noted earlier, most authors attribute the recent rise in the Japanese divorce rate to a combination of the decline of the traditional Japanese family system (which also applies a notion of semi-extended family structure and of marriage as a family obligation rather than individual choice), and to the direct effects of Western ideas concerning individualism and the notion of the nuclear and conjugal family (Goode, 1963; Hendry, 1987; Kumagai, 1983; Smith, 1983; Cornell, 1989, 1990). For example, Kumagai (1983) claims that since the middle of the 1960s there has been a shift in public attitudes towards conjugal marriage in Japan, as shown by public opinion polls and by the self-reported causes of divorce to the family court. This evidence seems to indicate that the rise in the divorce rate in Japan is related to changing value systems, particularly to the greater importance individuals now place on shared ideas and mutuality within marriage.

However other studies have also found strong evidence linking divorce in Japan with personal economic hardships, particularly those felt by women, and domestic violence. For example, it has been found that the majority of divorces are initiated by women, and furthermore, that most women who seek divorce claim personality conflict, financial problems, and domestic violence as their primary reasons (Japan, 1990). The significance of economic factors is also underlined by the result of a 1978 study which found that: (i) divorced men were 16.3 per cent more likely than non-divorced men to have low incomes, and 14.2 per cent less likely to have high incomes; and (ii) amongst men between the ages of 35 and 39 years – the age group which is most likely to get divorced – those who were divorced were 27.2 per cent more likely to have low incomes than their non-divorced counterparts (Tamura and Tamura, 1988; Sasaki, 1989). These findings point to the fact that while the individual expectations of a love marriage may influence the rate of divorce, the economic causes of marital dissolution should not be underestimated.

Yet despite the recent rise, the divorce rate in Japan is still very low compared with other countries discussed in this volume, other than Ireland. Currently, the divorce rate in Japan is about 13 per 1,000. Given this relatively low rate, it would therefore appear strange that the numbers of divorced lone mothers in Japan should be increasing so rapidly. The main reason for this is that lone motherhood is often considered a long-term condition in Japan. Despite the increasing public acceptance of the Western notion of conjugal marriage and individualism, dominant public attitudes are still resistant to cohabitation and remarriage for women. For example, recent opinion polls indicate that, on the one hand, over 50 per cent of men and women under the age of 40 believe that marriage is not necessary if one is happy being single; but on the other hand, less than 30 per cent of people in that age group supported the idea of cohabitation. The reality of individual reluctance towards remarriage for women is also evidenced by the low remarriage rate among divorced women in Japan, as compared with both Japanese men, and both divorced men and women in many Western countries. For example, in 1980 the per annum remarriage rate for divorced women in Japan was 1.1 per cent – about one-ninth of that of divorced women in England and Wales (9.1 per cent) and about one-fifth the rate for Japanese men (5.3 per cent). Moreover among those 1.1 per cent who remarried, the majority were under the age of 30 (Inoue and Ehara, 1992; OPCS, 1991). Clearly, unlike lone mothers in many Western countries, there is a much lower chance of lone mothers in Japan exiting lone motherhood through remarriage and repartnering.

Lone mothers in Japan tend to have fewer children compared with their two-parent counterparts. According to the 1988 national survey of lone-mother families, nearly 90 per cent had less than two dependent children (Japan, 1992b).[1] Between 1978 and 1988, the average age of lone mothers has declined from 42.7 to 40.8 years. This decline is largely due to a sharp drop in the overall population of lone mothers over the age of 50, most of whom were widows, and a steady increase in divorce among couples in their 20s and 30s.

Lone mothers and paid work

The employment rate of lone mothers in Japan is extremely high. In 1988, 86.8 per cent of lone mothers were in paid work, as compared with just 31.8 per cent of married mothers (see Tables 5.2 and 5.3). This high employment rate can be directly attributed to inadequate state income support provision for such families. The post-war Japanese social welfare system has been largely based on the idea of 'poverty measure' (*sochi seido*) or poverty assistance – a system built around highly stigmatizing and discretionary provisions and on the legal assumption of family mutual support. Although many lone-mother families are theoretically entitled to receive the basic public assistance (*seikatsu hogo*), the stigma of receiving this assistance is so high that in reality only about 15 per cent of lone-mother families receive such provision (Japan, 1993). *Seikatsu hogo* is the most basic means-tested benefit for low-income families in Japan. It may be considered roughly equivalent to Income Support in Britain or Aid to Families with Dependent Children (AFDC) in the USA. According to the 1990 National Houshold Survey, whereas 49 per cent of lone-

	Self-employed (%)	Ordinary employment (%)	Temporary & casual employment (%)	Family business & other (%)	Not working (%)
1973	23.6	43.5	7.9	8.9	16.1
1978	15.9	60.6	8.5	–	14.8
1983	10.5	55.1	7.6	11.1	15.8
1988	10.6	48.2	16.8	11.2	13.2

Note Ordinary employment: workers hired and paid on regular monthly basis. *Temporary and casual employment*: workers hired on temporary or daily basis, usually for low wages and with poor job security
Source Japan (1973–1988) National Survey of Lone Mother Families (Tokyo: Ministry of Health and Welfare)
Table 5.2 Lone mothers' employment status: Japan 1973–88

	1985	1986	1987	1988	1989	1990
Mothers in 2-parent families working (%)	29.7	29.8	31.0	31.8	32.7	34.0
Lone mothers working (%)	87.2	not known	not known	86.8	not known	89.5

Source Japan (1991) Special Employment Survey, The Prime Minister's Office
Table 5.3 Employment rates for coupled and lone mothers: Japan 1985–90

mother families had a total income low enough to qualify for *seikatsu hogo*, only 14.5 per cent were in receipt of the benefit (Ishida, 1994). Although there exist a number of special provisions for lone-mother families, such as the Child Rearing Allowances (*Jido Fuyo Teate*) – a small supplementary allowance primarily for low-income divorced and unmarried lone-parent families – special tax deductions for low-income families, Loans for Fatherless Families, homes for lone-mother families (*Boshiryo* – discussed later), and day-care support, all of these are now strictly means tested and none offer adequate financial support. As a result, most lone mothers have little choice but to take up paid work and/or depend on financial support from their families.

There has been a noticeable change in the types of work taken up by lone mothers over the last couple of decades in Japan. As shown in Table 5.2, between 1973 and 1988 the proportion of lone mothers in self-employment fell by nearly half; at the same time, those in temporary and casual employment rose two and a half times. The proportion of lone mothers in ordinary employment remained relatively constant. It is difficult to tell from the Ministry of Health and Welfare survey how fully employed these lone mothers were, since the data in the category of 'ordinary employment' include both full and part-time work.[2] The Tokyo Metropolitan Government survey of lone mothers' employment has found that, in 1984, 28.5 per cent of all lone mothers were in part-time, temporary, or daily employment, while 53.8 per cent worked full time (Tokyo, 1985). In another Tokyo study, conducted in 1986/87, it was found that amongst all working lone mothers surveyed, 41.9 per cent worked part time (Tokyo, 1987). It appears that a little over half of all lone mothers work full-time.

Lone mothers' income

Despite their high labour-market participation rate, lone-mother families in Japan have a significantly greater risk of being poor compared with other types of families. For example, in 1988 lone-mother families were the lowest income group of all family groups: their average income was Y2.02 million (approximately £8,000), or 39.4 per cent of the average two-parent family income (Y5.13 million or about £20,000). Amongst lone-mother families, the average annual income of those headed by a widowed lone mother was about a third higher than those headed by divorced lone mothers, at Y2.42 million (£9,600) and Y1.85 million (£7,400) respectively (see Table 5.4). This difference is largely accounted for by the social insurance benefits provided to widows (the Widows and Survivors' benefits). Furthermore, the relative proportion of lone-mother families' income in relation to two-parent families shows a steady decline since the end of the 1970s, falling from 46.4 per cent of the average two-parent family income in 1978 to 45.0 per cent in 1983, and just 39.4 per cent in 1988 (Japan, 1992b). The worsening of lone mothers' economic status has been attributed to the fact that, unlike other families, they were not able to

	Two-parent families	All lone-mother families	Widowed lone-mother families	Divorced lone-mother families
Average size	3.31	3.19	3.44	3.09
Average employed family members	1.63	1.22	1.38	1.15
Average annual income	5,130,000	2,020,000	2,420,000	1,850,000
(as % of two-parent families)	(100)	(39.4)	(47.2)	(36.1)
Average annual income among lowest quartile	2,520,000	1,070,000	1,350,000	980,000
(as % of two-parent families)	(100)	(42.5)	(53.6)	(38.9)
Average annual income among second quartile	4,350,000	1,680,000	2,000,000	1,520,000
(as % of two-parent families)	(100)	(38.6)	(46.0)	(34.9)
Average annual income among third quartile	6,660,000	2,520,000	3,080,000	2,340,000
(as % of two-parent families)	(100)	(37.8)	(46.2)	(35.2)

Sources Japan (1988) National Survey of Lone Mother Families (Tokyo: Ministry of Health and Welfare); Japan (1988) The 1988 National Basic Family Survey (Tokyo: Ministry of Health and Welfare)

Table 5.4   Average annual income of two-parent families and lone-mother families: Japan 1988

benefit from the country's economic growth during this period. For example, between 1976 and 1988, the average income of two-parent families rose by 63.2 per cent in absolute terms, while that of lone mother families rose by only 29 per cent (Shoya, 1990).

The most important contributing factor to Japanese lone mothers' low income is their low level of earning. This is partly because of the marginalization of women within the labour market (Cook and Hayashi, 1980; Shinozuka, 1992; Ishida, 1994). This is, however, not limited to lone mothers but affects most women in Japan. The Japanese economy and labour market is based on a dual system in which a small core sector, dominated by large firms, operates on the basis of generous company benefits and a life-time employment system for men, supported by a large peripheral sector consisting of medium and small firms, which operates in a similar manner to the Western liberal free market model.[3] Thus a comparison of lone mothers' and women's work generally, by type of industry, shows little difference between the two; unlike men, more than 80 per cent of both lone mothers and women generally are found in manufacturing, retail, and service sector industries (constituting over three-quarters of the total employment in 1987). In addition, the majority of women are found in small firms of less than 100 employees, while most men are found in larger firms (Ishida, 1994). Overall, women are found in workplaces with low wages and low security jobs.

In addition to the marginalization of most women in sectors of the labour market with low wages and low job security, the wage system in Japan is also strongly based on a male-breadwinner model. For example, despite rising average incomes over the last few decades, the average Japanese women's wage relative to men was still just 60.7 per cent in 1992 (Tokyo, 1994). Not only do men and women start at different wage levels, but salaries in Japan are also generally tied to the length of steady employment. Since women are often forced to leave the labour market after marriage or after the birth of the first child, this means that most will not be able to keep their jobs long enough to earn a high income (Cook and Hayashi, 1980; Ishida, 1994). Indeed, data show that the average length of continuous employment for women in Japan was less than 60 per cent that of men, at 7.2 and 12.4 years respectively in 1990 (Japan, Ministry of Labour, 1990). Given such employment practices, Japanese women are seldom able to enter into career positions, and furthermore, are generally given lower status and lower paid positions compared with men regardless of company size and educational qualifications. For lone mothers who have the responsibility of maintaining their families, this implies significant economic difficulties.

Given their low income it is not surprising that in addition to their employment income many lone mothers in Japan depend on incomes from their children's work, support from their own families, and the fathers of the children, as well as the less stigmatizing public benefits such as child rearing allowances. Family support, particularly the maintenance allowance from children's fathers is, however, highly unreliable. For example, the 1988

	Wages/ salaries	Self- employment	Transfer payments	Other sources (including family)	Total
	(%)	(%)	(%)	(%)	(%)
Lone-mother families	81.5	1.4	11.3	5.9	100
Two-parent families	94.5	1.0	2.1	2.3	100

Sources Japan, Prime Minister's Office (1990)

Table 5.5 Income package structure of lone-mother families and two-parent families: Japan 1990

national survey found that three-quarters (75.4 per cent) of divorced lone mothers reported that they had *never* received maintenance support from the fathers of their children, while 10.6 per cent claimed to have received only some, and only 14.0 per cent reported to have been in receipt of regular support. On the other hand, the majority of Japanese lone mothers to take up the less stigmatizing child rearing allowance programme (*Jido Fuyo Teate*).

Lone mothers are more likely to depend on their earnings from work than on either transfer payments or private support. On average, in 1990, lone mothers derived 81.5 per cent of their income from wages and salaries (see Table 5.5). This is not far below the average of 94.5 per cent of income from wages and salaries for two-parent families, in substantial contrast to countries such as Britain and Germany (see chapters 3 and 7 in this volume).

3. Discourses Around Lone Motherhood in Japan

The dominant political and popular discourses around lone motherhood over the last decade and a half show an interesting parallel with the discourses around what is now commonly accepted as the 'Japanese-style welfare regime' or the 'Japanese-style welfare society' (*Nihongata fukushi shakai*). This neo-conservative rhetoric argues that, unlike other industrialized countries in the West, Japan should not aim to establish a *welfare state* but should rather see its objective as creating a uniquely Japanese-style *welfare society* founded on the principles of 'mutual and self-help' and 'independence' (Baba, 1979; Asahi Shinbun, 1983c; Institute of Social Science, 1985; Zenkoku Shakai Fukushi Kyogikai, 1989) – an analysis on which I expand later.

This Japanese-style welfare society discourse, which dominated public and political debate in Japan since the mid-1970s, has clearly had a powerful influence on discourses about the ideal family structure, mothers' paid work, and hence also about lone mothers. These discourses can be divided into three stages:

(i) *1980–86*, the first phase of welfare reform and a period of discourse on the declining family and attacks on lone mothers;

(ii) *1986–90*, a period of muted discourses on lone motherhood and an increasing focus on the second phase of welfare reform, including the introduction of the Gold Plan in response to the 'aging society'; and

(iii) *post-1990*, the period of a new policy emphasis on family support for 'traditional' two parent families in the wake of declining birth rates and a rapidly aging society, culminating in the introduction of the Angel Plan in response to the declining birthrates.

Before I go on to discuss these periods, however, it is important to describe the economic and political background to the emergence of the discourse on the Japanese-style welfare society.

Origins of the Japanese-style welfare society discourse

The 'Japanese-style welfare society' discourse first emerged as a theoretical alternative to the welfare state in response to the external and domestic pressures experienced in the wake of the 1973 oil crisis, and its subsequent recessionary effects. Domestically, the decline in economic growth combined with rising unemployment immediately after 1973, and the fiscal crisis of 1975, led to a radical shift in public opinion. General support for the progressive expansion of a universal welfare system was replaced by a reassessment of the direction and the nature of welfare (Shinkawa, 1990; Tabata, 1990; Hiwatari, 1993). Externally, the supposed 'crisis' of welfare states in the West during this time also gave Japanese critics of further welfare expansion significant ammunition to assert their case. The political debate during this period reveals a steady shift away from a more social welfare-oriented policy to a more fiscally conservative policy (Hiwatari, 1993). In the public forum, right-wing scholars took a dominant position in public and political discourse. They emphasized the problems associated with the Western welfare states, the so-called 'English Disease' (*Eikokubyo*) of uncontrollable welfare expenditure and a high welfare dependency rate combined with a decline in economic performance – as supposedly seen in Britain since the 1970s (Shinkawa, 1990). One consequence of this debate was the establishment of the Ad Hoc Commission on Administrative Reform in 1981. The main objective of the Commission was to carry out complete administrative and welfare reform in order to achieve smaller state provision and greater self-reliance through welfare cuts.

This notion of the Japanese-style welfare society was premised on the idea of economic rationality and moral imperative. Economically, not unlike the neo-conservative fiscal policies introduced by many of the western countries in the 1980s, the Japanese Government saw low taxes and welfare cuts as the solution to a growing government deficit. This was achieved through political compromise between the government (particularly the Ministries of Finance, Health and Welfare, and Labour), the trade unions and business, with the implementation of deficit reduction and a cross-subsidization of welfare schemes across the parties in order to achieve a parity of costs and benefits. In addition, the government also played a key role in coordinating the new labour market arrangements (Hiwatari, 1993: 26). For example, with the support of the government, big businesses and the trade unions agreed on wage restraint and cooperation with necessary technological advances; in exchange, the business sector assured the workers of employment security. In order to maintain the labour-market policy of low unemployment and the welfare policy of containing costs (particularly those of pension benefits), businesses were urged, with financial support from the Ministry of Labour, 'to retain workers after retirement age, to retrain elderly workers, to assist them to find secondary jobs, and to extend the retirement age' (Hiwatari, 1993: 27).

Morally, the Japanese-style welfare society discourse introduced two new important concepts to the notion of welfare in Japan. First, as its name indicates, the discourse argued that Japanese society was by nature not conducive to becoming a 'welfare state', as might be the case for other industrialized nations but, rather, could only become a 'welfare society'. Welfare obligations were to be shared by *all members* of society, and not left to the state. The reason, so the argument went, was that Japanese culture is so implicitly rooted in the idea of the family and mutual aid that any attempt to artificially install state welfare would not only go against Japanese cultural sensibility but would also damage the family and society as a whole.

A second dimension introduced by the Japanese-style welfare society discourse was a new definition of the concepts of work, welfare and individual autonomy (i.e. economic independence). This was achieved by linking the post-1973 welfare crisis directly to the issue of the aging society. For example, at the time of the so-called welfare crisis in Japan in 1975, the proportion of Japanese people of the age of 65 and over was only 8.8 per cent, one of the lowest in the industrialized nations (Japan, 1993). However, by the end of the 1970s, the issues of the aging population and the future welfare burden of the aged were already publicized to the extent that it was generally accepted that Japan had already become an 'ageing society'. The government sought to reduce the cost of welfare by cutting pension payments through an aggressive employment extension policy for elderly people. The policy was put forward on the grounds that paid work was not only beneficial to both the individual and society, but furthermore, that it was implicit in the Japanese value system (e.g. Japan, 1983).

The importance of emphasizing work rather than welfare as the rightful option for elderly people in Japan is that it sets out the basic principles of mutual and self-reliance and family economic independence (i.e., non-welfare dependence) for all. Here, it is also important to emphasize that within the framework of the Japanese-style welfare society discourse, the idea of work is defined not as an individual right in the sense of a fundamental universal right, nor even as a citizenship obligation; rather it is defined as a rightful option for Japanese people, partly because it springs from the individual's need to achieve autonomy and self-realization through work; and partly because their work is also conducive to the common good of society. Moreover, it is assumed that the Japanese people's propensity to work also implies their general antipathy to welfare, and hence to the Western model of welfare and early retirement. Given this framework, the appropriate role for the state with respect to welfare would then be to enable and encourage individuals to participate in employment and thereby achieve economic independence, and escape welfare dependence.

In summary, the Japanese-style welfare society discourse has been redefining the notion of welfare in Japan to emphasize, first, welfare pluralism by revising the earlier trajectory of progressive expansion of the state welfare of the pre-1973 era and refocusing on the roles played by the family and community, and secondly, the importance of the labour market and the sanctity of the individual and family self-reliance as solutions to the problems of welfare.

The impact of the Japanese-style welfare society discourse on lone-mother families

1980–86: the declining family and attacks on lone mothers

The first half of the 1980s saw intense public and political preoccupation with what many of the government White Papers called the problems of 'loosening of family ties and the crisis in family relationships' (Japan, 1985). With the implementation of the first phase of the welfare reform (*Fukushi Kaikaku*) by the Ad Hoc Committee on Administrative Reform in 1981, the issues of rising divorce rates and increasing numbers of lone-parent families, as well as increasing juvenile delinquency, were highlighted. At the same time the supposedly adverse effects of internationalization, such as excessive individualism and egotistic behaviour, were singled out as the main causes of these social ills.

The actual pattern of public discourse, however, was less straightforward. For example, while there was a growing public acceptance of the importance of women's paid work, at the same time mothers' labour-market participation, and women's changing attitudes towards marriage and family, were also identified as contributing to the decline of the 'traditional' family and the arrival of new social problems. Hence, when the national divorce rate in Japan rose above 1.5 in 1983, it was hailed by the media as the '1.5 crisis', while divorced couples were attacked for their excessive egotism and irresponsibility (Asahi Shinbun, 1985a). The Annual Report on National Life was also quick to point to the 'loosening of family ties and the crisis in family relationships' by linking divorce and lone motherhood to such social problems:

Declining mutual assistance and broken family relationship have caused many problems for children, who are in the weakest position in

the family. The first problem is the increase in juvenile delinquency
. . . A second problem is an increase in the number of abortions
among young people . . . [and] a third problem is an increase in
juvenile runaways. This suggests that there are problems in their ties
with their families.

(Japan, 1985: 163–5)

Conceptions of the 'problem' of divorce and the loosening of family ties and
relationships were also shaped by the image of the long-suffering father in the
American movie, 'Kramer vs. Kramer', which became one of the most popular
movies in Japan in 1982. The film portrays a divorce case in which husband and
wife fight over the custody of their child, and where the father's case is
presented highly favourably. A cynical interpretation of such public attention
to the plight of lone-*father* families is that this, first of all, raised the public
consciousness about divorce as something which adversely affected both men
and women, and secondly, helped concentrate the public and policy attack
on just one gendered target group – mothers who walk out of marriage.
Throughout 1982 to 1984, lone-father families, rather than the more numerous
and economically marginal lone-mother families, became the main topic of
media and government investigation. For example, in 1982 a number of
prefectural and local governments initiated their own surveys of lone-father
families in response to the 'Kramer' phenomenon (Asahi Shinbun, 1982;
Kumamoto Nichinich, 1982; Tokyo Shinbun, 1982). The following year, for
the first time in history, the Ministry of Health and Welfare also included lone-
father families in their national survey of lone-mother families (Asahi
Shinbun, 1983a, 1983b; Yomiuri Shinbun, 1983). In all cases, it was found that
the majority of lone fathers were due to recent divorce or 'run-away' mothers.
It was also found that, while in relatively better economic circumstances
compared with lone-mother families, lone-father families were nevertheless in
a desperate condition because of lack of child care and domestic help. The
public and policy focus on the child-care and domestic problems faced by lone
fathers highlights the pervasive assumption that men's 'double burden'
(employment and home) was a problem – whereas women's was not. The
hardships experienced by lone fathers were further highlighted when the
media sensationalized a case of a murder/suicide involving a lone father and his
three daughters in 1984 (Nishinihon, 1984; Sankei, 1984; Shinno-mainichi,
1984; Mainichi Shinbun, 1985). The public and political response to the case
was an outcry of sympathy for lone fathers, and, ironically, a severe criticism of
divorcees and lone mothers. The media criticized the supposed high welfare
dependency of lone-mother families, while paradoxically claiming that many
of the country's orphanages were crowded with the unwanted children of
unmarried and divorced lone mothers (Kahoku Shinpo, 1983; Sankei, 1984b;
Asahi Shinbun, 1985b; Mainichi Shinbun, 1985). The government also
highlighted the rapid increase in the numbers of lone mothers dependent on
the child rearing allowance, the income supplement allowance primarily for

non-widowed lone mothers. It was during this period that the government proposed an overall review of the existing income support programme for divorced and unmarried lone-mother families, and moved towards introducing what it called 'the Kramer Measures' (*Kramer taisaku*) to ensure parity of welfare support between lone-father and lone-mother families (Asahi Shinbun, 1983b; Yomiuri Shinbun, 1984).

Following the 'Kramer' period, 1985 and 1986 saw some important changes in government policy towards lone-mother families in Japan, particularly affecting divorced and unmarried lone mothers. In 1985, the government introduced a new Child Rearing Allowance Law, which significantly tightened the eligibility criteria for the allowance and also extended ex-husbands' obligation to pay maintenance. The new law proposed to disallow divorced lone mothers from receiving allowance assistance if the annual income of their ex-husband exceeded 6 million yen per year; they should seek child support from their ex-husband, not the state. Another proposal was to disallow unmarried lone mothers from receiving the child rearing allowance.

The legislative change to the Child Rearing Allowance Law and the government policy proposals to disallow unmarried lone mothers from receiving child rearing allowance were criticized by the National Association of Lone Mother Families and women's groups; however, their voices were marginal. The fact that the National Association of Lone Mother Families was largely dominated by widowed lone mothers also did not help the group establish a strong and clear position from which to mount an effective attack on the government. In the end, the new Child Rearing Allowance Law was passed without much effective opposition, while the proposal to deny unmarried lone mothers welfare entitlement was rejected by the government. On the other hand, the welfare entitlements of lone-father families were extended to the same level as lone-mother families (except for the widows pensions schemes) through the 'Kramer Measures'.

1986–90: public silence on lone-mother families

After the legislative change of 1985/86, the dominant political and popular discourses around lone motherhood fell into near silence. Rather, welfare debates shifted to the issues of the elderly and community care and the declining birth rate. The two main annual government White Papers, the White Paper on National Life (*Kokumin Seikatsu Hakusho* – published by the Ministry of Finance) and the White Paper on Health and Welfare (*Kosei Hakusho* – published by the Mininstry of Health and Welfare), reveal a consistent emphasis on these topics. Since these papers outline the respective Ministry's policy and fiscal objectives, they also serve as barometers for the direction of research and debate in Japan. The sudden disappearance of lone-mother families from the public and policy discourses in Japan contrasts quite markedly with the case of lone mothers in countries like Germany, where the

Year	Aged households (%)	Lone-mother families (%)	Households with sick or disabled person (%)	Other households (%)	Total (%)
1970	31.4	10.3	35.9	22.4	100.0
1975	34.3	9.5	46.1	10.2	100.0
1980	32.6	12.6	43.5	11.3	100.0
1985	32.5	14.4	43.6	9.5	100.0
1990	39.3	11.7	41.1	7.9	100.0
1991	41.0	10.9	50.4	7.7	100.0

Source Health and Welfare Statistics in Japan, Ministry of Health and Welfare, Japan, 1993
Table 5.6   Distribution of public assistance by type of household: Japan 1970–91

Year	Receiving public assistance (%)
1975	18.9
1980	21.2
1985	22.5
1990	11.9

Source Ishida (1994)
Table 5.7   Percentage of lone-mother families receiving public assistance: Japan 1975–90

issue of declining birth rate was associated with a more positive valuing of lone mothers.

In reality however, the cuts in welfare support for divorced and unmarried lone mothers continued as the state strengthened its policy emphasis on lone mothers' economic self-reliance. The rates and numbers of lone mothers dependent on public assistance (*seikatsu hogo*) also declined steadily from 1985, as shown in Tables 5.6 and 5.7. Lone mothers, as a proportion of all families receiving public assistance dropped from 14.4 to 10.9 per cent between 1985 and 1991, while the proportion of lone-mother households receiving assistance halved, from 22.5 per cent to 11.9 per cent between 1985 and 1990.

The tacit policy vis-à-vis lone-mother families during this period therefore can be understood as an official non-recognition, as the state-strengthened its support for the traditional two-parent and multi-generational family mode.

Post-1990: the resssertion of the traditional two-parent family ideal

The relative silence on lone-mother families during the second half of the 1980s, did not however imply public or political condoning of these families. Rather, the discourse on lone-mother families was submerged into an implicit criticism through the public reassertion of the 'traditional' two-parent family structure during this period. This became even more evident in 1992 when the government introduced the 'Angel Plan', a family preservation and support policy plan aimed at addressing the problem of the declining birth rate. It aims to minimize the rapid aging of the population by actively promoting child bearing and family preservation. The Angel Plan locates the problem of the declining birth rate in Japan over the last few decades firstly, in the changes in the functioning and the structure of Japanese families, and secondly, in the changes in women's lifestyles and expectations. Examples of changes associated with women's behaviour that are commonly singled out are higher educational achievement and increased labour-force participation rate, and an increased average age of first marriage. These all point to a decline in the likelihood of women marrying at a younger age, and hence a lesser likelihood of them having a large family. In addition to this, from the point of view of welfare state and housing issues, high housing costs, the small size of living spaces, and the high costs associated with child rearing and education have also been singled out as having an adverse effect on family planning among couples of child bearing age.

The Plan is progressive in the sense that it attempts to support the two-parent family by simultaneously encouraging mothers to participate in the labour market and to strengthen the functions of the family. At a formal level, it recognizes and emphasizes the importance of women's labour-market participation and the double burden this has placed on women, in terms of the expectation that women will manage both earning and caring roles within the family. The recent political discourse around the family and women's dual role also suggests a reappraisal of the Western models of welfare policy. Over the last few years, for example, the European Union's family policies have been identified as exemplary models of successful societies, and Sweden's family policy has been particularly singled out for its progressiveness and effectiveness in raising the national birth rate (now the highest in the Western Europe). The current Japanese Government response is to selectively adopt some of these ideas. In terms of rhetoric, it is admirably positive. As Prime Minister Miyazawa stated in his administrative policy speech in January 1992, 'In a truly advanced nation, women are able to realise their potential both at work and in the home . . . It is now necessary to develop further an environment for women to make the most of their abilities and expertise' (Nikkei Business, 1992: 11).

The Angel Plan urges the importance of enhancing and supporting the positive functioning of the family, through active co-ordination between the state and the labour market to help working mothers combine paid work and child rearing. However, it offers little in the way of real substantial policies aimed at changing existing labour market practices towards women. For example, while the Plan emphasizes the importance of men's participation in child rearing and suggests that business provides child-care leave for parents, shortens working hours, and provides child-care services within the workplace, none of these have actually been supported by legislation. Instead, most of the Plan's policies have been focused on providing extra help for working mothers through increased public and private day-care spaces, and offering tax relief and child allowances to encourage young families to have more children. As a total package, therefore, the Plan fits quite well with the overall policy framework of preparing for and alleviating some of the damaging consquences of the aging society. However, in terms of actual labour-market co-ordination, it falls short of offering real alternatives to existing labour-market functioning and structure. Hence the basic market assumption of the male-breadwinner model and gender asymmetry remain unchanged and unchallenged.

Public discourse has been generally supportive of the Plan, while at the same time, being critical of its failure to exert more pressure on business. For example, the Plan has been criticized as not doing enough to make business change employment practices so as to allow fathers to participate in child care (Nihon Keizai, 1994; Sankei, 1994; Yomiuri Shinbun, 1994). Here, the Swedish and EU cases have been also widely used as exemplars to criticize government policies. At the same time, concerns about the declining birth rate and increasing divorce rate have resulted in unconditional support for any policy which aims to support family preservation. For example, in 1993 when the national birth rate fell below 1.5 children per woman, the media was quick to draw a connection between the rising average age of first-time mothers and the rising average age for first-time marriage, and at the same time, to contrast this with the record level of divorces – particularly amongst those married for less than a year (Kobe, 1994).

4. The Japanese Welfare State Regime and Lone Motherhood

As discussed in the previous section, since the end of the 1970s the welfare regime in Japan has been strongly shaped by the concept of the Japanese-style welfare society. This regime has affected the policy approach to lone-mother families in two ways: (i) a policy emphasis on the idea of lone mothers' economic independence and self-reliance through paid work; and (ii) policy support for the 'traditional' two-parent model.

In terms of policies for lone-mother families, there had been a series of cuts in welfare provision since the mid-1980s. For example, total government expenditure on welfare for lone-mother families was cut by about 15 per cent between 1985 and 1990 (Japan, Ministry of Health and Welfare, 1990). This particularly affected divorced and unmarried lone-mother families. The most significant changes were seen in three areas:

(i) restructuring of the functions of homes for lone-mother families (the *Boshiryo*), the largest item in the welfare expenditure for lone mothers;

(ii) changes in the Child Rearing Allowance legislation in 1985; and

(iii) a shift in emphasis from income support to a loans programme for lone mothers.

The provision of homes for lone-mother families (the *Boshiryo*) is the oldest and the largest welfare programme for lone-mother families in Japan. The original aims of the homes were to provide needy lone mothers and their children with a safe and secure living environment, and institutional support to help them overcome their personal hardships. Although the actual proportion of lone-mother families dependent on *Boshiryo* is very small, they are nevertheless an important institution particularly for younger and new lone mothers who are most likely to have greater need for housing and financial support.[4] In the 1980s, these homes came under criticism from the government for their failure to encourage greater self-sufficiency among lone mothers.

A series of government-led enquiries into the future role of *Boshiryo* resulted in the introduction of new objectives to encourage lone mothers to achieve economic independence and self-sufficiency through in-house skills training, personal guidance, job counselling and placement, and child care. This expansion of service provision meant that the nature of these homes for lone-mother families changed from primarily long-term housing support to a transitional residential programme linking lone mothers to the labour market (Zenkoku Shakai Fukushi Kyogikai – Boshiryo Kyogikai, 1992).

In the 1980s, income maintenance support for lone-mother families also came under the 'welfare reform' emphasis on self-reliance and independence. In 1985, the main income supplement provision for non-widowed lone-mother families, the child rearing allowance, was significantly altered in response to the increasing number of divorced lone-mother families. The new Child Rearing Allowance Law (1985) introduced the idea of a two-tier system of income testing, and also the ex-husband's child support obligation. The ceiling for the income cut-off is set so low that only those with near poverty level income qualify for the allowance. In 1990, for example, the income cut-off level for a lone-mother family with two children was Y1.93 million per year, Y20,000 less than the Ministry of Health and Welfare's official poverty line (*Seikatsu Hogo Kijun*) (see Table 5.4 for the incomes of lone-mother families). As a result, the number of lone mothers receiving the child rearing allowance has been declining since 1985, despite the steady increase in the total number of lone-mother families (Ishida, 1994). For many lone mothers who are denied the allowance, the economic impact is enormous, resulting in an average drop in their total income of about 25 per cent.

In addition to the introduction, for the first time, of a two-tier means-testing system for child rearing allowance, the idea of the husband's child support obligation was also introduced in the 1985 Child Rearing Allowance Law. Maintaining that husbands have a legal obligation to support their children and that the Japanese welfare society is premised on the mutual support of family members not the state, the new law also made divorced lone mothers, at least for the first year, ineligible to receive child rearing allowance if the income of their ex-husband exceeded 6.0 million yen per year. Given that over 86 per cent of divorced lone mothers claim to receive no regular child support from their ex-husbands, the new legislation has meant considerable economic hardship for divorced lone mothers. This legislation was later amended so that if a divorced lone mother did not receive any support from her ex-husband for a year, she would be able to apply for the child rearing allowance.

In the place of income supplement provision, however, much emphasis has been placed on the Loans for Lone Mother Families Programme (*Boshi Fukushi Shikin Kashitsuke*) as a way of 'guaranteeing the healthy and sound growth of children through stabilizing family income and encouraging self-efforts of families to improve their situations' (JNC-ICSW, 1990: 57). For example, the overall budget for the loans programme increased over 7.5 fold between 1953 and 1980 (Tarukawa, 1982). The Loans for Lone Mother Families Programme was originally established in 1953 to help lone mothers gain economic independence, primarily by starting small businesses. The government at the time was particularly interested in supporting lone mothers to open tobacconists, and there was a special loan programme for starting such a business. By 1982, the Loans for Lone Mother Families Programme had become the second largest programme within the lone mother welfare system, after the *Boshiryo* (Soeda, 1982). The policy emphasis on economic independence through the loans programme has been criticized as an attempt to legitimate the government's denial of its basic welfare obligation to lone mothers (Tarukawa, 1982). However, many Japanese scholars are supportive of the idea. For example, Soeda (1982) regards the Loans for Lone Mother Families Programme as a positive step in lone mother policy. Arguing for the 'vital effectiveness of developing individual (economic) independence as a precondition for achieving full social welfare policy and practice', Soeda considers the Loans for Lone Mothers as not only economically pragmatic but also a positive social investment for the future (Soeda, 1982: 2).

A closer analysis of the expenditure for the Loans for Lone Mother Families Programme, however, shows a continuing reduction in the relative amount of money allocated to starting and operating businesses, in contrast to a significant increase in the proportion allocated to special financial loans for such expenses as children's education. Since the budget allocation reflects demand, it suggests that these loans – rather than promoting economic independence of lone-mother families by helping them establish their own business or gain entry into the labour market – have become a way for lone mothers to supplement the cost of their children's educational expenses. In other words, loans have become a replacement for income supplement support.

The Japanese welfare regime, centred on self-sufficiency for lone mothers, reveals an obvious gap between the state's idea of 'the lone mother problem' and the reality of lone mothers' labour-market participation. For example, studies consistently show that despite their high labour-market participation rate, there has been a steady decline in lone mothers' relative income in comparison with all other families (Shinozuka, 1992; Ishida, 1994). As Ishida (1994) points out, poverty among lone-mother families in Japan is not due to their lack of labour-market participation or their high dependence rate on welfare, as government policies often assume. Rather, it is a result of a labour-market structure based on the male-breadwinner model. This model is premised on women's dependence on men, and thus justifies unequal treatment between men and women within the labour market. Women are not able to enter the labour market on an equal footing with their male counterparts, both in terms of wages and working conditions. Furthermore, women are often denied opportunities to continue paid work after marriage or childbirth as it is assumed they are to fulfil their primary roles of wives and mothers. In addition, social welfare arrangements also have been premised on the idea of women's dependence on men. Hence, for example, while widows and their children are entitled to the relatively generous survivors' pension schemes (in addition to being exempt from public and political criticism), divorced and unmarried lone mothers are expected to rely on their ex-husbands or ex-partners for support or to gain self-reliance through paid work.

5. Labour Markets

The national labour market

As already discussed in the previous section, the labour market structure in Japan is highly discriminatory against women. For lone mothers the existing labour market structure disadvantages them from achieving full economic independence because of three distinct features:

(i)   a family wage system based on a male-breadwinner model;
(ii) patriarchal corporate-style employment arrangements; and
(iii) a growing polarization of working hours between men and women as a result of recent labour market restructuring.

The male-breadwinner family wage model

Since the end of the Second World War the Japanese economic and labour market systems have followed what may be described as the male-breadwinner family wage model. This model assumes that men should be able to earn an adequate family wage to support their families, while women should devote themselves to the tasks of the primary carer and unpaid worker at home. This model, in turn, rationalizes women's subordinate role and marginal status within the labour market: women are not only systematically assigned low-skill and low-status jobs with low wages, but they are also relegated to the smaller subsidiary industries and service sectors – in other words, women are generally consigned to the periphery of the labour market (Nakagawa, 1995). For example, as mentioned earlier, despite the generally high rate of female labour-market participation (48.4 per cent of all female population over the age of 15, in 1990), the average female wage has remained at only about 60 per cent of that of the males for the last two decades (Tokyo, 1994).[5] The average length of continuous employment for women is also much lower than that of men, at 7.2 and 12.4 years respectively, suggesting that women's careers are often cut off (Japan, Ministry of Labour, 1990). Over the last couple of decades, there has also been a noticeable increase in the concentration of women in the tertiary industrial sectors, such as wholesale, retail, and service industries, and also in part-time work (Tokyo, 1994). Today the labour market age-participation pattern for women shows a deepening of the 'M-shape' (as opposed to its reduction in most other industrialized countries). This indicates a mass exit of women from the labour market after marriage and/or the birth of the first child, and a re-entry after child bearing.

Patriachal corporate employment arrangements

The type of male-breadwinner family wage model in Japan is, however, distinct from those found in many of the industrialized countries in the West in that it is also based on a corporate labour market arrangement premised on the traditional patriarchal Japanese family system (*kafuchosei*) Osawa (1993), for example, argues that this patriarchal corporatist structure not only structures the highly gendered division of labour and wage system, but also the seniority-based wage system (for men) and the system of sub-contracting arrangements between the large firms and the medium- and small-size enterprises. The reality of the gender relationship evident in such patriarchal corporatist arrangement is that men are concentrated in the corporate sector, which not only dominates economically but can also provide higher wages and life-time employment, while women are confined to the medium- and small-size subsidary enterprises where the wages are low and jobs are less secure.

The increasing polarization of work hours based on gender

The recent structuring of the labour market in Japan has also led to a growing polarization of working hours between men and women. Under the new labour market structure, businesses are under increasing pressure to abandon the traditional practice of life-time employment and seniority systems, and take on the Western-style free market model of labour arrangements. In addition, given Japan's high labour cost in the international market, companies are also forced to cut costs by making full-time workers work longer hours and employing more part-time workers. Male workers are therefore expected to work longer hours, while women are increasingly channelled into part-time work. The polarization of work hours by gender implies a further entrenchment of the male-breadwinner arrangement by making it less possible for men to spend time at home, and restricting women's full-time employment. Furthermore, this has also dovetailed with the state's growing expectation of women's role in unpaid work within the family and the community.

In summary, the labour market structure presents a formidable barrier against lone mothers achieving economic self-sufficiency. Lone mothers experience difficulties in the labour market in at least two ways: as women, they are discriminated against because of their gender, and as lone mothers they are further discriminated against because of their marital and social status. Thus lone mothers earn much less than male breadwinners in two-parent families. In addition, recent studies show that, compared with other women workers, lone mothers are still more likely to experience discrimination in the workplace and to change jobs more frequently (Sasaki, 1989; Japan, Ministry of Health and Welfare, 1992b).

Local labour markets

The above section discussed some of the major national labour market barriers to lone mothers gaining employment. However, in addition to these factors, there is also a noticeable neighbourhood effect on lone mothers which closely relates to the nature of the local labour markets, as well as to community networks. For example, it has been observed that there is a proportionally higher concentration of lone mothers in cities as compared with smaller communities because of the availability of jobs, a greater sense of anonymity, and more access to public services such as job training, day care, and public housing (Peng, 1995; Betania Homu, 1986). Within large cities, also, there are certain districts where lone mothers are more likely to live and work. For example, certain local districts in Tokyo, such as Nerima-ku, tend to attract more lone-mother families because: (i) these districts tend to have more 'progressive' local governments and thus provide more support, such as job training and job opportunities, public housing, and public child-care facilities; (ii) lone mothers tend to work near their home because of child-care arrangements; and (iii) there are good networks of local lone-mothers' support groups. Local districts with a growing population, like Nerima-ku, have been very active in recruiting lone mothers to work in the public sector. Ironically, today these jobs are highly sought after by lone mothers because of the job security, relatively flexible hours, and the public sector workers' pension plan.

6. Neighbourhood Case Study: Constraints and Opportunities for Lone Mothers

In this section, I use the case study based on Nerima-ku in Tokyo to describe the effects of neighbourhood on lone mother families. In 1992, I carried out an in-depth study of the social and economic conditions of lone-mother families in

Japan. The study was motivated by the apparent disjunction between the strong public criticism of lone motherhood and the steady increase in their numbers. This suggests that, despite the public admonishment, the social and economic reality for many women in Japan is such that lone motherhood in some cases is still preferable to remaining in marriage. What makes women decide upon lone motherhood? How do lone mothers negotiate their living and work arrangements? The study was based on in-depth interviews with 24 lone mothers living in Tokyo. It examined in detail some of the constraints and opportunities faced by Japanese women within marriage and as lone mothers.

The ages of the lone mothers interviewed ranged from the early 20s to late 50s. They included three widowed, eighteen divorced/separated, and two unmarried lone mothers. The research participants were selected through a snowballing process, which relied on chains of acquaintanceship and networking from one individual to another. There are very few 'official' entry points from which one could make contact with lone-mother families in Japan, and their stigmatization as 'deviant' families can make other means of contacting them extremely difficult.

The research participants differed not only in terms of age, but also in terms of their family backgrounds. Of the 24 lone mothers, about half were born and raised in middle-class families, while the other half were from working-class backgrounds. About half of the lone mothers were living in a district of Tokyo called Nerima-ku, known for its progressive local council and relatively inexpensive private housing, while the other half came from the rest of metropolitan Tokyo.

The interviews aimed to:

   (i) find out the reason for the women's lone motherhood;
  (ii) identify economic and social constraints and opportunities; and
 (iii) gain information concerning their paid work and support from the state, family, and friends and neighbours; in other words, their income packaging structures.

Constraints and opportunities

The interviews revealed some striking commonalities in the experiences of these lone mothers, despite their different backgrounds. These commonalities can be organized into three themes: (i) the preconditions for lone motherhood; (ii) their experiences with regard to paid work and housing; and (iii) their experiences with regard to public attitudes and concern for their children.

The preconditions for lone motherhood

The preconditions for lone motherhood were remarkably similar for most of the women interviewed. First, most of the lone mothers experienced much financial and emotional hardship in their marriage before they became lone mothers. Because of this, with the exception of the widows, all but one claimed that they had actively chosen to become lone mothers rather than having the condition imposed onto them. Given that most of these women had had negative experiences in their marriage, most of them therefore claimed that they were quite happy being lone mothers, or that they felt personally much happier after becoming lone mothers, despite the fact that they became considerably worse off economically and socially compared with most two-parent families as a result. (Interestingly, this sense of emotional relief and personal happiness upon becoming lone mothers was shared by the widowed as well as the non-widowed lone mothers.) Moreover, almost all of the women also claimed that they felt little or no desire to remarry or to find a new partner. For divorced and separated lone mothers the most common causes for them opting out of marriage were one or, more often, a combination of the following: the failure of the husband/partner to live up to the social norms implicit in a male-breadwinner society; and the failure of the husband/partner to assume expected male behaviour.

The failure of the husband or the partner to fulfil their male-breadwinner role, or more precisely, the failure to earn an adequate income and/or to share their income with their wife and children, was the most commonly cited reason for women to decide to divorce or separate. For example, the majority of the divorced/separated lone mothers reported that their husbands either did not provide them with any support while they were still together or, if they did, not enough for the family to live on. As a result, many of these women had to take part-time jobs or piece-work at home in order to supplement their family income, while others had to rely on relatives – usually their own parent or parents-in-law – for regular financial support. For many of these women, lone motherhood was the only option available in order to escape from the objective poverty they experienced within their marriages. Indeed, most of these lone mothers found that although their total family income had declined after leaving their husbands, nevertheless their financial situation in reality improved because they were then able to gain control of all the family income.

Related to the issue of the failure of the husband/partner to live up to the male-breadwinner role, many of the lone mothers also claimed that their husband/partner was unable to assume expected male behaviour; that is to provide 'husbandly' leadership within the marriage. The husband's excessive (financial and emotional) dependence on their wife was an example of such behavioural problems. Many felt that an excessively dependent husband was a serious problem because it implied, first, financial hardship for the family (as such a husband was often unable to provide adequate economic support for the family), secondly, an additional emotional burden for the wife. As some of the lone mothers claimed, it was like 'having another child at home'.

The above points to a rather different interpretation of lone motherhood to that which public and political discourses would suggest. In contrast to the general view of lone mothers and lone motherhood as 'problems', these women regarded lone motherhood rather as a *solution* to economic and emotional problems associated with the structure of marriage, strongly premised as it was on the male-breadwinner model. The experiences of these women illustrate, first, that rather than being passive victims, most of them chose lone motherhood because, given their economic and emotional circumstances, it was preferable to marriage. Secondly, their experiences also suggest that these women made this choice not because they supported the idea of lone motherhood, but rather because they subscribed to the ideal of the traditional two-parent family male-breadwinner model. For these women, the traditional two-parent family, male-breadwinner model implied a household economic arrangement whereby women's housewife role within the home should be complemented by the husband's obligation to look after the family's economic welfare. Hence, when it became evident that their husband was not able to fulfil his expected obligations, economic imperatives dictated that they should leave the marriage. For these women, lone motherhood was therefore a logical solution to the *failure* of men to uphold the expected male-breadwinner role. This suggested that it is worthwhile considering the issue of lone motherhood in Japan in terms of the contradictions in the structure of the marriage model premised on the notions of gender role asymmetry and male breadwinning. The study's findings reveal that in direct contrast to government attempts to reassert the 'traditional' family, too great an adherence to the male-breadwinner model may promote rather than help reduce lone motherhood.

Lone mothers' experiences of work and housing

All of the lone mothers interviewed in this study were in employment at the time of the interview. Almost all of them, however, also claimed that they experienced considerable difficulties at work. The greatest difficulty cited was in finding paid work in the first instance. Many employers would not hire a lone mother or, if they were already working before becoming lone mothers, they were eventually forced to leave because of employer harassment or because of a bad 'human relationship'. The unmarried lone mothers were particularly badly treated as their pregnancy was strongly criticized by both their employers and their trade unions. Both the unmarried lone mothers interviewed were forced to quit: one because both her employer and her union claimed they could not support an unmarried lone mother, and the other because her co-workers and the management made it personally too uncomfortable for her to remain in her job.

Other lone mothers, including the widows, also found it very difficult to find jobs because of the time conflict with child-care arrangements. Most public day care is only open from 9am to 5pm, and therefore mothers are expected to arrange their paid work hours to fit day-care hours. Both male and female full-time workers in Japan are expected regularly to work overtime beyond normal working hours. This implies that, in most cases, working mothers will not be able work full time or to work too far away from their home and/or day-care centre. The constraints posed by day-care arrangements meant that most lone mothers had to settle for available employment in the local area. Most lone mothers in the study reported that they had to change jobs several times before they settled in their current one, and also often had to take less well paid or inappropriate jobs just so that they could be near their homes or day-care centre.

The older lone mothers (i.e. those who became lone mothers in the 1970s and the early 1980s) were more likely to have low-status public sector jobs, for example as cooks, secretaries and traffic attendants in state schools. Many claimed that they were actually 'assigned' to these jobs by the welfare office or by the *Boshiryo* when they first became lone mothers, as a part of the government's job link programme. The younger lone mothers were more likely to be found working in the private sector as office workers, cooks in restaurants, and factory workers. While these low-status and low-paid jobs are still available within the private sector, very few of the lone mothers regarded them as permanent employment. Most claimed that they were in search of more secure and better paying employment. Except for the few lone mothers who had professional skills like nursing, most of them were paid between Y2.0 to Y3.0 million per year, barely above the 1990 poverty level income for a lone-mother family with two children of Y1.95 million.

In terms of housing, about one-third of lone mothers interviewed lived in public housing (most in Nerima-ku), while the rest mainly lived in privately rented flats. One widowed and two divorced lone mothers owned their own home. For most of the lone mothers in private rented flats, finding housing was very difficult. Aside from the high cost, which in many cases came to about 60 per cent of their total income, many also claimed that they were discriminated against by landlords and neighbours because of their lone-mother status. A few of the women reported that they had to move out of their home after they became lone mothers because of landlord harassment.

Lone mothers' experiences of public attitudes and concern for their children

Most of the lone mothers, including widows, found that their status was a liability for them at work and in finding housing, and also in developing social relationships. Not only did many of them claim that they felt discriminated against and stigmatized by their neighbours and friends (as some of them called it, '*shiroi me de mirareru*' – to be looked at with disdain), several also said that they were rejected and/or disowned by their own families. For example, most of the divorced lone mothers had temporarily to sever their relationships with their family while they worked out their problems. One divorced lone mother, for instance, reported that when she left her husband, her family did not want her around and treated her 'as if [I] were a big sour or mentally ill'. The two unmarried lone mothers also reported that they were disowned by their family when they chose to keep their children. One of them had a daughter who was 9 years old at the time of the interview and who had still not met her grandparents.

On the other hand, other lone mothers, particularly the younger divorced women from middle-class families, were given relatively good support from their families. For example, many of the middle-class divorced/separated lone mothers in their 30s reported that their decision to leave their husband was supported by their own families, and in some cases also by the family of their ex-husband. In addition, many of them continued to receive material and financial support from their family after the divorce/separation. Family support is, in most cases, dependent on the initial cause of the marital break-up. In the case of the husband's failure to uphold his male-breadwinner role, there was much family sympathy and support for the lone mothers (and often from both sides of the family). Again, this suggests that, contrary to public and policy thinking, too much emphasis on the male-breadwinner model can actually legitimate the formation of lone-mother families.

Neighbourhood context

The above findings illustrate that there is a significant neighbourhood effect on lone mothers in terms of access to day care, housing, and paid work. The study shows that Nerima-ku district, with its relatively large supply of public housing flats, progressive local government and the availability of work, is clearly a 'preferred' neighbourhood for lone mothers in Tokyo. The availability of public housing in this neighbourhood is largely a result of the fact that it is located in a newly developed residential area of the city. Although public housing allocation in Tokyo has changed to a lottery basis in recent years (aside from a set income condition), lone mothers are still given special consideration in this district. For many of the lone mothers, public housing meant not only cheaper rent but also a better living environment for them and their children. For example, the cost of a flat in public housing was in most cases about a third that of regular flats in the private market. Moreover, there are no extra charges associated with moving into public housing flats, as is the case for most private housing.[6] Given that lone mothers can pay up to 60 per cent of their total income in rent in the private market, public housing made a considerable difference to their total household income.

Public housing also offered a better living environment for many of the lone-mother families because it gave them a secure residency, and also a community in which they could meet other families in similar situation. Many of the lone mothers who lived in public housing, for example, claimed that they felt that not only were they accepted by their neighbours but also that they were able to develop social relationships with other families – particularly with other lone-mother families – who lived in the area. Moreover, many of the lone mothers also expressed some positive effects for their children of living in the public housing complex. Several lone mothers, for example, reported that having other lone-mother families in the area meant that their children did not have to feel excluded or suffer from discrimination and bullying at school.

It is important to stress that the attitudes of neighbours, and of school and day-care teachers, are extremely important considerations for lone mothers. For example, many of those interviewed claimed that having support from their children's teachers or day-care workers made a real difference to the well-being of their families. In Japan education is one of the most crucial factors determining individual success in adulthood, and there is considerable pressure on mothers to ensure that their children do well in school. Doing well in school, however, implies not only excelling academically but also being well-liked and accepted by school authorities and other students. Lone mothers are therefore particularly sensitive to the fact that their marital status might disadvantage their children both socially and academically. Indeed, almost all of the lone mothers interviewed reported that their greatest concern was that their children might suffer discrimination at school. These concerns are not unjustified, as several lone mothers complained that their children were not given the same kind of attention from their teachers as other children, or that they had been punished by their teachers for things they did not do. A few lone mothers, who were themselves children of lone-mother families, also reported that since they had personally experienced discrimination at school and in employment, they feared that their children would also face a similar problem when they grew up. In Japan it is very common for employers to review the family background of potential employees. The Japanese family registry (*koseki*) is an official and public document which contains, among other personal information, the family structure, birth legitimacy and any criminal record of each individual in a family. Finally, several lone mothers also claimed that they had to spend more money than most two-parent families on clothes and material things for their children because they did not want people to look down on them.

These findings suggest that the social support in neighbourhoods – housing, neighbours and schools – makes a significant difference to the economic independence and well-being of lone-mother families. Not only are direct and indirect economic support, in the form of public housing, day care and job training, important in helping lone mothers become, and remain, economically 'independent', but these provisions also create a social environment which provides important social network support for lone-mother families.

7. Conclusion

This chapter has looked into lone motherhood in Japan. The first half examined the situation of lone mothers nationally and analysed the discourses around lone motherhood since the beginning of the 1980s, while the second half examined the various neighbourhood constraints and opportunities for lone mothers based on an original study of lone mothers living in Tokyo. The discourse analysis suggests a sustained public and political criticism of lone motherhood in Japan over the last decade and a half. These criticisms are primarily rooted in the assumption that lone-mother families are a source of social and welfare problems, which are in turn reinforced by the development of the idea of the Japanese-style welfare society premised on family mutual support and individual economic independence. The pervasive public and policy position towards lone-mother families in Japan is thus to discourage the formation of such families by asserting the traditional two-parent family based on the male-breadwinner model.

The interview survey of lone mothers, on the other hand, shows that despite these negative discourses, there exist certain imperatives which lead women to choose lone motherhood over marriage. For example, a strong expectation of the male-breadwinner model of marriage on the part of women can actually facilitate the formation of lone-mother families when their husbands fail to uphold their breadwinner role. This suggests that the Japanese social structure, premised on gender asymmetry and the male-breadwinner model, can be both a source of constraint for women and the cause of lone motherhood. Finally, once women do opt out of marriage and choose lone motherhood, their economic and social situation can be very hard. Nevertheless many find it a positive experience. For lone mothers, the nature of the local community and labour market is crucially important. The case study of lone mothers in Nerima-ku shows that lone mothers' work and living arrangements are strongly affected by the availability and nature of employment, housing, child care, and their acceptance by neighbours in the local area. The neighbourhood effect, as this study has illustrated, may serve both as a constraint and, at the same time, a source of support and opportunity.

Notes

1 The 1988 national survey, published in 1992, is the most recent official government survey of lone-mother families in Japan. The survey is conducted by the Ministry of Health and Welfare every five years. The survey began in 1953, and examines the demographic, social and economic circumstances of lone-mother families in the country. Information concerning lone-mother families was included in the survey for the first time in 1983.
2 'Part-time' work in Japan is defined as less than 35 hours per week.
3 Since the collapse of the bubble economy in Japan after 1990, the core sector has been gradually restructuring its employment system to reflect a more free market-oriented approach. This includes the termination of the life-time employment system, termination of automatic pay rise according to seniority, and introduction of a wage system based on meritocracy for male workers.

4   In 1992 there were 325 *Boshiryo* across the country with an admission capacity of 6,412 lone-mother families, or 0.75% of all lone-mother families (Japan, 1993).
5   In firms with 30 or more employees, women's average income was only about 50 per cent that of male employees (Japan, Ministry of Labour, 1990).
6   In Japan, it is not uncommon for the owner of a privately rented flat to demand up to 6 months' worth of rent up front when a new tenant signs the rent contract. This amount is normally divided into: 1 month in equivalent for the real estate as the service charge; 2 to 3 months worth in non-refundable key money; and 2 months worth in deposit.

References

ASAHI SHINBUN (1982) *'Hirogaru "chichi to ko" no fukei: fushikatei 1472 setai'* 20 June (Akitaban).
ASAHI SHINBUN (1983a) *'Komatte imasu, jaji to kyoiku: fushi katei – ken ga jittai chosa'* 8 April 1992 (Naganoban).
ASAHI SHINBUN (1983b) *'Zenkoku ni 12-man setai: fushi katei – seibetsu ga 6 wari'* 21 June 1983.
ASAHI SHINBUN (1983c) *'Genzai no Katachi: nihongata fukushi – sanin senkyo ni atatte'* 8 June 1983.
ASAHI SHINBUN (1985a) *'Ego marudashi: Musekinin na oya'* 27 December 1995 (Kanagawaban).
ASAHI SHINBUN (1985b) *'Nihon no dokokade mainichi 6 nin mo'* 31 March 1985.
BABA, KEINOSUKE (Ed.) (1979) *Shakai Fukushi no Nihongata Tenkai*, Tokyo: Shakai Fukushi Hojin.
BETANIA HOMU (1986) *Shogaikoku ni Okeru Hirorioya Katei no Doko to Fukushi*, Tokyo: Fukushi Hojin.
BRINTON, M. C. (1993) *Women and the Economic Miracle: Gender and Work in Postwar Japan*, Berkeley: University of California Press.
CORNELL, L. L. (1989) 'Gender differences in remarriage after divorce in Japan and the United States', *Journal of Marriage and the Family*, **51** 2, pp. 457–63.
CORNELL, L. L. (1990) 'Peasant women and divorce in preindustrial Japan', *Signs*, **15**, 4, pp. 710–32.
COOK, A. H. and HAYASHI, H. (1980) *Working Women in Japan: Discrimination, Resistance, and Reform*, New York: Cornell University Press.
GOODE, W. (1963) *World Revolution and Family Pattern*, New York: Collier Mac-Millan.
HATANAKA, M. (1992) *'Boshi Katei no Shakai Hosho'*, *Kikan – Shakai Hoshu Kenkyu*, **28**, 3, pp. 270–8.
HAYASHI, C. (1978) *'Sengo ni Miru Boshiryo no Ayumi to Kadai: Showa 20-nen kara 40-nen made'*, *Boshi Kenkyo*, **1**, pp. 126–38.
HAYASHI, C. (1980) *'Sengo ni Miru Boshiryo no Ayumito Kadai'* in Yoshida Kyuichi (Ed.) *Boshikatei* (special edition of *Gendai no Esupuri*) No. 142, pp. 201–23.
HAYASHI, C. (1990) *'Fuetsuzukeru Boshisetai no Jittai'* in *Sekai o Hiraku Jidokenri Hosho*, Tokyo: Metropolitan.
HAYASHI, C. (1992) *'Hinkon no Joseika to Boshiryo'* (unpublished paper).
HENDRY, J. (1987) 'Marriage and the Family in Modernising Japan' (Sounderdruck aus

SAECULUM XXXVIII, Heft 1; Verlag Karl Alber Freiburg/Munchen) Germany, conference paper.

HIWATARI, N. (1993) 'Sustaining the welfare state and international competitiveness in Japan: the welfare reforms of the 1980s and the political economy', (paper presented at the 1993 Annual Meeting of the American Political Science Association, Washington DC).

HOKKAIDO (1993) '*Fushikatei kaigonin seido: riyou wa hotondo zero*' 19 June 1983.

IMAMURA, A. E. (1987) *Urban Japanese Housewives*, Honolulu: University of Hawaii Press.

INOUE, T. and EHARA, Y. (1992) *Josei no Deta Bukku* (Women's Data Book), Tokyo: Yukikaku.

INSTITUTE OF SOCIAL SCIENCE, UNIVERSITY OF TOKYO (1985) (Ed.) *Fukushi Kokka, 6: Nihon no Shakai to Fukushi*, Tokyo: University of Tokyo Press.

ISHIDA, Y. (1994) '*Boshisetai no Kakei to Shotokuhoshyo*', *Kokumin Seikatsu Kyenkyu*, **34** (2), pp. 1–14.

JCN-ICSW (1990) *Social Welfare Services in Japan*, Tokyo: JNC-ICSW.

JAPAN (1980) *Scenarios, 1990*, report of General Policy Committee of Social Policy Council, Social Policy Bureau, Economic Planning Agency, Ministry of Finance, Japan.

JAPAN (1983) *Japan in the Year 2,000: Preparing Japan for an Age of Internationalisation, the Ageing Society and Maturity*, report of Long-term Outlook Committee, Economic Council, Economic Planning Agency; printed by the Japan Times.

JAPAN (1984) *Annual Report on National Life, 1983*, Tokyo: Ministry of Finance.

JAPAN (1985) *Annual Report on National Life, 1984*, Tokyo: Ministry of Finance.

JAPAN (1986) *Annual Report on National Life, 1985*, Tokyo: Ministry of Finance.

JAPAN (1987) *Historical Statistics of Japan* (Volume 5), Tokyo: Statistics Bureau.

JAPAN (1992a) *Vital Statistics*, Tokyo: Ministry of Health and Welfare.

JAPAN (1992b) *S-68 Nendo Zenkoku Boshisetai Jittai Chosa*, Tokyo: Ministry of Health and Welfare.

JAPAN (1992c) *The 1988 National Survey of Lone Mother Families*, Tokyo: Ministry of Health and Welfare.

JAPAN (1993) *Health and Welfare Statistics in Japan*, Tokyo: Ministry of Health and Welfare.

JAPAN, MINISTRY OF FINANCE (1994) *Kokumin Seikatsu Hakusho* Tokyo: Okurasho.

JAPAN, MINISTRY OF HEALTH AND WELFARE (1988) *Showa 63 nendo Jinko Dotai Tokei*, Tokyo: Ministry of Health and Welfare.

JAPAN, MINISTRY OF HEALTH AND WELFARE (1990) *Heisei 2 nendo Jinko Kotai Tokei*, Tokyo: Ministry of Health and Welfare.

JAPAN, MINISTRY OF HEALTH AND WELFARE (1991) *Heisei 3 nendo Jinko Kotai Tokei*, Tokyo: Ministry of Health and Welfare.

JAPAN, MINISTRY OF LABOUR (1990) *Fujin Rodo no Jitsujo*, Tokyo: Ministry of Labour.

JAPAN, PRIME MINISTER'S OFFICE (1990) *Kokumin Seikatsu ni Kansuru Yorochosa*, Tokyo: Prime Minister's Office.

JAPAN, THE SUPREME COURT (1987) *Showa 61 nendo Shiho Tokei Nenpo* (The 1986 Annual Judicial Statistics), Tokyo: The Supreme Court.

JAPAN, THE SUPREME COURT (1991) *Heisei 2 nendo Shiho Tokei Nenpo* (The 1990 Annual Judicial Statistics), Tokyo: The Supreme Court.

KAHOKU SHINPO (1983) *'Seikatsu hogo setai 5-nen de 3-wari zo: boshikatei wa nibai ni'* 28 December 1983.

KOBE (1994) *'Shussanritsu saitei no 1.46nin: heisei 5-nen jinkodokotokei, rikon saiko no 19-man gumi'*, 24 June 1994.

KUMAGAI F. (1983) 'Changing Divorce in Japan', *Journal of Family*, (Spring), pp. 85–107.

KUMAMOTO NICHINICH (1982) *'Fushikatei 5-nen mae yori 2.6 baizou'*, 18 March 1982.

KUMAZAWA, M. (1995) 'Nihonteki Keiei to Joseirodo', in Kisokeizaikagaku Kenkyujo (Ed.) *Nihongata Kigyoshakai to Josei*, pp. 43–83, Tokyo: Aoki Shoten.

LEBRA, J., PAULSON, J. and POWERS, E. (Eds) (1976) *Women in Changing Japan*, Boulder: Westview Press.

LEBRA, T. S. (1978) 'Japanese women and marital strain', *Ethos*, **6**, 1, pp. 22–41.

LEBRA, T. S. (1984) *Japanese Women: Constraint and Fulfillment*, Honolulu: University of Hawaii Press.

MAINICHI SHINBUN (1985) *'Minkon no hah fue, sono ko wa . . . – Nyujiin no 4 nin ni hitori'*, 6 January 1985.

MOROSAWA, Y. (1985) *'Ningen toshiteno "Mikon no Haha"'*, in Suzuki Naoko (Ed.) *Shiryo: Sengo Bosei no Ikikata*, pp. 169–79, Tokyo: Domesu.

NAKAGAWA, S. (1995) *'Nihongata Kigyoshakai ni okeru Josei no Rodo to Kazoku'*, in Kisokeizaikagaku Kenkyujo (Ed.) *Hihongata Kigyoshakai to Josei*, pp. 13–41, Tokyo: Aoki Shoten.

NIHON KEIZAI (1994) *'Shasetsu: Ikujitaisaku niwa Shakai Zentai ga Sekinin o Motte'*, 25 June.

NIKKEI BUSINESS (1992) *'Tsutometsuzukeru Onna: Tsukaenu Kigyo niwa Myonichi ga Nai'*, July 6th Edn, pp. 10–23.

NISHIDA, Y. (1990) ' "Reassessment of welfare services" and the trend of welfare policy for the disabled', *Annals of the Institute of Social Science*, **3**, pp. 115–54.

NISHINIHON (1984) *'Aah, Fushi Katei'*, 7 February (evening edition).

OPCS (1991) *Marriage and Divorce Statistics*, London: OPCS.

OSAWA, M. (1993) *Kigyochushin Shakai o Koete: Gendai Nihon o Gender de Yomu*, Tokyo: Jijitsushinsha.

PAULSON, J. (1976) 'Evolution of the feminine ideal' in Lebra, J., Paulson, J. and Powers, E. (Eds) *Women in Changing Japan*, pp. 1–24, Stanford, CA: Stanford University Press.

PENG, ITO (1995) 'Boshi Katei: A Theoretical and Case Analysis of Japanese Lone Mothers and their Relationship to the State, the Labour Market, and the Family, with Reference to Britain and Canada', PhD thesis, London School of Economics.

SALAMON, S. (1974) 'In the Intimate Arena: Japanese Women and their Families', PhD thesis, University of Illinois, Champaign.

SANKEI (1984a) *'Jichitai: fushikatei ewa teusuna enjo'*, 21 February 1984.

SANKEI (1984b) *'Seso han'ei, ijo na "manpai": kateihokai ya rikon, mikon no haha fue'*, 4 March 1984.

SANKEI (1984c) ' *"Ichitai: Fushi Katei hewa Teatsu na Enjo"'*, 21 February.

SANKEI (1994) *'Kosodate ni Shakaitekina Shien o'*, 25 June.

SANKEI (1985) *'Jido fuyo teate kaisei: mikon no hahajogai wa hitsuyo'*, 10 March 1985.

SASAKI, M. (1989) 'Stress and Coping Among Divorced Single Women Living in Homes for Single Mothers and Children in Japan: A Decriptive Study', DSW Dissertation for the School of Social Work, Columbia University.

SHAKAIFUKUSHI KENKYUJO (Ed.) (1983) *Boshifukushi – Fushifukushi no Kenkyu*, Tokyo: Shakaifukushi Hojin Koseikai.

SHINKAWA, T. (1990) *The Political Economic of Social Welfare in Japan*, PhD thesis, University of Toronto, Department of Political Science.

SHINNO-MAINICHI (1984) '*Fushi Katei nimo Atatakai Enjo o*', 15 February.

SHINOZUKA, E. (1992) '*Boshisetai no Hinkon o Meguru Mondai*', *Nihon Keizai Kenkyu*, **22**, pp. 77–118.

SHOYA, R. (1990) '*Boshisetai no Hinkon*', in Joseish Sogo Kenkyukai (Ed.) *Nihon Josei Seikatsushi*, pp. 133–66, Tokyo: University of Tokyo Press.

SMITH, R. J. (1983) 'Making village women into "good wives and wise mothers" in prewar Japan', *Journal of Family History*, **18**, 1, pp. 70–84.

SMITH, R. J. and WISWELL, E. L. (1983) *The Women of Suye Mura*, Chicago: University of Chicago Press.

SOEDA, Y. (1982) '*Boshifukushi Shikin Kashitsuke Seido no Shomondai: Hajimeni*', *Boshi Kenkyu*, **5**, pp. 1–4.

SOEDA, Y. (1990) 'The development of the public assistance system in Japan, 1966–83', *Annuals of the Institute of Social Science*, **32**, pp. 31–66.

TABATA, H. (1990) 'The Japanese welfare state: its structure and transformation', *Annals of the Institute of Social Science*, **32**, pp. 1–30.

TAIRA, K. (1967) 'Public assistance in Japan: development and trends', *Journal of Asian Studies*, **27**, pp. 95–109.

TAMURA, K. and TAMURA, M. (1988) *Rikon no Ningengaku*, Tokyo: Shisutemu Faibu.

TARUKAWA, N. (1978) '*Boshifukushiseisaku no Kosei to Doko*', *Boshi Kenkyu*, **1**, pp. 1–17.

TARUKAWA, N. (1980) '*Boshi Fukushi Seisaku no Kosei to Doko*', in Yoshida Kyuichi (Ed.) *Boshi Katei*, **22**, pp. 143–65.

TARUKAWA, N. (1982) '*Boshifukushi Shikin Kashitsuke no Rekishi*', *Boshi Kenkyu*, **5**, pp. 5–27.

TOKYO (1985) *Tokyo-to ni ikeru Tanshinkazoku no Jokyo to Tanshinkazoku Taisaku no Genjo*, Tokyo: Tokyo Metropolitan Government.

TOKYO (1987) *Tokyo-to Hihogosetai Seikatsu Jittai Chosa: Kekka Hokokushu (Showa 61-nendo)*, Tokyo: Tokyo Metropolitan Government.

TOKYO (1992) *Heisei 3 Nen Hitorioya Katei no Shiori*, Tokyo: Tokyo Metropolitan Government.

TOKYO (1994) *Tokyo Josei Hakusho*, Tokyo: Metropolitan Government of Tokyo.

TOKYO SHINBUN (1982) '*Fushikatei ni Nakano-ku ga enjo no te o*', 7 February 1982.

VOGEL, S. H. (1978) 'Professional housewife: the career of urban middle class Japanese women', *Japan Interpreter*, **12**, pp. 16–43.

YOMIURI SHINBUN (1983) '*Ganbaru fushikatei*', 17 June 1983.

YOMIURI SHINBUN (1984) '*Koredemo "teate" kirunoka*', 5 May 1984.

YOMIURI SHINBUN (1994) '*Sasetsu: Akachan no Heru Kuni to Fueru Kuni*', 25 June 1994.

YOSHIDA, K. (1980) *Boshi Katei: sono seikatsu to fukushi* (Special Edition, Gendai no Espuri, Vol. 142, May).

YUZAWA, N. (1991) ' "*Yitakasa*" *Jidai no Boshisetai no Genkyo*', *Koteki Fujo Kenkyu*, **142**, pp. 13–24.

ZENKOKU SHAKAI FUKUSHI KYOGIKAI (1989) *Fukushi Kaikaku*, Tokyo: Shakai Fukushi Hojin.

ZENKOKU SHAKAI FUKUSHI KYOGIKAI – BOSHIRYO KYOGIKAI (1979) '*Arubeki Boshiryo no Sugata*', *Boshi Kenkyu*, **2**, pp. 171–91.
ZENKOKU SHAKAI FUKUSHI KYOGIKAI – BOSHIRYO KYOGIKAI (1992) *Dai 35-Kai Zenkoku Boshiryo Kenkyu Taikai*, Tokyo: Shakai Fukushi Hojin.

Chapter 6

Single Mothers in Australia: Supporting Mothers to Seek Work

Marilyn McHugh and Jane Millar

1. Introduction

The labour-market participation rate for single mothers in Australia – typically referred to as sole mothers[1] in Australia and throughout this chapter – currently stands at just over 50 per cent; a figure that has not much changed since the late 1980s. Compared with many other countries – as various chapters in this book show – this is not a particularly high level of economic activity. It is also lower than the participation rate for Australian married mothers, currently at just under 60 per cent. On the basis of these figures Australia could be characterized as a country where sole mothers are as likely to be 'mothers' as they are to be 'workers'. The nature of the income support available to, and received by almost all, sole mothers seems to reflect this. The 'sole parent's pension', first introduced in the early 1970s, provides a weekly benefit payable as long as there are children under the age of 16. There is no 'work test' attached to the benefit and the support it offers is therefore conditional on the mothering, rather than the employment, role. The benefit levels received, while not generous (for a sole mother with one child equivalent to about 35 per cent of average male earnings: ABS, 1994b), do allow women to be full-time mothers.

However, this benefit is only part of the support offered to sole mothers in Australia. In the late 1980s the introduction of new policies designed to give sole mothers access to employment training and to financial support from ex-partners reflected a changing view both of the role of sole mothers and of the obligations of policy towards them. Instead of replacing male earnings, as the sole parent's benefit was largely intended to do, recent policy has been geared towards encouraging sole mothers to take paid work and to enforcing the financial obligations of fathers. Australia can be characterized as a country in transition where the answer to the mother/worker issue is apparently changing, with a shift in focus from supporting sole mothers at home to seeking to offer more support for employment. This chapter analyses changing patterns of employment for sole mothers in Australia and the changing material, policy and social context of these. The focus is on recent change and on policy development and changing attitudes over the past 15 to 20 years in particular. This has been a time of rapid change, in both family structure and employment patterns. In addition, as in many other countries especially in the English-speaking world, the mid-1980s was a period when social security and income maintenance systems were under government review, not least as a result of concerns about projected future costs. The Australian Social Security Review, established by the Labour Government in 1986, focused in particular on the implications for state benefit provisions of changing employment and family patterns (Cass, 1986). The Review is thus central to analysing recent policy changes, including provisions for sole parents, and is discussed further below. First, however, we describe the growth in sole motherhood and the changing patterns of women's employment trends.

2. Sole Mothers in Australia

Numbers and characteristics

As Table 6.1 shows, the proportion of families headed by a sole parent has roughly doubled over the past 20 years, from 9 per cent in 1975 to 18 per cent in 1994. As is usually the case, the vast majority of these sole parents are women. There is little information available on the ethnic background of sole parents, but a recent survey of Aboriginal and Torres Strait Islanders (ABS, 1994) found that about 29 per cent of those families were headed by a sole parent – much higher than the rate for families in general. However, patterns of family and kinship structures in Aboriginal communities are not generally centred around the nuclear family (Collard et al., 1994) and thus the concept of a 'sole parent', which is defined in relation to a 'couple', is unlikely to carry the same meaning as for non-indigenous Australians. Based on data from the mid-1980s, Cass, Wilkinson and Webb (1990) found that the incidence of sole motherhood tended to be higher among English-speaking Australian-born women than among non-English-speaking women born overseas. They estimated that only about 10 per cent of all sole mothers fell into the latter group.

Year	All sole parents	Sole mothers (%)	All families with children (%)
1974	183,000	86	9
1985	316,000	89	14
1994	424,000	88	18

Source Millar and Whiteford (1993) Table 1 and ABS (1994), Tables 24 and 25.
Table 6.1 Sole-parent families: Australia, 1974, 1985 and 1994

The main routes into sole motherhood are through marital breakdown, widowhood, breakdown of cohabitation, and breakdown of non-cohabiting sexual relationships. Marital breakdown is the most common way to become a sole mother, with the divorce rate at about 12 per 1,000 marriages (ABS, 1995b), and with about two-thirds of all sole mothers being divorced or separated women. This figure remained fairly constant throughout the 1980s, although over the same period the proportion of never-married mothers increased (from about 19 per cent to about 25 per cent) while the proportion of widows fell (from about 14 per cent to about 8 per cent). Births outside marriage increased from 9 per 1,000 in 1971 to 23 per 1,000 in 1991 (ABS, 1994a). Never-married mothers now make up about a quarter of the total. The available statistics do not indicate the extent to which these never-married women are ex-cohabitants or not. In general, however, they are not very young women. Teenage sole motherhood remains relatively uncommon with only about 3 per cent of sole parent pensioners being teenagers (Walshe, 1994).[2] In general sole mothers are slightly older than married mothers, and the average age of sole parent pensioners[3] has increased from 28 in 1975 to 33 in 1994 (ABS, 1995b).

Table 6.2 shows the marital status of sole-parent pensioners from 1980 to 1994. This provides a fairly reasonable estimate of the changing marital status of all sole parents, since the majority (over three-quarters) do receive some pension income. This shows that the proportion who are unmarried has remained fairly constant at 17 to 18 per cent of the total. Widows have fallen from 14 per cent of pension recipients in 1980 to just over 2 per cent in 1995. Formerly married women make up the vast majority of the total throughout.

As Table 6.3 shows, sole mothers tend to have smaller families and older children than married mothers. The one-child family is especially common among sole mothers: half have just one child compared with a third of married mothers. On the other hand, however, sole mothers are also more likely to have larger families: 16 per cent have three or more children compared with

Year	Unmarried (%)	Ex-married (%)	Widowed (%)	Total
1980	18	68	14	100
1982	19	71	10	100
1984	19	72	9	100
1986	19	74	7	100
1988	20	75	5	100
1990	20	76	4	100
1992	18	79	3	100
1994	18	79	3	100
1995	18	80	2	100

Sources 1980–93 Department of Social Security (DSS) Annual Reports (various); 1994 and 1995: DSS, Management Information Section, Canberra

Table 6.2   Marital status of female sole-parent pensioners: Australia, 1982–95 (percentages)

	Sole mothers (%)	Married mothers (%)
Number of children		
One	50	34
Two	34	59
Three plus	16	7
Total	100	100
Age of youngest child		
0–4	38	50
5–9	31	27
10–14	31	23
Total	100	100

Source Number: Bradshaw et al. (1996), Table 2.10. Youngest: ABS (1994a) Tables 13 and 25
Table 6.3 Sole and married mothers: number of children and age of youngest child: Australia, 1994

only 7 per cent of married mothers. About 38 per cent of sole mothers have a youngest child of under four (under school age) compared with 50 per cent of married mothers, and sole mothers are correspondingly more likely to have teenage children (31 per cent compared with 23 per cent). These characteristics reflect the fact that the group defined as 'sole mothers' includes women whose previous experiences of partnership, marriage and motherhood are likely to have been very different. Nevertheless two main groups predominate and their family and individual characteristics are important in understanding how they are likely to be placed in relation to the labour market. The first, and largest group, are the older, divorced or separated women with two or three children of school age, including adolescent children. For these women, marriage and motherhood have been a central part of their adult lives[4] and have already had a significant impact on their employment patterns. The second largest group are the younger, never-married, women who usually have just one child, but that child is often of pre-school age. In addition to acting as sole parents, these women are also experiencing the impact that the birth of a first child has upon women's employment, regardless of her marital status.

Mothers and employment

As in most of the industrialized economies, Australia has seen a rapid increase in the numbers of women, particularly married women with children, joining the labour force. In 1966 about 31 per cent of married women were economically active. By 1992 this had doubled to 61 per cent (Cass, 1994a). However, it was in the 1980s in particular, under a Labour government which placed a high policy priority on job creation, that women increased both their participation rates and their share of total employment (Brennan, 1994; Cass, 1994a and b; McCreadie, 1994). Brennan summarizes the key trends:

> The expansion of job opportunities for both men and women between 1983 and 1989 was one of the major achievements of the Hawke government. More than 1.5 million new jobs were created in those years and 56 per cent of them were filled by women . . . women accounted for 46 per cent of full-time employment growth and 77 per cent of part-time employment growth . . . the total number of women employed rose by 600,000 or 27 per cent, and women's rate of workforce participation rose from 42 to 51 per cent . . . women were also recorded as having declining rates of unemployment . . . and the number of women classified as hidden unemployed or discouraged job seekers was also substantially reduced . . . women were undoubtedly the star performers in the Australia labour market . . .
>
> (1994: 169)

The growth in women's employment brought more women of all types into the labour market, but some of the largest increases were found among married mothers of pre-school-age children. In just four years between 1984 and 1988 the participation rate for these women rose by almost one-third (32 per cent) compared with one-fifth (19 per cent) for all women with children. Although these women have lower employment rates than women with older children, nevertheless almost half of these mothers are now active in the labour market and as many as 20 per cent of all married women in the labour market have children aged under four (Brennan, ibid.). Thus for married women with children, including those with young children, there was a relatively steady rise in participation rates throughout the 1980s. However, this has not continued through into the 1990s when, as Table 6.4 shows, there has been no continuing increase in participation rates.

Year	Sole mothers (%)	Married mothers (%)
1975	48	na
1980	43	46
1985	41	51
1990	52	61
1994	52	61
With youngest child aged 0–4		
1985	28	37
1990	37	48
1994	31	48

Source 1975 and 1980 from Social Security Review (1986), others from ABS (1994a and b)
Table 6.4 Sole and married mothers' labour-force participation rates: Australia, 1970s to 1990s

Table 6.4 also shows that the pattern of employment participation over time has been slightly different for sole mothers compared with married mothers. From the 1970s into the 1980s sole mothers' participation rates actually fell and only started to rise again in the mid-1980s. Rates then rose faster than for married mothers, but from 1989, when the participation rate reached 52 per cent, there has been no further increase. For sole mothers with young children (under five) participation rates have again fallen in the 1990s.

Table 6.5 compares the current employment rates of sole and married mothers in more detail. Sole mothers divide into two more or less equal groups, of 'workers' and 'mothers', with 52 per cent defined as economically active and 48 per cent outside the labour force. For married mothers the split is more 60/40 than 50/50, with 61 per cent of married mothers economically active and 39 per cent not. Among the economically active, there are also differences between sole and married mothers: similar proportions work full time (23 per cent and 24 per cent respectively) but many fewer sole mothers are in part-time employment (20 per cent compared with 32 per cent) and more are unemployed (9 per cent compared with 4 per cent).

Employment status	Sole mothers (%)	Married mothers (%)
Full-time*	23	24
Part-time	20	32
Unemployed	9	4
Not in labour force	48	39
Total	100	100

* full-time workers: employed persons who usually work 35 hours or more per week; part-time defined as under 35 hours per week.
Source ABS (1994b).
Table 6.5 Sole and married mothers, employment rates: Australia, 1994

Of course, it is not really the case that sole mothers can be divided into two equal-sized but distinct groups: the workers and the mothers. This may be the impression that the cross-sectional statistics give, but in reality, if we could track employment patterns over time, they would reveal movements into and out of employment. This movement is connected, at least in part, with family responsibilities. Life-time employment patterns for Australian women tend to follow the line of full-time employment up to birth of first child, usually followed by a break in employment while there are pre-school-age children, a return to part-time employment while caring for school children, and full-time employment when children reach their teenage years (Cass, 1994b).[5] There are no longitudinal data to track these movements in detail, but Table 6.6 shows this through a cross-sectional analysis of employment rates in relation to age of youngest child. The table reveals both similarities and differences between sole and married mothers. For both there is a clear rise in labour-market participation as children get older, and an increased likelihood of full-time, as opposed to part-time, work. Thus 72 per cent of married mothers with a youngest child aged 15 to 20 are economically active compared with 48 per cent of those with a youngest child under five. Those with children 15 plus are more than twice as likely to have full-time jobs as mothers of the under fives (38 per cent compared with 15 per cent). Similarly, for sole mothers, 75 per cent of the mothers with a youngest child of 15 to 20 are economically active compared with 25 per cent of those with a youngest child under five. The sole mothers with older children are four times as likely as those with young children to have full-time jobs (42 per cent compared with 10 per cent).

The broad pattern is thus similar for the two groups of women. However it is also clear that there are some important differences. Unemployment is more of a problem for sole mothers, especially those with older children.[6] Part-time work is much less common for sole than for married mothers, whatever the age of their children. This gap in the extent of part-time work accounts for much of the overall differences in employment rates: if sole mothers had the same rates of part-time working as married mothers then the two groups would have almost exactly the same participation patterns. It is this fact, then, that requires investigation – what is acting to keep sole mothers out of the part-time employment market? High effective marginal tax rates (EMTR – a measure of the proportion of income that is lost to income tax and means tests when a sole mother increases her income) are often suggested by social policy analysts as a

	Sole mothers (%)	Married mothers (%)
Youngest child 0–4		
Employed full-time	10	15
Employed part-time	15	29
Unemployed	6	5
Not in labour force	69	52
Youngest child 5–9		
Employed full-time	22	25
Employed part-time	23	37
Unemployed	10	5
Not in labour force	44	33
Youngest child 10–14		
Employed full-time	30	34
Employed part-time	24	34
Unemployed	9	4
Not in labour force	37	28
Youngest child 15–20		
Employed full-time	42	38
Employed part-time	21	32
Unemployed	12	2
Not in labour force	25	28

Source ABS (1994b).
Table 6.6 Sole and married mothers, employment rates by age of youngest child: Australia, 1994

disincentive to enter part-time work. In an overview of the distribution of EMTRs faced by actual or potential employed persons across the Australian population, it appears that sole mothers have the highest proportion of individuals with EMTRs of over 60 per cent (Polette, 1995).

Employment rates and income levels are closely correlated. The overall employment rate of just over 40 per cent for sole mothers means that about six in ten of these families have no income from employment but are reliant upon state benefits, usually entirely but sometimes in combination with other income, for example child support payments. By contrast, among married couples with children, only 24 per cent have no employment income and almost half (47 per cent) have two earners. Thus, not surprisingly, as Table 6.7 shows, family income tends to be much lower for sole-parent families compared with couples. About 41 per cent of sole parents have income in the lowest quintile compared with 17 per cent of couples with children. Only 6 per cent of sole-parent families get into the highest quintile compared with 22 per cent of couples. If there are no earners in the family, then the sole parents and the couples have rather similar income distributions. But where there are earners, the single sole-parent earners are worse off than the single two-parent earners and are very substantially worse off than the two-earner two-parent families.

The difference between one-earner sole parents and one-earner couples is due to the fact that the former are mainly women while the latter are mainly men. Women's full-time weekly average earnings are equivalent to about 83 per cent of men's (McCreadie, 1994). In two-earner couples, the addition of the woman's wage, even if she is in part-time work, makes a significant addition to the total family income. For part-time work, women's earnings add an additional 24 per cent to family income, for full-time work this amounts to an additional 40 per cent (Cass, 1994a). As Cass points out, women's earnings reduce both within-family income inequalities (by giving women direct access to a greater share of family income), and between-family wealth inequalities (by giving more families the opportunity to become home-owners). Neverthe-

Quintiles	All sole parents (%)	All couples (%)	No earner sole (%)	No earner couple (%)	One earner sole (%)	One earner couple (%)	Two earner couple (%)
lowest	41	17	57	54	16	8	4
second	26	19	23	27	33	27	7
third	17	21	11	10	25	30	20
fourth	10	21	6	5	16	19	32
highest	6	22	3	4	9	15	36
(-000s)	(596)	(3884)	(289)	(732)	(246)	(947)	(1844)
% of family type	(100%)	(100%)	(54%)	(21%)	(46%)	(27%)	(52%)

Source ABS (1994b), Table 12

Table 6.7 Income quintiles by family status: Australia, 1992

less, the growth of the two-earner family has meant an increasing gap between the incomes, and thus living standards, of sole-mother families and those of two-parent families.

Poverty rates among sole mothers are particularly high, with numerous studies demonstrating that sole-parent families are far more likely to be in poverty than other family types, with their poverty rate at least three times that of couples with children (ABS, 1992). For example, 44 per cent of sole parents were estimated to be in after-housing poverty in 1990 compared with 24 per cent of two-parent families. Sole parents are much more likely (44 per cent compared to 18 per cent) to be living in rented accommodation than couple families. In the states of Victoria and Queensland around one-quarter of emergency relief applicants were sole parents (Brotherhood of St Laurence, 1994; Thornwaite, Kingston and Walsh, 1995). On an international basis sole parents are considered a vulnerable population, and among a group of 13 OECD countries Australia, along with Canada and the USA, was found to be least effective in reducing poverty levels of sole-parent families by tax and transfer policies (Forster, 1993).

3. Discourses around sole motherhood in Australia

Sole motherhood does not seem to have attracted the negative construction in Australian policy that has been increasingly characteristic of the UK or the USA. This is apparent, for example, in the evolution and objectives of the recently introduced 'child support' legislation. As Millar and Whiteford (1993) point out, both Australia and the UK have sought to enforce much higher levels of child support from separated parents, by changing the way in which such payments are calculated and collected. However, the Australian legislation was developed in the context of debates about child poverty and the best way to support sole parents. The UK legislation, by contrast, emerged in a context of debate over 'irresponsible' parenthood and the need for government to enforce parental obligations which, it was suggested, would otherwise be ignored.

It may be that lack of overt hostility to sole mothers reflects both the lack of a racial dimension to the issue, as well as a more general lack of interest in the concept of the 'underclass' in Australia (Mann, 1994). The race issue, and fear of a growing underclass, have fuelled the strong negative constructions of sole – or more accurately, single – motherhood in the USA and to a lesser extent, in the UK, as discussed in the relevant chapters in this volume. There has been some debate over whether benefits have encouraged sole motherhood. For example, Swan and Bernstam (1987a and b), noting the rapid increase over time in take up of sole parent pension, argue that the availability of welfare payments for sole mothers has encouraged the growth in their numbers. This is despite the evidence that it is the breakdown of relationships and divorce which are the main routes into sole parenthood for Australian mothers, and the fact that their dependence on benefits impoverishes women and children and leads to poverty. In addition, a small but vocal number of post-divorce men's groups, with concerns over family law issues, lobby government sub-committees on issues of access, custody and the perceived inequities of the child support scheme. They are featured on talk-back radio shows and reported in the media. To date their success in effecting policy change has, however, been minimal.

Looking further back, in their account of unmarried motherhood in Australia between 1850 and 1975, Swain and Howe (1995) argue that unmarried mothers were not only economically deprived but were also stigmatized by society, at a time when 'the survival of single mothers and their children depended on their silence' (p. 5). They argue that the 1970s marked a time of change, reflected in a growing self-awareness and self-help movement among the women themselves, and in legal and policy reform. These included the abolition of the legal status of 'illegitimacy' in 1975; extensive and radical changes to family law, including no-fault divorce resolution; and the extension of the supporting parent's benefit to unmarried mothers (see below for further discussion of the latter). Compared with earlier times, the unmarried mothers of the 1960s and 1970s were older, more middle-class, better educated, and more likely to view themselves as people with rights and choices. They were both willing and able to begin to confront the practical difficulties of sole motherhood and to push for policy and legal change. The establishment of National Councils for the Single Mother and her Child in many states at this time reflected these changes, and these and other groups were central to policy change:

> The decade from 1965–75 had shown that women were able to influence family policy and to lobby the state to provide the income maintenance that they needed to achieve independence. Their right to have a family without a husband had been given public recognition.
>
> (Swaine and Howe, 1995: 206)

However this does not mean that there is general acceptance of a right to unconditional public support for sole mothers. Instead Walshe (1994) argues that there is a long-standing expectation that sole mothers are more 'deserving' of state support if they also make efforts to support themselves. She suggests that the Councils for the Single Mother and her Child won support for more positive policies for sole mothers in the 1960s and 1970s by stressing that 'the best interests and welfare of the ex-nuptial child . . . whether the single mother's pregnancy was deliberate or accidental . . . [depended on] whether single mothers were willing to support themselves through employment' (1994: 57). Attitudes hardened again during the economic recession of the 1980s but today the policy emphasis on encouraging employment is better able to 'mirror community attitudes that suggest that parents should be responsible for their children and be willing to help themselves . . . it seems that sole parent families are seen to deserve support most when they are willing to help themselves' (ibid. 65).

This is also part of changing views about the duties and responsibilities of mothers more generally. As described above, over the space of a relatively short period of time, mothers – married and sole – have entered the Australian labour market in significant numbers and there are now about 1.5 million employed mothers, out of a total workforce of 13 million. The impact of this has been somewhat contradictory. On the one hand, women's additional role as paid worker has not led to any significant re-distribution of domestic labour within the family, and men continue to leave the bulk of domestic work to their partners. Time-budget studies show that a husband whose wife has a full-time paid job does no more than a man whose spouse does no paid work; that the average time spent by husbands in unpaid work is less than half that of their partners; and that men have not increased their hours of domestic work as more women have entered paid work (ABS, 1988 and 1992; Bittman and Lovejoy, 1993; Rimmer and Rimmer, 1994). At work, many employers continue to resist making provisions for their workers as parents as, for example, the continued opposition by employers' associations to family and parental leave and maternity benefits shows (McCreadie, 1994). On these two fronts, therefore, practical support from partners and from employers to help women to combine their caring roles and their employment roles seems to have been less than forthcoming.

On the other hand, among women themselves, and in their capacity to influence public policy, there have been some significant advances. Cass argues that the impetus for the rise in female labour-market participation in the 1980s came very much from women themselves:

> job growth and child care services provided opportunities necessary for women to realize their aspirations with somewhat less struggle than their forebears. Public policies did not create these aspirations but they did create the climate in which women could redefine their identities and spheres of activity.
>
> (1994a: 116)

Survey evidence on women's attitudes shows that the majority strongly support the view that women should have the right to combine motherhood and employment. However, that is not to say that these roles are seen as equally important. Rather the order is very much 'mother and worker' and not 'worker and mother' since, for the majority, the needs of children for care are placed above access to employment. Thus there is support for mothers to stay at home with young children but to go to work as children grow older.

This can be seen more generally in attitudes to women's employment over the life cycle. A nationwide survey of over 2,000 respondents found that the majority of Australians (84 per cent) think that women should work full time after marrying and before there are children. When there is a child under school age many (65 per cent) feel that women should stay at home, though one-third (31 per cent) support part-time work. Even after the youngest child starts school, most (73 per cent) thought mothers should only work part time and less than a fifth (16 per cent) felt full-time work was appropriate. After children had left home around two-thirds see full-time work and one-third part-time work as the ideal for women (Evans, 1995). King and McHugh (1995) and King, Bradbury and McHugh (1995) report similar findings for two particular groups of women: the wives of men receiving disability pension and the wives of men receiving unemployment benefit.

Women themselves have played a central role in defining their needs and in influencing social policy in a way that makes Australia unusual compared with many other countries. The Australian 'femocrats' – women with feminist agendas operating within bureaucracy and government – were a particular force during the 1980s (Sawer, 1990; Watson, 1992; Dowse, 1983). Bettina Cass, influential herself as chair of the Social Security Review team, argues that, while assumptions about women's financial dependency on men have shaped Australian policy in the past, and continue to do so, nevertheless:

> assumptions of women's dependency are being challenged in several ways: (1) women's increased labour force participation, (2) assertion of their market rights, (3) growth of women's employment in the public sector, and (4) more feminists in decision-making roles in government women's bureaus. . . . As a result, some public policies, albeit uneven in their development and implementation, are promoting the idea that women should assume the responsibilities and earn the equal rewards of labour force participation.
>
> (1994a: 111)

Brennan (1994), in her analysis of the development of child-care policy in Australia, makes a convincing case that feminist activism in the bureaucracy and in national and local politics was the driving force behind the development of child-care policy during the 1970s and 1980s. Further she argues that the fact that women played such an important role in shaping policy in this area has led to a system of child care which, while not as comprehensive as that found in the Nordic countries for example, has expanded very rapidly and meets about two-thirds of the demand for work-related care (with a government commitment to meeting all such demand by 2001). Child care is now defined as a central element of the 'social wage', and the rights of both parents and children to have access to child care are well established.

It is clear that women as mothers *and* workers is now the dominant construction in policy. Much of the Australian debate around the International Year of the Family in 1994 centred on issues of how to develop policy further to integrate employment and caring roles for parents (Inglis and Rogan, 1994; Wolcott and Glezer, 1995). Farrar (1994) argues that much of current policy reflects a reconstruction of the relationship between the state and families.

Discussing policy measures such as the new Parenting Allowance (see below), the expansion of child-care provision, and moves to introduce family leave, he suggests that 'here, perhaps, we are seeing a redefinition of the maternal role, one which no longer rests on women's presumed role within the family as carers' (ibid. 22). He points out, however, that other policies – especially policies of 'community care' and cuts in support to young people – are actually increasing dependency on the family for certain groups. Cass (1994a) also points to the ambiguities of policy: in many areas moving away from a construction of women as dependent wives but still resisting a reconstruction of the meaning of 'independence' as it applies to men: 'Women cannot be economic, political and social citizens until men accept their full social obligations and responsibilities for care-giving work' (ibid. 121).

4. The Australian Welfare Regime

The Australian social security system is almost unique among the industrialized countries in never having adopted the social insurance approach, in which access to benefits is dependent on contributions made (Castles, 1985; Mitchell, 1991; Bryson, 1992, 1995). Almost all benefit in Australia are income-tested and asset-related. Australia is therefore something of an anomalous case in terms of the sort of criteria that are usually adopted for classification into 'welfare regimes', since these often depend upon weighting 'insurance' benefits above 'assistance' benefits. However, Castles and Mitchell (1990) and Mitchell (1991) argue that the Australian focus on income-related benefits and central wage controls means that the impact of policy is generally redistributive, and thus to view Australia as a welfare 'laggard' or as a 'liberal' welfare regime is misleading.

Cass (1994a) argues that the Australian system, whereby entitlement to benefits is based on a combination of current status (e.g. unemployed, elderly, sick, and so on) and of family income level, has created something of a contradiction for women. On the one hand, benefit entitlement is not tied to previous labour-market participation, and so women have never been excluded from claims because of their different, that is non-male, employment patterns (as happens in the UK and many other countries with social insurance schemes: Millar, 1989; Lewis, 1992). On the other hand, the means-tested nature of the benefits is based on the construction of the family as a single unit, in which men and women share their income, and this has tended to exclude married women from receipt of benefits in practice, unless their partners were also claimants. Thus women have always had rights to claim benefits as individuals but their actual receipt of state support was very dependent on their family status. In addition, the centralized Australian approach to wage bargaining and industrial relations was also based on the concept of the 'family' as a single unit. In the *Harvester* decision of 1907 the Commonwealth Court of Conciliation decreed that basic wages for unskilled workers should be set by the income needs of a man with a dependent wife and three children (Bryson, 1992; McCreadie, 1994). Thus the concept of a 'male breadwinner' earning a 'family wage' was made quite explicit in both social security policy and in wage bargaining in the public and private sectors. In this sense then, Australia could be characterized as a 'strong breadwinner' welfare state, to use Lewis's (1992) classification; or as a country with a 'gender contract' based on a 'housewife' role for women (Duncan, 1995).

However, in recent years, there has been quite a significant shake-up of the social security system, specifically with the intention of making the structure of benefits fit better with family and labour-market change. Recent policy has thus moved away from this 'family' based approach, particularly with a series of changes introduced by the Commonwealth Government in 1994–95 (although the groundwork for these changes was arguably laid by the mid-1980s social security reviews). The 'Parenting Allowance' was introduced in 1995[7] and has two components. The basic core payment is made to any parent at home with children and with minimal personal income. The additional payment is made to certain benefits recipients, in particular women married to unemployed men. These women, if they are childless and aged under 40, are no longer eligible for benefits simply as 'dependent wives' of their partner. Instead they have to establish their own eligibility (including being available for work) and make their own claim. Those with children and older women are exempt from this and can receive either a 'Partner Allowance' (older women) or an 'Additional Parenting Allowance' (mothers). For all women one of the most significant aspects of these changes is that women now receive their benefit entitlement themselves rather than through an addition to the man's benefit. Age and marital status still play a part in determining how women will be treated in social security but women receive their benefits directly rather than through their partners. Since it is usually the woman who also receives Family Payments in respect of children this means that, in unemployed families, the woman will be the one with the greater share of joint income.[8] The benefit system has thus made some significant shifts towards treating women as individuals rather than as dependants of their male partners, within the context of a means-tested system. Benefits for sole mothers have also been recently reformed.

Social security support for sole mothers

The first Commonwealth pensions for widows were introduced in Australia in 1942 (Raymond, 1987). They were specifically intended to enable widows with dependent children to stay at home and care for their children rather than go out to work, and for widows aged over 50 on the grounds that they would find it difficult to enter the labour force. The status of 'widow' was defined very broadly, to include also 'deserted' wives, divorced women and de facto widows (if they had been cohabiting for at least three years). Divorced and deserted women first had to seek maintenance from their former partners, and they also had to wait six months before they could make a claim. State welfare assistance could be claimed during that time. In 1973 the introduction of 'supporting mother's benefit' extended eligibility to unmarried mothers, deserted de facto wives, prisoners' de facto wives and other separated women who were not eligible for the widow's pension. In 1977 this became 'supporting parent's benefit' as sole fathers were brought into the scheme. From 1980 the six month qualifying period was withdrawn. The widow's pension and the supporting parent's benefits were subject to income and asset tests and paid at the same rate – so that in effect all sole parents received the same levels of state support. There were no work tests or requirements, so sole parents could receive state financial support for as long as required provided that they had a child aged under 16 or who was a full-time student under 25.

The Social Security Review, set up in 1986, paid particular attention to sole parents and especially to issues of employment, producing a number of papers on barriers to work (Frey, 1986) and employment prospects (Jordan, 1989) and an 'Issues' paper that set out policy recommendations (Raymond, 1987). This paper starts by placing the issue of support for sole parents firmly in the context of increased employment among women:

> Over the past 20 years there has been a marked shift in attitudes towards the participation of married women and women with children in employment. . . . In the past it had been assumed that women should become financially dependent on their husbands when they married and their careers should be devoted to the rearing of children. It was this philosophy which was behind the introduction of the widow's pension in 1942. . . . In recent years, however, with the rapid growth in the numbers of sole parent pensioners there has been concern on a number of fronts that there should be increased incentives and opportunities for sole parents to participate in the labour force. There has been a view that sole parents, like married mothers, should participate in the labour force, particularly if their children are of school age.
>
> (Raymond, 1987: 3)

The recommendations put forward thus focused on how to improve employment incentives and opportunities, including the introduction of a single sole-parent benefit for all sole parents and an increased level of family allowance for children in sole-parent families. Alongside the review of social security provisions the government also set up a special committee to look at the operation of child maintenance. As a consequence three major changes were made to support for sole parents:

- 1988: the Child Support Act was passed, with the aim of increasing child maintenance payments from separated parents.

- 1989: the Sole Parent Pension was introduced, replacing the Supporting Parent's Benefit and Widow's Pensions for widows with children.
- 1989: the JET (Jobs, Education and Training) scheme was introduced, intended to offer support and training to help sole parents into employment.

These measures add up to a new 'package' of support for sole parents in which employment incentives play a significant role. The sole-parent pension consists of a basic amount payable to any sole parent with at least one child aged under 16.[9] This is set at the same level as the single rate of the Age Pension. Sole parents are also entitled to payments for their child or children. These are the basic family payment (of a flat-rate amount per family) and an Additional Family Payment. The latter includes an amount per child (which varies with age) and a Guardian Allowance in recognition of the additional costs that they face. Assistance with housing costs, and medical and pharmaceutical costs may also be available. Separate income tests are applied to maintenance income and to earned income. In 1994 there were about 314,000 sole parents receiving the pension, 94 per cent of them women, and it is estimated that about 72 per cent of all sole parents receive a pension. About 22 per cent of sole parents pensioners also have some earnings (up from only 9 per cent in 1983). All sole parents claiming the sole-parent pension are required to take action, through the Child Support Agency, to obtain child support. The proportion of pensioners receiving child support has increased from 26 per cent in 1988 to just over 41 per cent in 1994 (DSS, 1994).

The JET scheme has been central to the objective of improving employment opportunities. This is a national voluntary programme for sole-parent pensioners which provides assistance with education, training and finding work and with child-care placements. The scheme is jointly administered by the Departments of Social Security, of Employment, Education and Training, and of Human Services and Health. JET advisers in DSS interview clients (sole-parent pensioners) for an assessment of education, training and employment needs. Clients may then be referred to JET contact officers at the Commonwealth Employment Service who advise of available employment and training programmes or registration for employment. Three groups of sole parents are specifically targeted in the JET scheme: those on pension over 12 months with a child aged 6 or more; those within two years of losing pension because their youngest child is turning 16, and those who are teenage sole parents.[10]

Department of Social Security statistics (DSS, 1995) show that between 1989 and 1994, 157,700 sole parents participated in the JET scheme and 45,700 (29 per cent) found paid employment. Employment outcomes in 1994 from the JET programme indicate that the proportion of JET clients with earnings was significantly higher (31 per cent) than for the sole-parent pensioner population as a whole (22 per cent). The average earnings of $222 per week for employed JET clients was higher than for the total sole-parent pensioner population of

$159. Of all JET clients approximately one half (46 per cent) have participated in a training course. Between 1989 and 1994 approximately 39,500 (25 per cent) of JET clients undertook an education course either at school, technical college or university. JET clients also took up 73,500 labour-market programme placements between 1989 and 1994 (Jordan, 1994). Over 80 per cent of JET placements in these training schemes were in three specific programmes – Jobtrain, which places people on 8–10 week training courses (41 per cent); Skillshare, which offers community-based training for long-term unemployed people (23 per cent); and Jobstart, which is wage subsidy payable for up to 26 weeks (16 per cent).

While the JET scheme is regarded by the DSS as a great 'success' (DSS, 1995), the problematic nature of defining success is worth considering. Nominating the standards against which the 'success' of policy outcomes are to be judged needs to be clarified. For example, there is the problem of whether the improvements in the participation in education, training and employment can actually be attributed to the programme. As Shaver et al. (1994) point out, given the voluntary nature of JET, it is possible that these results reflect self-selection in take-up, with the programme being used most readily by those sole parents most likely to become employed in any case. Jordan also cautions against:

> the practice of reporting of employment and further education or training as positive outcomes of participation in the program where the one is or can be the intended final result and the other no more than a stage in a process whose outcome is still unknown.
>
> (1994: 70)

Success could be seen as the employment the sole mothers gained through JET, but the types of employment and hours worked by the JET sole parents is not discussed in the DSS evaluation report (DSS, 1995). Alternatively, the extent to which overall employment rates for sole mothers have risen could be seen as indicative of the success, not just of the JET scheme, but of the general drive to encourage and support more paid employment. As Table 6.8 shows, in

Year	Full-time (%)	Part-time (%)	Unemployed (%)	Total in labour force (%)
1989	25	21	5	52
1990	26	19	7	52
1991	24	19	7	51
1992	23	20	9	52
1993	23	20	9	52
1994	23	20	9	52

Source ABS (various years)

Table 6.8 Sole mothers' labour-market participation rates: Australia 1989–94

the five years from 1989 to 1994, full-time employment among sole mothers has fallen slightly and part-time employment has remained at about the same rate. Unemployment, however, has risen significantly, from about 5 per cent of all sole mothers in 1989 to 9 per cent in 1994. This gives an unemployment rate of almost 17 per cent of those economically active, much higher than the rate of nine per cent (December 1994) for women in general (ABS, 1995d). In addition, the average duration of unemployment among sole mothers has risen from 39 weeks in 1989 to 61 weeks in 1994 (ABS, 1994c). Thus it could be that the initial effect of the policies aiming at encouraging work has been successful in getting sole mothers to seek work, but their chances of actually finding work clearly remain problematic. The next sections explore some possible reasons for this.

5. Sole Mothers in Labour Markets: Opportunities and Constraints

The labour market that women in Australia face is gender segregated. Nationally, although women have increased their participation in employment (as described above), the employment experiences of women remain very different from those of men. Women are concentrated into a limited number of occupations and industries, and gender segregation in employment appears to be becoming more entrenched (Brennan, 1994). Women are also much more likely than men to work in part-time jobs. Growth in part-time employment was very significant in the 1980s, with the number of part-time jobs rising from 1.1 million in 1983 to 1.6 million in 1994 – from 17 to 23 per cent of all jobs (McCreadie, 1994) – and part-time work tends to be concentrated in those occupations that provide 'women's jobs' (Cass, 1994a). Three-quarters of all part-time workers are women. However, not all women are equally likely to have part-time jobs. Rather it is women with family, especially child-care, responsibilities who are most likely to work part time. In 1993 about 10 per cent of all employed men worked part time, compared with 42 per cent of all employed women and 60 per cent of employed women with children; and men's average weekly hours of work have risen from 36.7 in 1980 to 40.5 in 1990 (Cass, 1994b).

Gender segregation also shows up in the JET programme, in which there is a tendency to provide training in 'women's jobs'. An evaluation of JET conducted by the Department of Social Security (DSS, 1990) found that the previous workforce experience of JET clients was predominantly in the areas of work traditionally undertaken by women – work with limited skills, low pay, few career prospects and poor job security. Over half of the sole mothers were either undertaking labour-market programmes in office-skill courses or were in subsidized employment in clerical occupations. Others were in training courses for retail work and the hospitality trade. Sole mothers completing courses, as well as those who did not require training, entered employment in traditional female occupations – office, hospitality, retail and factory sectors – occupations offering low wages, low status and insecure and casual employment (DSS, 1990).

A fieldwork survey with 243 older sole mothers (Shaver et al., 1994) provides information from a group of women who are one of the target groups of the JET scheme – women with their youngest child about to turn 16 and about to lose entitlement to the sole-parent pension. The study found that approximately three months before they were to lose their pension some 22 per cent had no knowledge of JET and a further 7 per cent were aware of the programme but had had no contact with it. Women of non-English speaking backgrounds were generally the least well informed. About half the women in the sample had undertaken some form of education or training in the last five years, with by far the largest number in computing, office skills and business training (accounting for more than half of all courses taken). The next largest group had training in the service sector: courses included nursing assistant, pharmacy assistant, child and aged person care, first aid, family planning, community organization and hearing and sign language for the deaf. Only a small number completed courses in the 'non-traditional' areas of car maintenance and bricklaying. Several women took language courses, mainly to learn spoken and written English.

For those who found employment, this was heavily concentrated in the areas of office work and sales and service jobs, but there were also a substantial number in unskilled work. Not all who found employment were secure and financially better off. Employment for these women can be a tenuous state – women lost jobs as well as found them and most of the jobs the women held were on a casual basis, with more than half carrying no entitlement to paid sick leave. Some women were patching together two or more such positions. There was also underemployment, with women unable to get as much employment as they wanted or needed. Nearly a year after cessation of pension almost a third of the sample still had no paid work and more than half the women in the study reported lower incomes after the transition from pension than before.

These findings, and those of the DSS evaluation of JET, seem to bear out the concerns expressed by McHugh (1989), in a review of the employment patterns of sole and married mothers as JET was introduced. She concluded that sole mothers would most likely find positions in low-status occupations, characterized by predominantly part-time employment and a low level of income. So while these outcomes were probably to be expected they hardly provide a satisfactory or successful outcome for sole mothers, when little is achieved but a movement from dependency on a minimal but secure income support from benefits, to minimal income from an insecure labour market job with all the associated costs involved. One of the emerging reasons that JET clients return to claiming sole-parent pension is that they face great difficulties in remaining in jobs that lack family-friendly work conditions, especially paid leave for sick children (Zanetti, 1994).

Access to JET schemes was found to be particularly difficult in rural areas.

JET works on the co-ordination of officials in the departments of social security and employment, with women referred to the employment service after an interview with a DSS JET Adviser. In country areas the distance between the two can be 100 to 200 kms. Access for sole mothers and liaison between staff is highly problematic and places additional constraints on the type of education, training or employment options available.[11] In general, rural areas suffer higher levels of unemployment and have much more restricted job opportunities for women than urban areas. While there is immense diversity in rural areas in Australia, in many of the smaller towns populations are declining and economies stagnating. In the 1980s and 1990s policies of regional centralization, amalgamation of government services, reduced commodity prices, and the introduction of high-tech farming have adversely affected employment opportunities for both women and men in many small to medium size rural areas, and led to increasing levels of unemployment (Dawson, 1994). Continuing cutbacks and removal of government services from small and medium rural towns has resulted in a decline in women's traditional jobs in hospitals and schools and other service areas, and a reduction in essential health, medical, community and child-care services crucial in assisting low-income families such as sole mothers.

Job opportunities for those able to afford to relocate are occurring in larger service centres in country areas. In the last two decades there has been an increase in the rates of rural married women's labour-force participation, particularly in part-time work that fits with domestic, child-care and farm responsibilities. Many farmers' wives have been forced by current economic conditions to seek employment, often travelling considerable distance to their closest town to take poorly paid, casual work, to help support their families. However in some areas employment opportunities are non-existent (Gibson, Baxter and Kingston, 1990).

For women, especially sole mothers, attempting to find or return to paid work there are barriers specific to non-urban areas. Distance, transport costs, isolation, and lack of educational resources (there are no tertiary or technical educational institutions in many small to medium rural towns) discourage women from external studies, and for Aboriginal women seeking employment prejudice is still a feature in country towns. Among the most disadvantaged in rural communities are sole parents. In the 1980s Dempsey (1992) found over 60 per cent of separated, divorced or widowed women were in the lowest income bracket, and overall this group had the lowest average annual income.

Frey (1986), in her study based in three different areas, showed how local labour-market variations affected the employment possibilities for sole mothers. She found that the types of jobs non-employed sole mothers thought that they could get were not generally the types of jobs that were available locally, 'probably indicating a lack of knowledge of local job market opportunities' (p. 10). She also found significant differences in employment patterns and education and training levels across the three areas (a rural farming and tourist area, an outer suburb of Sydney, and an area of inner-city Sydney).

Each of the three areas presented different types of employment opportunity. In the first there was high unemployment and the few vacancies available were casual part-time jobs in the service sector. In the second, most available jobs were in Sydney itself and therefore required quite substantial travelling times each day and also child care that could cover such long hours of combined travel and work. In the third area jobs were relatively plentiful but were full-time jobs, usually requiring high levels of skills and experience.

Thus the three labour markets were very different, but all, in their own ways, illustrate the difficulties facing sole mothers. In all three areas, however, it was child care that the women highlighted as a key problem: getting care that was affordable but flexible enough to cover irregular working hours, before- and after-school care, school holidays, sick children, and travel times raised problems in all three areas. Transport was also an important issue, not only in the rural areas but also in the two Sydney areas. Problems with transport, and with housing, were also found by Cass et al. (1990) in their study of non-English-speaking sole mothers living in Sydney. These women were from three main groups: Vietnamese, Turkish and Spanish speaking, and the majority were not employed. They faced 'formidable barriers' to employment, including their 'perceptions of their responsibility to care for their children', especially in a society in which they felt they did not have a secure base. That non-English-speaking sole mothers have particularly high levels of use of the JET scheme (DSS, 1990) is probably also indicative of their greater need for help in gaining access to paid work.

6. Sole Mothers in Neighbourhoods

The skills that sole mothers have, the benefits they can receive, and the job opportunities open to them are all important factors in the access of sole mothers to employment. But these are still only part of the picture and it is also important to consider the extent to which there is family and community support – both practical and attitudinal – for employment. Jordan suggests that there remains much ambivalence in this respect:

> Women have become less likely to prefer the option of staying out of employment, and the community less likely to support it, but neither women, their families, nor the institutions of the community have fully adjusted to those historic changes.
>
> (1989: 12)

Everingham (1994), in her study of mothers in one area of New South Wales, shows how mothers in different areas tend to construct similar ideas and expectations about their 'mother/worker' roles and that these shared expectations themselves act as constraints upon what is considered acceptable. Thus the women in the 'suburban' area (mainly middle-class and married) tended to see paid work as something that was very much second to, and fitted around, their mothering obligations. Paid work thus meant part-time work. Women in the 'kinship' area (working-class, including more sole mothers) tended to view paid work as incompatible with motherhood and most were full-time mothers. Women in the 'alternative' area ('counter-culture', middle-class and mix of partnership status) were less likely to hold one particular view and women here included both full-time workers and at-home mothers. This would suggest that within the overall group of 'sole mothers' there is likely to be substantial variation in attitudes to mothering and employment.

The available evidence is somewhat limited. Jordan (1989), interviewing sole mothers in Melbourne, concluded that, for the vast majority of the sole mothers, there was a preference for employment ('the welfare of their families probably suffers more from insufficient encouragement than from unreasonable pressure to work', p. 65) but that many sole mothers nevertheless found it difficult to take up work. Some suffered problems of ill-health (themselves or their children) and many lacked any qualifications or training. In addition, a significant minority of the mothers (about 27 per cent) were so socially isolated that their capacity to access training, child care, or jobs was very limited. These included in particular women from non-English-speaking backgrounds who also, as migrant women, lacked family and neighbourhood networks of support. More generally, Jordan points to a problem of low aspirations:

> Limits are imposed by their own vision of feasible futures. Many can see no further than part-time work in secondary occupations. . . . It is one thing to help them to act on their present intentions, another for them to redefine their place in the world.
>
> (ibid.: 111)

Older sole mothers are also likely to be wary about a full-time employment role. A recent study of sole mothers who were about to lose their entitlement to benefits due to their youngest child turning 16 years of age (Shaver et al., 1994) showed that these sole mothers tended to see themselves as mothers first and workers second – despite the fact that they were facing the necessity of having to seek paid work. When first interviewed (just before their sole-parent pensions were withdrawn) two-thirds of the women described themselves as either a 'mother' (44 per cent) or a 'home-maker' (20 per cent), compared with one-fifth who described themselves as 'paid worker' (12 per cent) or 'unemployed' (5 per cent). Interviewed again 12 months later (when they were no longer receiving benefits as sole parents), two-fifths continued to describe themselves as either 'mother' (24 per cent), 'home-maker' (10 per cent), or 'home-maker/mother' (8 per cent) while one-quarter described themselves as either 'paid worker' (15 per cent) or 'unemployed' (12 per cent). At both interviews about one in five (17 per cent) described themselves as having joint roles. Thus, for these older mothers, the dominant image was that of 'mother/home-maker' and not 'worker' or even 'mother/worker'.

Child-care constraints and opportunities

Child care is one of the most important single problems for sole mothers seeking work. In 1993 about half (49%) of all children under 12 were involved in some form of child care (ABS, 1994b). Of these, informal care was more common than formal care (38 per cent using the former compared with 19 per cent using the latter and 8 per cent using both). There was little variation in use of child care across states, although usage rates were slightly higher in the Australian Central Territory (i.e. the capital Canberra and surrounding region). Children were more likely to be in some form of child care if their parents were employed: 76 per cent of employed sole mothers use child care, compared with 62 per cent of two-earner couples and 35 per cent of one-earner couples. Employed sole mothers were more likely than couples to rely on a combination of formal and informal care (28 per cent compared with 18 per cent of two-earner couples), perhaps indicating their need to juggle care from different sources.

As discussed above, child-care provision has expanded rapidly over the past 20 years. In 1993 there were more than 200,000 Commonwealth subsidized places with around 300,000 children attending each week (Brennan, 1994). Much of the demand for work-related care is met but there are problems in accessing care for those who want care for other than work-related reasons. In addition Brennan points to a shift from the non-profit, community-based sector to the private sector. Most new places, especially for pre-school children, have been in the private sector, especially in the urban areas of New South Wales and Victoria (including Sydney and Melbourne). Community-based services do remain the largest single sector but the growing importance of the private sector may mean that the child-care needs of employed parents become increasingly separated from issues of the best interests of children and the sort of care provision that best meets their needs. A final concern that Brennan expresses is the move away from locating new services in areas of greatest need to a more market-orientated approach. Commercial operators choose where to set up but they can receive Commonwealth financial aid wherever they do set up. Such providers may also be reluctant to take very young children and babies, so that community-based services end up providing more of this, relatively expensive, area of care.

Access to child care for women on JET schemes is a particular problem for those in rural areas (ACOSS, 1991). Centre-based child care, which is regarded as offering a more stimulating environment for children, is less likely to be available to mothers in rural or semi-rural areas. For JET mothers with school children there are problems in gaining places for after-school care and fee relief is not adequate to cover costs. Affordable school vacation care is not always available and mothers commented that the 'better' ones fill up quickly. Even with fee relief the costs for excursions connected to care programmes plus the basic fee are beyond the reach of most sole mothers. Mothers with older school-age children reported resistance from their children in attending both forms of care.

Wolcott and Glezer (1995) reporting on the Australian Living Standards Study, point out that mothering roles and child care are the main reasons that both married and sole mothers give for not being employed outside the home. Of the sole mothers, over half said that they were not in work because their children were too young or they preferred to care for their children themselves (57 per cent), while one-fifth (21 per cent) said that child care was a problem. Finding jobs with suitable hours, close to home may have helped in this, but such jobs were very difficult to find. Overall Wolcott and Glezer conclude:

> there appear to be more similarities than differences between sole mothers and married mothers when participation in paid and unpaid work is examined. Being female and being a mother creates common denominators that contrast with being male and a father when work and family decisions of both sexes are compared.
>
> (ibid.: 131)

7. Conclusion

Australian women have done much to create and sustain new roles for themselves over the past two to three decades, and in particular women with children are participating in paid employment in increasing numbers. The impacts are, however, somewhat contradictory: women are more financially independent but they are still paid less than men, they mainly work in 'women's jobs', and they continue to bear responsibility for domestic work and child care. For sole mothers there are also many contradictions. As this chapter has described, sole mothers form almost one in five of all families with children, they are mainly White English-speaking women, ex-married, with one or two children. They are heavily reliant on state benefits, either as sole source of income or as an addition to low earnings and/or child support. They have a much higher than average risk of poverty. About half of all sole mothers have paid work and half do not. Barriers to work include lack of adequate and affordable child care, lack of suitable employment in the right locations, and lack of transport. However, policy towards sole mothers has increasingly stressed employment and sought to encourage and sustain this through a mixture of financial incentives and work training. The JET scheme is one of the most comprehensive and accessible employment training schemes for sole mothers anywhere, although as we have seen, it is difficult for the scheme to break away from gender segregation in the labour market and so sole mothers tend to be trained mainly for service-type jobs. The women themselves are not all alike in their attitudes to motherhood and to paid employment. Some, especially the older women, see themselves as primarily mothers and are reluctant to enter paid employment. Community attitudes sometimes support them in this. For others, their problem is how to be both mothers and workers when the support infrastructure needed for this, although much improved, is still short of meeting need.

There have been some far-reaching changes in the approach to social security benefits in Australia in recent years, with deliberate attempts to shift away from family-based and gender-differentiated provisions to more individual-oriented systems. How far this can be successful in the context of family-based means-tests is not yet clear, but the Australian experience may have resonance elsewhere: how far is it possible to combine individual entitlement with more targeted systems of support? For sole mothers a strong policy commitment to encouraging employment seems to have been met by a positive response among many sole mothers themselves. Sole mothers are ready and willing to work when there are suitable employment options that can accommodate their caring responsibilities. It is of course pointless to encourage employment if jobs are not available. The moves to increase levels of child support received by sole mothers may help to open up part-time opportunities for them, if they can put together an adequate income through a combination of part-time employment, social security benefits and child maintenance.

At the start of the chapter we suggested that Australia was a country in transition – from a situation where the main thrust of policy was to support sole mothers to stay at home to one where the focus is on encouraging sole mothers into employment. However, the future of sole-parent families mainly reliant on income support is bleak. At a time of continuing high national unemployment of over 8 per cent (1996), and with a new Liberal administration focusing on cutting back and tightening public spending in all areas, there is unlikely to be any relief through additional income support measures for sole mothers. Unless there are improvements in the economy resulting in substantial job growth the situation of poverty for many sole-parent families, compounded by the constraints that caring places on their labour-market participation, will continue. The picture from Australia reflects the ways in which policy, discourse and attitudes interrelate: there is cause for pessimism, especially in the failure to tackle continuing and widening inequalities in both labour-market opportunities and income levels; but also cause for optimism, especially in relation to women's capacity to influence and construct policies that meet their needs.

Notes

1 The issue of terminology raises many problems and the labels used to describe mothers living without current partners are far from neutral, but reflect current views and attitudes (Millar, 1994).
2 The rate of teenage births has fallen from 55.5 births per 1,000 of the population in 1971, to 21.9 in 1992 (Walshe, 1994).
3 About seven in ten sole parents receive this 'pension' (as it is termed in Australia), so this is broadly representative of all sole parents.

4   The average age at first marriage is 27 for women, which has risen from 21 in 1974 (ABS, 1994a). The divorced and separated sole mothers who are in their mid to late thirties now would probably have married at about age 24 (ABS, 1994) in the early 1980s.

5   CEC (1993) describes three main patterns of lifetime participation for women: (i) single-peak curve, with most women giving up employment with marriage and/or children; (ii) twin-peak curve, with most women giving up employment during child rearing years but returning thereafter; (iii) inverted U, with continuous high levels of employment throughout. Australia would fall into the second category.

6   These figures refer to registered unemployment and so their levels are at least in part a function of the rules governing such registration. Unemployment rates in recent years are discussed in more detail below.

7   There was a stepping-stone to this, in the form of the Home Child Care Allowance (HCCA) introduced in September 1994, to replace an income tax rebate paid to men with a dependent spouse and child. The HCCA was paid directly to the partner of a couple (usually the wife) at home with dependent children (under 16 years of age). There was a means test, relatively generous, on the claimant's income but not on that of her partner. This meant that, although couples were not financially better off, it was the woman, and not her spouse, who was the actual recipient of the payment. The HCCA was incorporated into the 'Parenting Allowance' in July 1995.

8   What effect, if any, this will have on intra-family equity or, to put it more plainly, on who will make the decisions about money management will be of interest to social researchers in the future.

9   The maximum age of qualifying children had been reduced from 24 to 16 in 1987.

10 In addition a series of pilot projects has targeted the most socially disadvantaged sole parents: those who have been more than five years on pension (long-term dependency) and parents with either Aboriginal and Torres Straits Islands backgrounds or who are non-English speaking (Zanetti, 1994).

11 Direct access through employment offices was made available to sole-parent pensioners in 1994 (Davis-Goff, National Director of JET, personal communication), but that does not necessarily solve the travel problem.

References

AUSTRALIAN BUREAU OF STATISTICS (ABS) (1988) *Time Use Survey, Sydney May–June 1987*, Catalogue No. 4111.1, Canberra.

AUSTRALIAN BUREAU OF STATISTICS (ABS) (1992) *Survey of Families in Australia*, Catalogue No. 4418, Canberra.

AUSTRALIAN BUREAU OF STATISTICS (ABS) (1993) *How Australians Use Their Time*, Catalogue No. 4154.0, Canberra.

AUSTRALIAN BUREAU OF STATISTICS (ABS) (1994) *Labour Force Status and Other Characteristics of Families*, Australia, Catalogue No. 6224.0, Canberra.

AUSTRALIAN BUREAU OF STATISTICS (ABS) (1994a) *Focus on Families: Demographics and Family Formation*, Catalogue No. 4420.0, Canberra.

AUSTRALIAN BUREAU OF STATISTICS (ABS) (1994b) *Focus on Families: Income and Housing*, Catalogue No. 4424.0, Canberra.

AUSTRALIAN BUREAU OF STATISTICS (ABS) (1994c) *Distribution and Composition of Employee Earnings and Hours*, Australia, Catalogue No. 6306.0, Canberra.

AUSTRALIAN BUREAU OF STATISTICS (ABS) (1995a) *National Aboriginal and Torres Strait Islander Survey 1994*, Catalogue No. 4190.0, Canberra.

AUSTRALIAN BUREAU OF STATISTICS (ABS) (1995b) *Marriages and Divorces 1994*, Catalogue No. 3310.0, Canberra.

AUSTRALIAN BUREAU OF STATISTICS (ABS) (1995c) *Recent Changes in Unpaid Work*, Occasional Paper, Catalogue No. 4154.0, Canberra.

AUSTRALIAN BUREAU OF STATISTICS (ABS) (1995d) *The Labour Force Australia*, Catalogue No. 6203.0, Canberra.

AUSTRALIAN COUNCIL OF SOCIAL SERVICES (ACOSS) (1991) *Survey of Community and Employer Attitudes to the Jobs, Education and Training Program*, ACOSS, Sydney, August.

BITTMAN, MICHAEL and LOVEJOY, FRANCES (1993) 'Domestic power: negotiating an unequal division of labour within a framework of equality', *Australian and New Zealand Journal of Sociology*, **29**, 3, pp. 302–21.

BRADSHAW, J., KENNEDY, S., KILKEY, M., HUTTON, S., CORDEN, A., EARDLEY, T., HOLMES, H. and NEALE, J. (1996) *The Employment of Lone Parents: A comparison of Policy in 20 Countries*, Family Policy Studies Centre/Joseph Rowntree Foundation.

BRENNAN, D. (1994) *The Politics of Australian Child Care: From Philanthropy to Feminism*, Australia and England, Cambridge University Press.

BROTHERHOOD OF ST LAURENCE (1994) 'The vulnerability of sole parents to poverty', in *Brotherhood Comment*, Melbourne: BSL.

BRYSON, L. (1992) *Welfare and the State: Who Benefits?*, London: Macmillan.

BRYSON, L. (1995) 'Two welfare states: one for women, one for men', in Edwards, A. and Magarey, S. (Eds) *Women in a Restructuring Australia: Work and Welfare*, Sydney: Allen & Unwin.

CASS, B. (1986) *The Case for Review of Aspects of the Australian Social Security System*, Social Security Review, Background/Discussion Paper No. 1, Canberra: Department of Social Security.

CASS, B. (1993) 'Caring work and welfare regimes: policies for sole parents in four countries', in Shaver, S. (Ed) *Comparative Perspectives on Sole Parent Policy, Work and Welfare*, University of New South Wales, Sydney: SPRC Reports and Proceedings No. 106.

CASS, B. (1994a) 'Citizenship, work and welfare: the dilemma for Australian women', *Social Politics*, **1**, 1, pp. 106–23.

CASS, B. (1994b) 'Reframing family policies', in Inglis, J. and Rogan, L. (Eds) *Flexible Families: New Directions in Australian Communities*, New South Wales: Pluto Press.

CASS, B., WILKINSON, M. and WEBB, A. (1990) 'Single parents of non-English speaking backgrounds', in Whiteford, P. (Ed) *Sole Parents and Public Policy*, SPRC Reports and Proceedings No. 89, Social Policy Research Centre, University of New South Wales.

CASTLES, F. (1985) *The Working Class and Welfare, Reflections on the Political Development of the Welfare State in Australia and New Zealand, 1890–1980*, Sydney: Allen & Unwin.

CASTLES, F. and MITCHELL, D. (1990) *Three Worlds of Welfare Capitalism or Four?* Canberra: Australian National University, Pubic Policy Discussion Paper No. 21.

COLLARD, D., CROWE, S., HARRIES, M. and TAYLOR, C. (1994) 'The contribution of Aboriginal family values to Australian family life', in Inglis, J. and Rogan, L. (Eds) *Flexible Families: New Directions in Australian Communities*, New South Wales: Pluto Press.

COMMISSION OF THE EUROPEAN COMMUNITIES (CEC) (1993) *Employment in Europe*, Luxembourg: Office of Official Publications of the European Commission.

COMMONWEALTH OF AUSTRALIA, DEPARTMENT OF SOCIAL SECURITY (DSS) (1990) *JET: Interim Evaluation Report*, Policy Research Paper No. 62, Canberra: Australian Government Publishing Service.

COMMONWEALTH OF AUSTRALIA, DEPARTMENT OF SOCIAL SECURITY (DSS) (1994) *Annual Report 1993–94*, Canberra: Australian Government Publishing Service.

COMMONWEALTH OF AUSTRALIA, DEPARTMENT OF SOCIAL SECURITY (DSS) (various years) *Annual Reports*, Canberra: Australian Government Publishing Service.

COMMONWEALTH OF AUSTRALIA, DEPARTMENT OF SOCIAL SECURITY (DSS) Unpublished data on sole parent pension receipt, courtesy of Management Information Section.

COMMONWEALTH OF AUSTRALIA, DEPARTMENT OF SOCIAL SECURITY (DSS) (1995) *Sole Parent Program Branch, Memorandum*, Canberra: Australian Government Publishing Service.

DALY, A. (1994) 'Employment and social security for Aboriginal women', in Edwards, A. and Magarey, S. (Eds) *Women in a Restructuring Australia: Work and Welfare*, Sydney: Allen & Unwin.

DAVIS-GOFF, G. (1994), National Director of JET, Department of Employment, Education and Training, personal communication, Social Policy Research Centre, February.

DAWSON, B. (1994) 'Rural employment in Australia', *Rural Society*, **4**, 2, pp. 14–21.

DEMPSEY, K. (1992) *A Man's Town: Inequality between Women and Men in Rural Australia*, Melbourne: Oxford University Press.

DOWSE, S. (1983) 'The women's movement's fandango with the state', in Baldock, C. and Cass, B. (Eds) *Women, Social Welfare and the State*, Sydney: Allen & Unwin.

DUNCAN, S. (1995) 'Theorizing European gender systems', *Journal of European Social Policy*, **5**, 4, pp. 263–84.

EVANS, M. D. R. (1995) *Norms on Women's Employment over the Life Course: Australia, 1989–93*, Worldwide Attitudes, Canberra: Research School of Social Sciences.

EVERINGHAM, C. (1994) *Motherhood and Modernity*, Buckingham: Open University Press.

FARRAR, A. (1994) 'Reconsidering the family and the state', in Inglis, J. and Rogan, L. (Eds) *Flexible Families: New Directions in Australian Communities*, New South Wales: Pluto Press.

FORSTER, M. (1993) *Comparing Poverty in 13 OECD Countries: Traditional and Synthetic Approaches*, LIS Working Paper No. 100, CEPS/INSTAD, Luxembourg.

FREY, D. (1986) *Survey of sole parent pensioners' workforce barriers*, Background Paper No. 12, Social Security Review, Department of Social Security, Canberra.

GIBSON, D., BAXTER, J. and KINGSTON, C. (1990) 'Beyond the dichotomy: the paid and unpaid work of rural women', in Alston, M. (Ed.) *Rural Women*, Key Papers Number 1, Centre for Rural Welfare Research, Charles Sturt University-Riverina, NSW.

INGLIS, J. and ROGAN, L. (Eds) (1994) *Flexible Families: New Directions in Australian Communities*, New South Wales: Pluto Press.

JORDAN, A. (1989) *Lone parents and wage earner? Employment prospects of sole parent pensioners*, Background Paper No. 31, Social Security Review, Department of Social Security, Canberra.

JORDAN, A. (1994) 'Labour market programs and social payments', *Social Security Journal*, December, pp. 60–78.

KING, A. and McHUGH, M. (1995) *The wives of disability support pensioners and paid work*, SPRC Reports and Proceedings, Social Policy Research Centre, University of New South Wales, Sydney.

KING, A., BRADBURY, B. and McHUGH, M. (1995) *Why do the Wives of Unemployed Men have Such Low Employment Rates?*, SPRC Reports and Proceedings, Social Policy Research Centre, University of New South Wales, Sydney.

LEWIS, J. (1992) 'Gender and the development of welfare', *Journal of European Social Policy*, **2**, 3, pp. 159–73.

MANN, K. (1994) 'Watching the defectives: observers of the underclass in the USA, Britain and Australia', *Critical Social Policy*, Issue 41, **14**, 2, pp. 79–99.

McCREADIE, R. (1994) 'I haven't had so much fun since the International Year of the Piano Tuner', in Inglis, J. and Rogan, L. (Eds) *Flexible Families: New Directions in Australian Communities*, New South Wales: Pluto Press.

McHUGH, M. (1989) *Sole mothers and labour force participation*, paper given at the third Australian Family Research Conference, Ballarat College of Advanced Education, 26–29 November, Victoria.

MILLAR, J. (1989) 'Social security, women and equality in the UK', *Policy and Politics*, **17**, 4, pp. 31–321.

MILLAR, J. (1994) 'Defining lone parenthood: family structures and social relations', in Hantrais, L. (Ed.) *Conceptualising the Family*, University of Loughborough: Cross-National Research Papers, ESRC/CNAF.

MILLAR, J. (1996) 'Mothers, workers, wives: cross-national policy approaches to supporting lone mothers', in Bortolia-Silva, E. (Ed.) *Good Enough Mothering?*, Hemel Hempstead: Harvester/Wheatsheaf.

MILLAR, J. and WHITEFORD, P. (1993) 'Child support in lone-parent families: policies in Australia and the UK', *Policy and Politics*, **21**, 1, pp. 59–72.

MITCHELL, D. (1991) *Income Transfers in Ten Welfare States*, Aldershot: Avebury.

MITCHELL, D. (1993) 'Sole parents, work and welfare: evidence from the Luxembourg Income Study', in Shaver, S. (ed) *Comparative Perspectives on Sole Parent Policy, Work and Welfare*, SPRC Reports and Proceedings No. 106, Social Policy Research Centre, University of New South Wales, Sydney.

POLETTE, J. (1995) *Distribution of Effective Marginal Tax Rates Across the Australian Labour Force*, Discussion paper No. 6, National Centre for Social and Economic Modelling, Australian National University, Canberra, NATSEM.

RAYMOND, J. (1987) *Bringing up Children Alone: Policies for Sole Parents*, Issues paper No. 3, Social Security Review, Department of Social Security, Canberra.

RIMMER RUSSELL, J. and RIMMER, SHELIA (1994) *More Brilliant Careers: The Effect of Career Breaks on Women's Employment*, Women's Bureau. DEET, AGPS, Canberra.

SAWER, M. (1990) *Sisters in Suits, Women in Public Policy in Australia*, Sydney: Allen & Unwin.

SHAVER, S., KING, A., McHUGH, M. and PAYNE, T. (1994) *At the End of Eligibility: Female Sole Parents Whose Youngest Child Turns 16*, SPRC Reports and Proceedings No. 117, Social Policy Research Centre, University of New South Wales, Sydney.

SOCIAL SECURITY REVIEW (1996) *Labour Force Status and Other Characteristics of Sole Parents, 1974–1985*, Canberra: Social Security Review, background paper No. 8.

SWAIN, S. and HOWE, R. (1995) *Single Mothers and their Children: Disposal, Punishment and Survival in Australia*, Cambridge: Cambridge University Press.

SWAN, P. and BERNSTAM, M. (1987a) 'Brides of the state', *Institute of Public Affairs (IPA) Review*, **41**, May–July, pp. 22–5.

SWAN, P. and BERNSTAM, M. (1987b) 'Support for single parents' in James, M. (Ed.) *The Welfare State: Foundations and Alternatives*, St Leonards: Centre for Independent Studies.

THORNWAITE, T., KINGSTON, C. and WALSH, P. (1995) *Drawing the Line on Poverty: An Assessment of Poverty and Disadvantage in Queensland*, Queensland: Queensland Council of Social Services (QCOSS).

WALSHE, R. (1994), 'Sole parents, the social security system and the community', in Inglis, J. and Rogan, L. (Eds) *Flexible Families: New Directions in Australian Communities*, New South Wales: Pluto Press.

WATSON, S. (1992) 'Femocratic feminisms', in Savage, M. and Witz, A. (Eds) *Gender and Bureaucracy*, Oxford: Blackwell.

WOLCOTT, I. and GLEZER, H. (1995) *Work and Family Life: Achieving Integration*, Melbourne: Australia Institute of Family Studies.

ZANETTI, C. (1994) 'Sole parents: trends and issues', *Social Security Journal*, AGPS, Canberra, ACT, pp. 92–102.

Chapter 7

Single Mothers in Germany: Supported Mothers Who Work

Martina Klett-Davies

1. Introduction

In Germany the number of single parents has doubled in the past two decades. Nearly all single-parent families (86.3 per cent in 1993) are headed by the mother.

In contrast to many other West European countries, and indeed to married mothers in Germany, single mothers (as a generic category) tend to be in paid employment (63 per cent) even though they often face extra obstacles in the labour market. Single mothers are also more likely to be in full-time employment than married mothers (65 per cent and 48 per cent respectively). And yet it is generally assumed that the 'conservative' German welfare state tends to treat single mothers more as mothers or wives rather than as workers (e.g. Esping-Andersen, 1990; Lewis and Ostner, 1994; Hobson, 1994).

In contrast to this 'traditional' view of the German welfare state some previously unpaid work has been accredited as a 'socially useful' activity. The government has introduced schemes which pay for child rearing and long-term care for relatives, work mostly done by women. While these schemes do not provide security comparable with that of full-time employment, they are nonetheless steps in the direction of a more inclusive social security system (Clasen and Gould, 1995). On the other hand these policies can be seen as conservative in that they are paying women to stay at home.

Another important theme in considering single motherhood is that although East Germany and West Germany – often referred to as the 'new Länder' and 'old Länder' after reunification (respectively German Democratic Republic, GDR, and Federal Republic of Germany, FRG, before reunification) – are now governed by one welfare state regime, single mothers' self-identification and economic behaviour still varies between the two former states. Until 1990, the states maintained two contrasting welfare state regimes. Throughout the chapter it will be important to keep this contrast in mind.

Section two begins with an overview of single motherhood in both the former GDR and the former FRG before reunification and what became the new and the old Länder after reunification. This is followed, in section three, by an examination of discourses on single motherhood. These discourses have developed in a quite different way from those in Britain and the USA. Section four discusses the validity of different welfare state theories for single motherhood in Germany. Welfare state theories tend to ignore inconsistencies between national and sub-national policies and this has significant implications for understanding single mothers' lives. Section five goes on to analyse the regional and national labour market situation for single mothers. Finally, section six will explore the influence of neighbourhood contexts on single mothers' positioning vis-à-vis the labour market. The overall aim of the chapter is to find out the factors relevant to single mothers' decisions about whether or not to take paid work.

2. Single Motherhood in Germany

The prevalence of single motherhood in Germany: two national trends

Germany is really two countries: the Berlin Wall was demolished in 1989 but – almost a decade later – economic and social walls continue to exist. The situation for single mothers in the new Länder is still quite different from that of their compatriots in the old Länder. Before reunification, citizens of the former GDR lived in a bureaucratic state collectivist system of welfare (Deacon, 1992). Single mothers thus grew up in a regime in which women were fully integrated members of a working society. In 1990 the GDR and FRG were reunited into one Germany, but under the West German understanding of the 'social market economy' (*Soziale Marktwirtschaft*). The FRG tended to maintain the bourgeois ideal of the male partner as breadwinner and the female partner as carer for the children and domestic worker in the household (Lewis and Ostner, 1994). Social policy in the new Länder is now quite opposite to that before reunification. It does not necessarily follow, however, that single mothers in the new Länder have simply responded to these policies as if they had no past. One cannot therefore speak of one national trend or of single mothers as a homogenous group in re-unified Germany.

In 1994 17.2 per cent of all families with children under the age of 18 were single parents in reunited Germany. The percentage of single parents in the former GDR tended always to be about 8 per cent higher than in the former FRG (see Table 7.1). Both show a steady increase in single parenthood, but the gap between the two has become wider over time, even during the four years since reunification and the advent of only one national social policy regime.

The overwhelming majority of single parents are women, German citizens and White. However, in 1994, 8.4 per cent of all single parents were

Year	Old Länder (%)	New Länder (%)	United Germany (%)
1980	10.3	18.0*	n/a
1990	13.4	21.3	15.3
1991	13.8	21.6	15.7
1992	14.1	22.2	16.0
1993	14.6	23.4	16.6
1994	15.1	24.5	17.2

* 1981 unmarried children living in household (Gysi, 1989)
Source Mikrozensus (sample: 1% of the population)
Table 7.1 Single-parent families as percentage of all families with dependent children under 18 years: Germany, 1980–94

not German citizens in the old Länder and just 1 per cent in the new Länder (Statistisches Bundesamt, 1996). The former GDR was virtually closed to and not very attractive to asylum seekers and other foreigners. After reunification their number is increasing.

Family structures and living arrangements

In Germany, as everywhere, it cannot automatically be assumed that a single mother lives alone with her children. The Mikrozensus (the most up-to-date and comprehensive sources of data) also records as 'single mother families' those where other persons such as partners or relatives live in the same household as long as they are not married to the mother. This is different from many other European countries in which cohabiting families are counted as a separate category. The cohabitation rate for single mothers has always been higher in the East. According to the Mikrozensus, in 1991 a fifth (20 per cent) of all single parents in the old Länder lived with relatives or other adults (Statistisches Bundesamt, 1996). In contrast, over a third of single parents in the new Länder lived with someone other than their children (Voit, 1993). A more recent survey estimates that half of all single parents have cohabited with a partner while being a single parent (Schneider, 1994).

In 1993, 86.3 per cent of all single-parent families in unified Germany were headed by the mother. The figure always tended to be somewhat higher in the former GDR and the now new Länder. After a divorce, mothers in the former GDR tended to receive full custody of the children, and therefore single-parent families are still more likely to be headed by a female (87 per cent) in comparison with the old Länder (83 per cent) (Statistisches Bundesamt, 1995).

Single parents tend to have fewer children than married parents. This is partly due to the lower age of single mothers, as well as financial constraints and lack of labour-market opportunities. Almost three-quarters (72 per cent) of all single parents had only one child in 1992. The first child seems to 'break or make' a relationship and single mothers generally have no more children during single motherhood. In contrast, less than half of all couples (47 per cent) had one child only, while 40 per cent had two children. Single-parent families are also much less likely to have three or more children (Statistisches Bundesamt, 1995). There is only a marginal difference in this between the old and new Länder.

Characteristics of single mothers by origin

In 1994 in the new Länder almost half (45 per cent) of all single mothers had never been married. In contrast, in the old Länder not even a third (30.4 per cent) had never been married (Statistisches Bundesamt, 1996). The post-war economic independence for women through employment, and a greater social acceptance of extra-marital relationships, are likely contributing factors to the higher percentage of never-married single mothers in the new Länder.

In the former FRG the proportional increase of single motherhood in the 1970s and early 1980s was the result of an increased number of divorces and separations (see Table 7.2). In contrast, the increase of single motherhood in the 1980s and 1990s is much more due to the rising number of never-married mothers. Their proportion is rising also as a consequence of the decreasing proportion of widows. In the former GDR the proportion of divorcees has always been especially high (49.2 per cent in 1981) while the proportion of never-married mothers was 30.4 per cent in 1981 (Gysi, 1989).

Route into single motherhood	1972 (%)	1980 (%)	1985 (%)	1990 (%)	1994 (%)
Never married	12	11	16	23	30
Separated/divorced	49	60	64	64	60
Widowed	40	28	19	13	10
Total	100	100	100	100	100

Note * from 1990 the Mikrozensus only includes the population living with their family. Until 1985 it included the population living in households.
Figures may not always add up to 100% due to rounding.
Source Mikrozensus, 1994, 1996*
Table 7.2 Route into single motherhood in the old Länder: Germany, 1972–94

Never-married mothers tend to be younger. Their rapidly growing number accounts for the fact that single parents are now on average younger than ever before. While single parents tend to have their first child early, married and cohabiting parents tend to delay child bearing (Peuckert, 1996). The proportion of single-parent families with children under the age of six has risen substantially, from 21 per cent in 1980 to 37 per cent in 1993 (Statistisches Bundesamt, 1996).

	Old Länder (%)	New Länder (%)	Unified Germany (%)
Under 25	7	13	9
25–35	40	49	43
35–45	40	32	37
45–55	11	5	9
Over 55	2	–	2
Total	100	100	100

Note Figures may not always add up to 100% due to rounding
Source Mikrozensus, 1996
Table 7.3 Single mothers with dependent children by age in old and new Länder: Germany, 1994

Single mothers' age may explain their lower vocational attainment (Gutschmidt, 1994a). Mothers who have their children under the age of 25 tend to have significantly fewer educational qualitfications (Drauschke et al., 1993).

Single mothers in the new Länder tend to be younger than in the old Länder. This can partly be explained by the higher percentage of 'never-married' mothers and the lower percentage of widows in the new Länder (Table 7.3). Youth in the former GDR generally had no post-adolescent, single adult phase. Women started child bearing and marriage there much earlier than in the former FRG (Buba et al., 1995).

Labour-force participation: two developments

Single mothers in Germany face various obstacles to taking up paid work, such as insufficient and inflexible child-care facilities, workplace inflexibility, lower vocational qualifications and the added difficulty of combining domestic, caring and paid work. However, they are more likely to be in paid employment than cohabiting and married mothers. The employment rate for divorced mothers was the highest in 1993 (70 per cent), followed by never-married mothers (61 per cent) and separated single mothers (60 per cent). Least likely to be in paid employment were widowed mothers (58 per cent). However, single mothers in any category are still more likely to work than married mothers (56 per cent) (Statistisches Bundesamt, 1995). In 1994, 12.3 per cent of single-mother families with dependent children received state benefits (*Sozialhilfe*) as a main source of income, and 11.5 per cent received unemployment benefits (Statistisches Bundesamt, 1996).

In other words, in 1992 20 per cent of all state benefit recipients were single parents, while as many as 35 per cent in the old Länder, and 16 per cent in the new Länder, were foreigners – mostly asylum seekers (*Frankfurter Allgemeine Zeitung*, 1995).

While the percentage of married mothers who work has marginally

	Old Länder		Unified Germany	
	Married mothers (%)	Single mothers (%)	Married mothers (%)	Single mothers (%)
1991	49.7	64.4	57.3	70.7
1992	51.8	65.3	56.6	67.7
1993	50.8	63.5	55.5	64.6
1994	–	62.3	56.2	63.4

Note * under 18 years
Source Mikrozensus
Table 7.4 Employment rate of married and single mothers with dependent children*: old Länder and unified Germany, 1991–94

decreased in united Germany and slightly increased in the old Länder, the changes in the number of single mothers in paid work are much more substantial (see Table 7.4). Firstly, fewer single mothers were in paid work in 1994 than in 1991. Secondly, while the number decreased by 2.1 per cent in the old Länder, it fell by a substantial 7.3 per cent in united Germany. It can only be concluded that single mothers in the new Länder have been hit hardest by the recession, rising unemployment and dramatic changes in the social welfare system (cf. Quack and Maier, 1994). These factors seem to have less effect on married mothers' employment rate. Never-married mothers' employment rate is decreasing most rapidly (by 9 per cent between 1990 and 1993), and this will have been particularly severe in the new Länder.

Since reunification single mothers in the new Länder have been able to take up the two-year state child rearing benefit (*Erziehungsgeld*), a three-year maternity leave (*Erziehungsurlaub*) and income support (*Sozialhilfe*). These new policies, in conjunction with the lack of opportunities in the labour market and worsening child-care facilities, may have contributed to the fall in single mothers' employment. Single mothers, especially never-married, may want to give up work and take the opportunities given by social policies to escape the double burden of work and motherhood and to spend time with their children – even if they are not forced to leave paid work by unemployment or cuts in child care.

Another contributing factor to the fall in single mothers' employment levels in the new Länder could be that some remain poor although they work. After reunification half of single mothers who were trained labourers, and 57 per cent of untrained labourers, claimed to have difficulties living on their income. These single mothers tended to feel worse off financially after reunification than before. Higher qualified single mothers tended to view their situation more positively (Meyer and Staufenbiel, 1994).

However, although the 1993 unemployment rate for women was higher in the new Länder (19.3 per cent) than in the old Länder (11.9 per cent), only 13.7 per cent of all single mothers in the new Länder were unemployed at that date (Drauschke and Stolzenburg, 1994b). It could be that single mothers in the new Länder are more oriented to paid employment than married mothers, and try to compensate for decreased job opportunities by being mobile and entering casual or temporary work (Berger et al., 1993).

Outright prejudice in the labour market against single mothers is not the only disadvantage single mothers face. Many single mothers, like married mothers, take up a different occupation when they re-enter paid work after child bearing. They either change their occupation entirely, or are often over-qualified in the new job after child bearing. This dequalification displaces other women with appropriate, but lower, qualifications. Single mothers with lower educational attainment and lower vocational qualifications are therefore more likely to be unemployed and receiving income support (Drauschke et al., 1993).

Although a high proportion of single parents are in paid employment, especially in the new Länder, they constitute one of the poorest family types. In 1994, 43 per cent of all single mothers in the new Länder had to make ends meet on a monthly net income of less than DM 1,800 (£800). Single mothers in the old Länder tend to be better off; only 27 per cent had to live on less than this amount (Statistisches Bundesamt, 1996). Most married couples with children, in both new and old Länder, had at least more than twice this monthly income (Statistisches Bundesamt, 1996; Meyer and Staufenbiel, 1994). Although single-parent households contain one less adult consumer, there are still fixed costs which remain (housing, heating etc.).

Many single mothers are likely to earn under DM 1,000 per month (£444) (14 per cent in the new Länder and 8 per cent in the old Länder). Very few single parents are found in high-income groups. However, in comparison with other countries Germany's single mothers are clearly not so badly off. According to the Luxembourg Income Study (LIS) of Western countries, German single mothers score highest on economic status after Norway and Sweden and above Australia, Britain, Canada, France and the USA. Germany's single mothers also show the least reliance on means-tested income after Sweden. Apart from demographic differences, it is labour-force participation rates and different social transfer levels which are mostly responsible for this different economic status (Wong et al., 1993). However, in 1984 single mothers in Germany scored highest in the poverty category (39.8 per cent) in contrast, for example, to the UK (15.8 per cent) and the Netherlands (3.8 per cent). This poverty line is defined as a household income of less than 50 per cent of the country's median adjusted household income (McFate et al., 1995, see also Neubauer, 1993a, 1993b).

Women in 'conservative' welfare states, if they work at all, are likely to be in part-time employment. This can be seen as a 'compromise' between women's increasing demands for fulfilment and independence through paid work, while at the same time maintaining dependence on a male breadwinner (Pfau-Effinger, 1994). This is supported by state policies and tax incentives. Single mothers cannot rely on a male breadwinner. They are thus not only more likely than married mothers to be in paid employment but they also work

	Less than 20 hours (%)	21–36 hours (%)	More than 36 hours (%)	Total (%)
Married mothers	34	18	48	100
Single mothers	17	18	65	100
All mothers	31	18	51	100

Note: Figures may not add up to 100 due to rounding
Source Statistisches Bundesamt, 1995 based on Mikrozensus, 1993; author's own calculations
Table 7.5 Hours worked by marital status of mothers with dependent children: re-unified Germany, 1993

longer hours. Less than half of married mothers in paid employment work full-time while two-thirds of single mothers work these long hours (see Table 7.5).

A single mother's life is likely to be harder than a married mother's, because she is most likely the sole earner and alone in combining paid employment with family responsibiities. She is more likely (a) to be in employment, (b) work longer hours and (c) to be poorer. The next section will examine where and how single mothers are positioned in public, political and academic discourses.

3. Discourses Around Single Motherhood in Germany

Single mothers as a social threat

So far in Germany single mothers have not been viewed as the social threat that they are supposed to pose in Britain and the USA (see chapters 3 and 4 in this volume). Hence German research, in contrast with much research in these countries, does not primarily focus on the 'negative' issues of single mother-hood, such as costs to the welfare state, poverty, juvenile crime and teenage pregnancies (Klett-Davies, 1996a). This is partly because German policies are pro-natalist, based on a concern with declining birth rates. In addition, policy discourses tend to view children as the future generation who should be integrated into society. Finally, Germany is not a 'liberal' welfare state regime – the type of regime in which a social threat discourse seems to make more sense.

However, in public discourse the notion of state-dependent single motherhood as a way of redefinition or 'escaping patriarchy' is slowly beginning to be seen as a social threat. There are single mothers who are being called 'egotistical feminists' because of their independence and pragmatism, in that they have supposedly given up on men (Niepel, 1994a). This notion can present a threat to a society created and mostly ruled by men. It is to be seen whether this view will become more widespread and lead to single mothers being scapegoated for high public expenditure. The proposed cuts in welfare spending to reduce debts in order for Germany to be eligible for the European single currency leads to the conclusion that this could become the case.

Single mothers as a social problem: the victimized mother?

The dominant popular discourse of single motherhood in Germany is that single mothers are poor, overworked and to be pitied (Heiliger, 1993; Schülein, 1994). However, this more sympathetic attitude entails patronizing as well as patriarchal elements.

For example, while single motherhood may no longer be viewed as an 'abnormal' family type in the media, it is still often regarded as 'incomplete' because of the missing, but essential, father figure for the child (e.g. Brinck, 1995a, 1995b; Brüning, 1996). Similarly, single motherhood is often seen as only a temporary 'emergency' solution which is to be pitied (Schülein, 1994). Although there is no data about the length of single motherhood status, empirical studies suggest that many single mothers do not plan to enter a close relationship or even to marry (Mädje and Neusüß, 1994a; Drauschke and Stolzenburg, 1994b; Klett-Davies, 1996b).

Another patriarchal element in this social problem discourse is that single mothers are generally seen as having a moral obligation to stay at home and raise their children. Not even a quarter (24 per cent) of the public feels that single mothers with young children should be in paid employment (Napp-Peters, 1983 and 1987). This of course is in some contradiction to the actual situation, discussed in section two, where single mothers are effectively forced to enter the labour market even if they do not want to do so, and indeed must enter it from a weak position.

This perception also assumes that single mothers cannot perform as well in paid work as women without children, or men. Single mothers are considered unpredictable because they have to stay at home when their children are sick. They are perceived as inflexible (Tietze, 1993). Such arguments are used to justify the unwillingness to employ single mothers. However, despite the attempt to keep single mothers out of the labour market, single mothers' participation rate remains relatively high.

This public perception is reinforced by the political discourse. The government periodically discusses how income support recipients can be encouraged to take up paid work. However, single parents are not included in this debate. Their working capability is regarded as limited (*Frankfurter Allgemeine Zeitung*, 1995). Nor are single mothers included in the debate on moonlighting or working 'cash in hand' while receiving state benefits. Single mothers only lose this status of 'immunity' from blame when children are no longer dependent, or when they enter a partnership with a man, who, in public and political perception, should maintain the family (see Schülein and Simsa, 1994).

Therefore single mothers do not feature particularly prominently in political and public debates around welfare spending. The public is rather sympathetic, if patronizing, and the image of single mothers is dominated by the perception that they lack adequate support and are impoverished as a result. This fits in quite well with the dominant 'conservative' image of traditional male-breadwinner families, and indeed can reinforce it.

Research on single parents in Germany began by focusing on the assumed negative effects of single parenthood, especially those affecting children. Within this, single mothers were treated as a homogenous group. Until the 1970s the patriarchal nuclear family was regarded as the ideal model (Bergler, 1964). This may not be the predominant view any more, but educational and social work studies especially tend to remain in this tradition. For example, single motherhood is seen as a negative outcome in itself and assumed to be related to the incapability of the mother's own father (Cierpka et al., 1992).

Connected to this social problem discourse is the work of some economists concerned with the question of how the labour-market participation of single mothers can be increased. Based on economic modelling, it is suggested that better schooling and training, improved child-care facilities and a different benefit system, would increase the probability of single mothers entering paid work (e.g. Laisney et al., 1993; Staat and Wagenhals 1993, 1994; Wong et al., 1993). These studies erroneously assume that single mothers are 'rational economic men' who want to maximize financial gain and who are not involved in wider social negotiations of what they should do as mothers singly responsible for their children (see Edwards and Duncan, 1996).

Lifestyle change

Since 1970 children born out of wedlock in the former FRG (and now in unified Germany) have the same rights as other children (this was always the case in the former GDR). With this new legal status, and also because of the women's movement, single motherhood has become more acceptable as an alternative family form. Reflecting this, there is a body of research focusing on the well-being of single motherhood, rather than on its assumed negative effects (e.g. Gutschmidt, 1986; Napp-Peters, 1983, 1987; Nave-Herz and Krüger, 1992; Nave-Herz, 1992a, 1992b, 1994; Frise and Stahlberg, 1992; Schöningh et al., 1991; Drauschke and Stolzenburg, 1994a, 1994b; Niepel, 1994b; Sander, 1993).

Seeing single motherhood as an alternative family type should not be confused with 'single motherhood by choice' (women consciously becoming pregnant and choosing motherhood without a partner); nevertheless, within this discourse, it is no longer assumed that single parenthood is just an emergency and short-term arrangement. It has also been found that once single parents, and especially single mothers, discover the advantages of this family form they often wish to continue in this family type (Nave-Herz and Krüger, 1992; Mädje and Neusüß, 1994a).

The influential sociological theory underpinning the view that single motherhood is a lifestyle change is modernization theory (Beck and Beck-Gernsheim, 1990, 1994). This is based on the idea that, consequent to industrialization and urbanization, there are more choices and negotiations about lifestyles available with progressing modernization. Women's access to education and the labour market, changes in divorce laws, and the women's movement, mean that marriage is no longer a constraining economic arrangement based on the traditional male-breadwinner/female-home-maker role. Women are no longer automatically assumed to be economically dependent on a man.

Within modernization theory individuals are viewed as liberated from traditional constraints and able to choose alternative lifestyles in a search for self-fulfilment. Traditional gender values and responsibilities are no longer universally valid and can no longer be taken for granted, but have to be negotiated. The result of all this is 'individualization'. The only constraint remaining is the labour market, with which any personal existence has to 'fit in'.

However, modernization theory ignores lack of choice. For example, German single mothers may be practically forced into the labour market – as discussed in section two. Individualization theory also does not sufficiently incorporate material circumstances, other than the labour market, which can inhibit lifestyle changes. It takes for granted that everyone in Western industrialized countries has a secure material existence. The theory conveniently forgets class, and assumes middle-class values in the seeking of self-fulfilment. More accurately, we should see single motherhood as a lifestyle change for mothers with children who live in varying social contexts which both constrain and enable (Klett-Davies, 1996a).

Escaping patriarchy

In opposition to both the 'social problem' and 'alternative lifestyle' discourses, a radical feminist view of single motherhood has gained considerable influence in German research. Here, single motherhood is connected with the liberation from domestic, as well as public, patriarchy. This view accepts the economic and social disadvantages faced by single mothers, but mainly focuses on the positive aspects for children, and its liberating effects for the mother. (Gutschmidt, 1994a, 1994b; Böhm, 1993; Meyer and Schulze, 1989; Mädje and Neusüß, 1994b). According to Heiliger (1993) children with single mothers receive more time, care and love, and they are more independent, less aggressive, and sometimes especially talented.

In this discourse women are no longer willing to subordinate themselves in relationships with men. Women's lives have become more independent and their expectations of men have changed. Most of the women can no longer imagine participating in a traditional division of labour. Men who share their expectations, however, seem to be difficult to find (Klett-Davies, 1996a).

For single mothers in the old Länder, economic dependence is no longer a barrier to escaping patriarchy, even if it means receiving state benefits. Moreover, in this discourse these state benefits are viewed positively and as an enabler. It has been argued that state dependency can contribute to the mother becoming very child centred, can knock her self-confidence and can give her a feeling of being locked into passivity. Female dependency on individual men can also be substituted with the equally strong and paralysing dependency on the '*Vater Staat*' (father state). Both are 'patriarchal structures' (Schultheiss, 1987).

I will now go on in section four to analyse the German welfare state regime and the way policies position single mothers as mothers, workers or as dependents.

4. Single Mothers in the German Welfare State: Supported Mothers, Workers or Dependants?

Germany's conservative welfare state: single mothers as mothers or workers?

Esping-Andersen (1990) has used Germany as a type case of the conservative corporatist welfare state. This is considered 'status conserving' in that it links workers' contributions with their entitlement to benefits. However, non-workers, such as single mothers who are unpaid carers and domestic workers, are not included in this analysis. Therefore this welfare state theory has been called 'gender-blind', and it is certainly 'single mother blind'. Leibfried (1993) developed the concept that citizenship in Germany's 'Bismarkian institutional welfare state' remains essentially *male* citizenship because it is oriented to the 'male form' of lifetime, continuous work.

Feminist researchers who look more explicitly at the position of women in the welfare states undertake a more differentiating approach which includes both women who are at work and those who are not. Hobson (1994) argues that the German welfare state regime supports the wives of working men and therefore the male-breadwinner/female-home-maker family (see also Meyer, 1994; Lewis and Ostner, 1994). Because the German benefit system is based on a contributory benefit system it supports workers or workers' wives rather than citizens (Wilson, 1993; Laisney et al., 1993).

However, Germany is no longer (if it ever was) a pure model of the conservative welfare regime. Recently a change towards a more 'modernized' approach has become clear. Firstly, women working part time have become more acceptable, and secondly, policies have been implemented to support previously unpaid caring work mostly undertaken by women.

A sort of compromise seems to have been reached for married women.

German men as well as women increasingly accept part-time working mothers. There is no strong movement towards full-time education for children and the majority of women seem to support the socio-cultural consensus that married mothers should be in part-time employment and continue to be dependent on male breadwinners (Pfau-Effinger, 1994). This view coincides with the Christian Democratic Government's preference for the integration of mothers into the labour force on a part-time basis: 'We need more family-friendly working hours, more part-time jobs – also for the qualified (skilled) professions, more kindergartens and child care facilities near work places' (Bundesministerium für Familien, Senioren, Frauen und Jugend, 1994: 12, translated by the author). The splitting of taxable income between husband and wife (*Ehegattensplittung*) fits into this view in that it encourages wives to have no or only a little income.

For single mothers the 'part-time' and the 'contributory' systems have not been altered and therefore we can agree with Hobson that:

> solo mothers have no policy domain either as full-time carers or as paid workers. Within the gender logic of the German policy constellation that is organised around marital status or paid work, solo mothers are a residual category.
>
> (1994: 182)

Single mothers clearly fall outside the 'wives of working men' category. Thus, the argument goes, if there is no male breadwinner in a family, single mothers should be encouraged to take up employment. However, unofficially, the Christian Democratic Government's welfare state regime is shaped by the Church and Christian beliefs in that it (a) takes on the role of the male breadwinner in part and (b) does not encourage single mothers to be in employment, especially if they have young children. This view is supported by public perception of single mothers and pro-natalist public policies (Napp-Peters, 1983, 1987; Bertram and Dannenbeck, 1991).

Whether the wider acceptance of part-time work, financial benefits for caring and a generous maternity leave, are a step towards more equality or whether they will help to conserve women's status as dependants, and therefore the 'conservative' welfare model is open to debate. One could argue that the German welfare state so far has been robust and that the accreditation of 'socially useful' activities reconfirms the traditional principle and characteristics of Germany's social market economy (see Clasen and Gould, 1995). Thus, on one hand reimbursement for caring in the home socially and financially acknowledges previously unpaid caring work, mostly conducted by women. On the other hand it may 'tie' women even more to caring work in the home, militating against their recent expanded role in the labour market.

Germany's conservative welfare state's policies: single mothers as dependants?

Since the beginning of 1996 every child over the age of three has a statutory right to a place in a Kindergarten (*Rechtsanspruch auf einen Kindergarten-platz*). It remains to be seen how local authorities can implement this law in practice. This legal right may enable mothers to seek paid employment although it can only really be seen as promoting part-time work because most Kindergartens close at midday. Only 10 per cent of all Kindergartens offer day-care facilities. It is thus difficult for single mothers to be in full-time employment and they are not able to live self-sufficiently as a consequence. In this way some mothers may be 'kept in place' (Brand, 1989). The government also seems to discourage women with children under the age of three from working at all. In the old Länder only 3 per cent of creches took children under that age (Laisney et al., 1993).

A major pro-natalist policy is the introduction of child rearing benefit (*Erziehungsgeld*). For children born after 1 January 1993, payments of DM 600 per month (£267) are made for 24 months. It is tax free and does not count as earned income for other state benefits.

A single mother who was employed before the birth of her child is also entitled to 36 months maternity leave (*Erziehungsurlaub*), with part-time employment up to 19 hours a week allowed during this period. Mothers' return to their previous job and position is assured, although this does not mean they can expect to work the hours that would suit them. After a three-year interruption mothers are also disadvantaged with regard to employment experience. Most mothers re-enter paid work at a lower qualification level. Gutschmidt (1989) sees this typical female employment biography as mainly responsible for single mothers' lower income.

In summary, although single mothers may not be catered for especially, the German welfare state regime treats them as child rearers during the first two years of their child's life. Mothers are able to live relatively comfortably on the benefits offered.

For the year the child is between two and three years old, single mothers are in 'no man's land'. The expiration of the two-year child rearing benefit represents an estimated 30 per cent fall in monthly public transfers if the single mother receives state benefits, although mothers are also still entitled to maternity leave. On the other hand state benefit policies state that only single mothers with a child over three years have to be available for paid employment, and the statutory right to child care is also only available when the child has turned three.

Mothers who receive benefits and whose children are over three years old are treated as workers in theory, but not in practice. State benefit offices have the right to force single mothers into paid work, but enforcement is handled laxly by regional offices and thus is not really an issue.

Single mothers who are not in employment are seen as family dependants.

It is characteristic of the German welfare system that family members, such as parents, grandparents, biological fathers and ex-spouses, are legally obliged to support the dependant. Only if this cannot be fulfilled is state benefit paid in full, and even then it can be recovered from the liable member of the family if their income exceeds certain limits (Hauser, 1992).

This policy, in addition to the other described benefits, reveals how single mothers are positioned as dependants more than as mothers or workers by social policy. In the German welfare state it is accepted that single mothers do not work and gain economic independence, and the state is prepared to pay the bill for this and to perform the male-breadwinner role. In doing so it does not jeopardize the traditional conservative commitment to the male-breadwinner/ female-home-maker role.

However, it seems that German social policy may have the opposite effect to the one it desires. Despite the public and social policy view that single mothers do not need to be in employment – despite the form of state benefits, the lack of a partner to rely on, inflexible child care, schools and shop-opening times – single mothers are more likely to be in employment and in particular to be in full-time employment than their married counterparts. Women are developing in a quite opposite direction to that intended by state policy. It could therefore be argued that individual attitudes and behaviour with regard to gender change are ahead of, or different from, the public gender attitudes and behaviour represented by the welfare state regime. Individualization may matter more than social policy (see Beck and Beck-Gernsheim, 1990). Women can decide how to live more independently – and not necessarily in line with policies which are based on traditional values – either deciding not to take up paid work and obtain benefits to support this, or viewing employment as a means to live self-sufficiently and independently.

Bureaucratic collectivism in the former GDR: single mothers who worked

Reunification has ended the post-war 'bureaucratic state collectivist system of welfare' that was exported from the Soviet Union, and which was especially well developed in the former GDR (Deacon, 1992). GDR welfare state policies clearly positioned mothers, married as well as single, as workers. Before reunification in 1988, 89 per cent of all single mothers were in full-time paid employment· in comparison to just 57 per cent in the former FRG (Walther, 1992).

Child care was available, flexible, free and open long hours (mostly from 6 am to 6 pm). As many as 80 per cent of all children under three years were cared for in nurseries in 1989, and 95 per cent of children between three and six went to Kindergarten. Mothers were eligible to one 'baby year' in which they continued to receive their income without working. Non-marital children always had the same legal rights as marital children. Divorce procedures were straightforward and cheap. Every working mother had special rights and single mothers received subsidies (Drauschke and Stolzenburg, 1994a, 1994b).

In the public discourse in the socialist former GDR, working single mothers were accepted and portrayed as 'super-women' who could manage everything: work, household and child care (Schwarz and Mieder, 1993). Nonetheless, the socialist ideal of a family was the nuclear family with two to three children, the parents in full employment and active in society. To be a single mother was considered acceptable as long as it was for a limited period only.

In the former GDR men and women had reached equal levels in education, vocational training and labour-market experience. However, women were paid less than men throughout the country's entire history even if they did the same job, and single mothers remained the poorest family type (although still faring better than their former FRG counterparts) (Sorensen and Trappe, 1995; Hauser et al., 1994).

Reunification has quickly changed the GDR's bureaucratic state collective system into a capitalist welfare system (Deacon, 1992). Single mothers in the East were almost immediately faced with the West German understanding of the social market economy. Full employment disappeared, unemployment increased, and employment became more insecure. Child-care facilities have deteriorated and are no longer free. While housing has become more expensive and subsidies are being cut, wages have not been increasing at the same rate. Liberal abortion and divorce laws are being reduced to traditional, West German conservative standards, and are increasingly influenced by the Church. For feminists this is considered an enormous 'backlash' (Behrend, 1995; Deacon, 1992).

The material position of single mothers, as discussed in section two, has also deteriorated – although of course both men and women originally welcomed the new-won freedom in the new Länder.

5. Single Mothers in Labour Markets

Economic restructuring and cultural continuity in the new Länder

The recession and the restructuring of the labour market in the new Länder since 1990 has seen a massive contraction in the typical male sectors. Men are now competing with women in former female work spheres. An increasing trend towards gender segregation can be observed (Hauser et al., 1991). Before reunification in 1990, women in the former GDR tended to work in light industries and in the service sector (e.g. the retail trade, post office, banks and insurance and 'other' services). However, after reunification these former female dominated sectors have developed more and more into mixed sectors, while previously mixed sectors have tended to become male dominated (e.g.

agriculture and processing trades). Former male-dominated sectors have become even more single sex (e.g. transport; mining; construction and manufacture) (Schenk and Schlegel, 1993: 375). Women, and single mothers in particular, may well be becoming the 'losers of reunification'.

The former GDR is a good example of the fact that high female labour-force participation, even with full-time work, does not automatically lead to egalitarian gender role attitudes or to increased social freedom for women (Sorensen and Trappe, 1995). The transformation of the socialist former GDR into part of capitalist unified Germany is a step into a 'new modernity'. This transformation is based on gender inequality, such as sex segregation and unequal pay, as well as gender equality. Gender equality and its values were prescribed and dictated by the socialist government. Even though this understanding of equality was accepted by 'everyday consciousness' it now appears that it was superficial and unstable, and moreover bore little relation to women's double burden at home and in labour markets.

Because paid work in the former GDR was obligatory, work was less valued as a means of self-fulfilment than in the former FRG, where women's paid employment was not mandatory and where the struggle for women's right to work has been fought in terms of individual freedom (Braun et al., 1994). This, together with traditional gender values, worsening labour-market conditions and increasing job segregation may have resulted in some mothers withdrawing from the labour market in the new Länder (Schenk and Schlegel, 1993). Reunification gave single mothers the opportunity to escape the double burden of motherhood and paid work by being able to rear their child themselves with support from modest state benefits.

Mikrozensus data in April 1994 shows that female employment in the new Länder has decreased and unemployment has increased. Married mothers in the new Länder are also more likely to be in paid work than single mothers there, unlike the old Länder (Statistisches Bundesamt, 1996). It remains to be seen whether these differences are due to labour-market discrimination against single mothers, or due to single mothers' decisions not to be in employment and to escape the double burden of paid work and unpaid domestic work.

In this respect, studies in the new Länder find that single mothers are still particularly motivated to be in paid employment and to stay in their jobs. Financial independence is still seen as very important and state benefits are disapproved of. Paid work is also seen as a means of integration in society, financially as well as socially. Single mothers in the new Länder are highly 'modernized' and have not changed their attitudes towards employment. However they are restricted by the economic recession and continuing segregation (e.g. Dannenbeck et al., 1995; Schneider, 1994; Bertram, 1995). Nevertheless, of all single mothers in employment, single mothers in the new Länder are about twice as likely to be in full-time employment (of 36 hours or more) than single mothers in the old Länder (Statistisches Bundesamt, 1996).

Economic restructuring and cultural continuity in the old Länder

As Duncan and Edwards argued in the introduction to this volume, welfare state theories tend to ignore sub-national differences. The geographical distribution of single mothers and their uptake of paid work in Germany has three dimensions: the north–south divide, the east–west divide and the rural–urban divide. I will discuss them in turn.

The north–south divide in the old Länder

Throughout the old Länder, single mothers as a proportion of all mothers with children under 18 years is fairly equal, and only marginally lower in the predominantly Catholic south (around 12 per cent) than in the Protestant north (around 14 per cent). The exceptions are the city Länder (*Stadtstaaten*) of Bremen (22 per cent), Hamburg (24 per cent) and Berlin (28 per cent), where the proportion of single mothers in the new Länder has always tended to be higher – as discussed earlier (Statistisches Bundesamt, 1996). The north–south divide is therefore not a factor in the different regional prevalence of single mothers.

However, as can be seen in Table 7.6, there is quite a substantial difference in the uptake of paid work between the Länder. Single mothers' labour-force participation in 1994 was highest in the south, and the region has therefore overtaken the rate of working single mothers in the new Länder. Participation is lowest in the northern and in parts of the old industrial west and in some city states.

Labour-market participation cannot be explained by labour-market factors alone. Rather the historical context has to be considered when trying to understand why women, and single mothers, in the south are most likely to be in paid employment – even though Bayern and Baden-Württemberg, with high single-mother participation rates, are states where the majority of citizens are Catholic (Bertram and Dannenbeck, 1991). Catholics tend to have a strong family orientation, with the male as a breadwinner and the female as a home-maker.

Historically, with industrialization, paid employment became removed from the home, which became purely a place for housework conducted by women. However, industrialization processes varied regionally, and as a result, female employment had, and still has, different meaning in different regions. This was reinforced by economic structures. For example, Baden-Württemberg combined agricultural sectors with the decentralized manufacturing sector and small businesses. These activities permitted the integration of employment and housework and could be adjusted according to the requirements of the family, where women's work outside the home was already favoured in this region (Sackmann and Häussermann, 1994).

	Married mothers working (%)	Single mothers working (%)
South		
Baden Württemberg	56	70
Bayern	60	72
North		
Niedersachsen	52	58
Schleswig-Holstein	50	56
West		
Hessen	51	67
Rheinland-Pfalz	53	65
Old industrial west		
Nordrhein-Westfalen	43	55
Saarland	42	47
City states		
Bremen	43	40
Hamburg	53	56
Berlin (East & West)	66	67
New Länder		
Brandenburg	73	68
Mecklenburg/Vorpommern	76	67
Sachsen	73	63
Sachsen-Anhalt	74	67
Thüringen	74	63

Source Mikrozensus data from April 1994 and author's own calculations

Table 7.6 Married and single mothers with children under the age of 18 by Land and labour-force participation: Germany, 1994

The majority of people in northern Germany are Protestant, and the divorce rate tends to be higher than in the south (Bertram and Dannenbeck, 1991). Nonetheless the participation rate for single mothers is much lower than in the south (or the former GDR). Historically, industrialization in Northern Germany started late, was poorly developed and was geared towards agriculture. Some women worked on farms, while some women who could not find work in agriculture emigrated into the cities and became servants but did not necessarily combine work with a family (Sackmann and Häussermann, 1994).

Nordrhein-Westfalen and Saarland were the core areas of German industrialization. However as Table 7.6 shows, single mothers' employment rates are lowest in these areas. This region became highly industrialized but was dominated by heavy industry and mining – neither of which employed many women. The service sector was also only poorly developed. In addition, the pace and nature of early industrialization in the locality emphasized women's domestic role (Sackmann and Häussermann, 1994).

Single mothers in the old Länder were more likely to be in full-time employment than their married counterparts, as discussed in section two. Within this however, their full-time participation rate also varied. As Table 7.7 shows, it was higher in the *Stadtstaaten* (city states) of Hamburg and Berlin. Schleswig-Holstein in the north and Baden-Württemberg in the south show the lowest full-time rates.

These regional differences in the role of women, especially mothers, combined with regional economic differences and their historical development, have significantly influenced women's oportunities to combine employment and housework (Sackmann and Häussermann, 1994).

However, the 'north–south divide' appears to be in contrast to traditional religious belief systems. The south is predominantly Catholic and traditional, and attitude surveys suggest that people in the south are not in favour of women entering the labour force in contrast to people in the more 'liberal' protestant north. Yet single mothers' labour-force participation rate is *higher* in the south than in the north. This disparity has been used to explain family

	Married mothers (%)	Single mother (%)
Deutschland	47	62
Old Länder	38	56
New Länder	75	82
South		
Baden Württemberg	37	49
Bayern	37	54
North		
Niedersachsen	33	50
Schleswig-Holstein	32	42
West		
Hessen	34	51
Rheinland-Pfalz	37	55
Old industrial west		
Nordrhein-Westfalen	38	53
Saarland	35	*
City states		
Bremen	35	*
Hamburg	35	61
Berlin (East & West)	63	72
New Länder		
Brandenburg	76	84
Mecklenburg/Vorpommern	75	79
Sachsen	73	80
Sachsen-Anhalt	76	83
Thüringen	72	84

* figures considered too low to be exact
Source Mikrozensus data from April 1994 and author's own calculations
Table 7.7 Full-time employment rate (26 hours or more) of single and married mothers with children under the age of 18 by Länder: Germany, 1994

orientation in the south and the more dominant work orientation in the north (Bertram and Dannenbeck, 1991; Dannenbeck et al., 1995). There seems to be a wide gap between attitudes (reflecting more 'official' religions), and practice in the form of historically developed negotiations between men and women in households.

Economic restructuring and cultural continuity in the old and new Länder – the east–west divide

The east–west divide is a new dimension in single mothers' regional employment rates. Tables 7.6 and 7.7 show this second geographical dimension for single mothers and their employment rate. As discussed above, single mothers are most likely to be in employment in the south of Germany, and they are least likely to be in employment in the north and west.

The similar rate of single mothers' employment for the old Länder and the new Länder in 1994 shows that the two Germanies are growing together quickly in this respect. The employment rate of single mothers in the GDR before reunification used to be about 90 per cent and most were in full-time employment (see Walther, 1992). Already, single mothers' employment rate in the new Länder is below that of the south and in line with some old Länder in the west (Table 7.6).

In contrast, married mothers' employment rates remained highest in the new Länder (72–76 per cent), while it is generally between 50 per cent and 60 per cent elsewhere. Again the early industrial regions of Saarland, Bremen and Nordrhein-Westphalia are the lowest, where married women's employment rates are under 50 per cent.

The decreasing number of single mothers in paid work in the new Länder is partly reflected in the unemployment figures: between 28 per cent and 31 per cent of single mothers were seeking work in April 1994. In contrast, the unemployment rate for single mothers in the northern Länder is only around 14–16 per cent, and even less in the old Länder (9–10 per cent in the southern old Länder and between 10 per cent and 12 per cent in the western old Länder) (Statistisches Bundesamt, 1996). This trend mainly correlates with labour market restructuring in the new Länder, in which single mothers tend to be the 'losers of reunification'. These figures also show that single mothers in the new Länder want to remain economically active and do not simply withdraw into single motherhood (Kaufmann, 1995; Quack and Maier, 1994).

Nonetheless, single mothers in almost every old Land are twice as likely to be unemployed, but are also more likely to be in employment than married mothers. In contrast, single mothers in the new Länder are 'only' between a quarter and a third more likely to be unemployed but are also less likely than their married counterparts to be in paid employment (Statistisches Bundesamt, 1996).

A 1989–90 opinion survey showed that men and women in the new Länder were less traditional than men and women in the old Land of Bayern. While 64 per cent of Bavarians thought that being a housewife and mother was totally fulfilling, only 34 per cent in the new Länder held this opinion. However, although there were surface differences in attitudes, they became similar when a closer look was taken. Both East Germans and Bavarians thought that full-time working mothers could not care sufficiently for their children (Dannenbeck et al., 1995).

Table 7.7 shows that more working single mothers in the whole of Germany tended to be in full-time work than married mothers in 1994. Furthermore, single mothers in the new Länder are much more likely to work 36 hours or more a week than single mothers with work in the old Länder. Thus, if mothers in the new Länder continued to be in employment after reunification they remained in the full-time work that was predominant in the former GDR. This is especially the case for single mothers.

Rural–urban divide

The third variable dimension in single mothers' uptake of paid work is the rural–urban divide. It has long been suggested that regional differences have not been sufficiently considered in academic social research (see Giddens, 1987). However, there are theories which incorporate urban 'modernity' and rural 'tradition' which support the 'distribution of modern lifestyles', such as single-mother families (see Duncan, 1995; Bertram and Dannenbeck, 1991).

According to small-scale studies in the former FRG and the old Länder, single mothers are much more likely to live in large cities than in rural areas and small towns, in comparison with coupled parents (Birg and Floethmann, 1994; Walther, 1992; Nauck, 1993). Single mothers from rural areas or small towns tend to move to larger cities because they fear prejudice and discrimination, or because of increased labour-market opportunities in cities (Napp-Peters, 1987). An additional explanation could be that higher divorce rates in cities create housing opportunities for single adults with children and better child-care facilities (Bertram and Dannenbeck, 1991). Single mothers living in cities are happier with their situation. Relative anonymity as well as more open-minded city attitudes may explain their feelings (Drauschke and Stolzenburg, 1994a).

Where the east–west divide meets the urban–rural divide, the number of single mothers is highest. The proportion of single mothers in East Berlin in 1994 passed the 30 per cent mark; it is now the state where single mothers form the largest proportion of families with children. All Stadtstaaten (East and West Berlin, Hamburg and Bremen) tend to have much higher proportions of single mothers than the other Länder, whether in the east or in the west (Statistisches Bundesamt, 1996).

However, although more single mothers tend to live and feel happy in cities, this does not mean that they are in employment and therefore financially independent. Table 7.6 shows that the employment rate was highest in Berlin (East and West), because of the traditionally high percentage of East Berliners in paid work. Only 56 per cent of single mothers in Hamburg and only 40 per cent in Bremen were in paid employment. This could only partly be explained by the higher unemployment rate in city-states (15 per cent in Hamburg and 19 per cent in East and West Berlin – no data is available for Bremen).

In terms of part-time labour-force participation it appears that mothers in Länder-capitals are more likely to work full time, while mothers in rural areas are more likely to work part time (Birg and Flöthmann, 1994). Table 7.7 shows that in the city-states of Hamburg and East and West Berlin single mothers' full-time employment rate is certainly higher than average for the new Länder (respectively 72 per cent and 61 per cent).

For single mothers the 'male-breadwinner/female-home-maker' model does not quite work in the same way as for married mothers. While the welfare state regime is prepared to substitute the missing male breadwinner to a certain extent and for a certain time, it might have a double-sided effect. In cities, the discourse of single motherhood as 'escaping patriarchy' might be more prevalent than in rural areas. The state may become the acceptable breadwinner and single mothers may not work at all for a limited time to be able to redefine their lives and to rear the child by themselves (Mädje and Neusüß, 1994b). However, if single mothers in city-states are in paid employment, they tend to be in full-time employment. Some single mothers may decide to be financially independent and identify themselves as a worker as well as a mother.

Pluralization of lifestyles is at a more advanced stage in urban areas and this is an effect of individualization (Beck and Beck-Gernsheim, 1990). This section has shown that local attitudes and behaviour in regard to gender are crucial for single mothers' decisions about whether to take up employment. Such sets of expectations and belief systems depend on historical and regionally developed processes (see Duncan, 1995).

6. Single Mothers in Neighbourhoods

Support networks – child care and neighbourhoods

Social networks have a major function in coping with single motherhood. With the onset of single parenthood, mothers' network often change; many relationships cease, especially if they are connected with the leaving partner. While single mothers are not isolated one cannot speak of *a* single-mother network (Niepel, 1994a, 1994b). Single mothers are not a homogenous group, although their social networks tend to be dominated by women – especially other single mothers – rather than family. In these networks there is much give and take support, for example exchange babysitting (Niepel, 1994b; Heiliger,

1993; Schülein, 1994). In a qualitative study carried out in East Berlin, single mothers were found to draw very much on 'Nachbarschaftshilfe', that is neighbourhood help. Many women had a good relationship with neighbours and shared child care (Drauschke and Stolzenburg, 1994a).

The empirical evidence for this section is based on the author's own study.[1] The analysis consists of 29 interviews with single mothers carried out in East and West Berlin in summer 1995. These semi-structured face-to-face interviews formed part of an empirical study into single motherhood discourses and employment in Britain and Germany (Klett-Davies, 1996a, 1996b). The interviews focused on the single mothers' biography, self-perception and opinions.[2] All those interviewed received state benefits, had at least one child born outside marriage and were not in employment.

The data from this study reveal that most single mothers feel socially supported. Many of their friends are other single mothers, who were easily met at institutions (e.g. while waiting in state benefit offices). Interestingly, the telephone is one of the most important mediums of communication. While not all women in East Berlin were connected to the phone, single mothers used the telephone to 'meet' their friends while looking after their sleeping child. The gym (often women only) also has an important function, not only for getting into shape but also as a meeting point. Benefit recipients get a discounted rate and creches are available at certain times.

However, single mothers in rural areas may not be as socially accepted as they are in cities, and may therefore be more socially isolated.

Turkish single mothers and cultural polarization

Race and ethnicity among single mothers in Germany has not yet been researched and has so far never been an issue in press or political debates. However in 1994 only 8.4 per cent of all single parents were not German citizens in the old Länder and just 1 per cent in the new Länder (Statistisches Bundesamt, 1996).

Berlin is characterized by its Turkish migrant population. My own study of single motherhood amongst women in Berlin shows that Turkish single mothers experience a variety of problems or 'clashes' with their traditional and religious families. A Turkish girl growing up in Germany learns and lives two opposing lifestyles. In the private sphere of her family she is taught traditional Muslim family values, while in Kindergarten, at school and at work in the public sphere she experiences more liberal ways of living. The two Turkish single mothers I interviewed had been 'officially' disowned by their father, cut off from their family and deserted by their older Turkish networks. However, they were often financially and practically supported in secret by their mother and sisters, rather than their German social network. For example, Burcu, a 24-year-old working-class single mother with minimal educational qualifications, has three children by three different fathers and lives on a large council estate on the outskirts of West Berlin. She has been disowned by her father and explains:

> It is difficult for [my father] to comprehend, to accept. He once said if I were married then it would not be a problem for him. Especially bad is that firstly I am not married and secondly that the children are from three different fathers. That is very difficult for him. Some fathers would accept it but the Turkish society, his friends, what they say about this, to have to defend this. They can't handle this. My mother is the same. . . . It is this way in every family who has this problem. That one child did something which does not agree with the tradition. Most can manage to iron it over or to hide it. My mother told everyone I was married and got divorced.

Burcu and other Turkish single mothers also tend to have their school and work biography frequently interrupted by their families. Parents often do not value education, training and work experience as an asset for their daughters, seeing them as contradictory to their traditional beliefs. The single mothers in my study had obtained hardly any educational qualifications and no vocational training. This makes it especially difficult for them to live self-sufficiently. However, the emotional strain of discrimination and disownment weighs heavily on these womens' shoulders, and they focus on the labour market as a way out of state and family dependence. For example, Meral, a teenage Turkish working-class single mother living on a large council estate in West Berlin, has no educational or vocational qualifications. She wants to enter an apprenticeship to enhance her future prospects, not just for herself but primarily for her child's material security:

> I need a job. I need a proper job, where I will be able to work later, where I can get an apprenticeship. I mean, I don't get child rearing benefit next year again. And I don't get advanced maintenance for ever, and child rearing benefit and this and that. I stop receiving child rearing benefit when the child is two years old and I want to be able to offer my child something later.

Social identities as mothers or as workers

From the earlier discussion in section five we could assume that single mothers in the old Länder identify themselves more as mothers than as workers, while single mothers in the new Länder clearly identify themselves as workers and not just as mothers. However, data from my own study do not confirm this.

In interviews with single mothers in East and West Berlin, some of the following discourses become obvious regardless of residency in East or West Berlin: (i) mothers who want to work but who face obstacles as workers; (ii) mothers who want to be full-time mothers for a certain time period; (iii) mothers who have certain requirements as workers that cannot be fulfilled; and (iv) workers who want to use the time to redefine their lives or to 'build a future'.

(i) Mothers who want to work but who face obstacles as workers

More 'economistic' social policy theorists sometimes assume that single mothers are in paid work only for a financial return (Laisney et al., 1993; Staat and Wagenhals, 1993, 1994). However, although it is not always cost efficient for single mothers to be in paid work many still continue to take up employment for a whole range of 'non-economic' gains, such as self respect and respect from others, feelings of independence, making friends and getting out of the home (Birg and Floethmann, 1994). Single mothers continue to view work as a means of integration into society, financially as well as socially. However, this has not always been made easy for them.

Susanne is a White working-class single mother and lives with her two daughters in a two-bedroom flat on a small, well-maintained council estate on the outskirts of West Berlin. She has no educational or vocational qualifications and has never been in permanent paid employment. When her first daughter was old enough to go into the Kindergarten she applied for work at the local chemist but was faced with changing times of work. Appropriate child care for the hours required would have been impossible to find. Germany's welfare state regime may have become 'modernized' by accepting mothers working part time, but it remains conservative in that it does not accommodate full-time mothers:

> At [name of the local chemist] I wanted to work. Because they were looking for people. But I would have faced a difficulty. . . . Because Kindergartens are not open in the afternoon and I would have had to do shifts. One week in the morning and one week in the afternoon. And I definitely would have faced problems, and my mum was in [name of town] and was not here. She lived there five years. I did not have friends as such, who I could ask to take care of my child while I had to work. . . . Childminders do also not work in the evening. They only work from 8 or 7 until midday 16 or 17 o'clock. That would have been difficult.

As with the other single mothers not in paid work, Susanne lists a variety of reasons to defend or justify her situation as a full-time mother. The reasons most often mentioned by the single mothers were: lack of flexible child care and support from family and friends, low wages, inflexible hours of work (shifts) and prejudice from potential employers. Susanne says:

I have registered with them [Catholic Kindergarten] every three months and after half a year I gave up. I also registered [my second daughter] and only the miniclub has offered a place. There she can go Tuesday, Thursdays and Fridays for three hours. And I do not get a Kindergarten place. It is really hard to get. You have to have a job first. When you can show that you have work you get a Kindergarten space. A friend of mine, who is also by herself, she can start on Monday [in her new job] and can only use the Kindergarten from Tuesday onwards. On Monday the grandma has to take care of the child. And I do not have this possibility. My mother is still young. She is 44 and not a pensioner but works part time. She could take the children sometimes but she does not do this.

(ii) Mothers who want to be full-time mothers for a certain time period

Some single mothers may decide to 'escape patriarchy', in that they decide not to rely on a male breadwinner's income and still have a child. Instead, the state becomes an acceptable breadwinner. Single mothers may identify themselves as mothers and not as workers despite the fact that they may be criticized for their state dependence. Their first priority is to rear the child by themselves and to be a 'good' mother.

As it happened, Susanne became pregnant again before she could start work. Her second daughter is now about three years old. She describes the decision-making process between work and full-time motherhood as a Catch 22. Living off benefits and committing herself to family life is not easy for her. Her mother would not help with child care and her father is not necessarily supportive either:

My father even. He once said to me: 'Think about it. I am working and you are living off me. I pay taxes for you to be able to receive state benefits'. Yes, this raises some thoughts, and one thinks how stupid this is. But somehow I wanted to be there for my children. It is a real Catch 22. You want to be there, but have to live off the benefit office to be able to stay at home. And, and then you are dependent and a parasite, that's what they say nowadays. It is difficult.

However, Susanne finds support for her decision to be a full-time mother elsewhere. Staff at the Catholic Kindergarten tell Susanne that she should be happy to be able to be a full-time mother and that she should enjoy this time:

Before I got [my second child] I have put [my first child] on the Kindergarten waiting list. I have never received a place. [My first child] was three years old and they [Catholic Kindergarten] said I should enjoy this free time at home, 'You do not have to go to work'.

Although mothers in the former GDR were supposed to be workers, these gender values were not always fully internalized. For example, Anne is a middle-aged middle-class woman who has been working for 15 years as a make-up artist for TV and film in the former GDR. She and her six-year-old son live either with her parents or in a one-bedroom unmodernized flat in an old purpose-built block in East Berlin. While she was working she saved up because she wanted to dedicate herself to full-time motherhood in the future. Her relationship did not last and she is not a single mother by choice:

> And I worked in my job and told myself, when I am at a certain age I want, if it works, a child and for this I save money. I prepared for this. During GDR times I would have not needed to go back to work for a long time. I needed to save because there you had no state support and I definitely wanted to be there for my child, about 5, 6 years. . . . Because I experienced so many negative things through my colleagues who had children and held on to a job. It is bad for the children when the parents are not at home. I did not want to do this.

(iii) Mothers who have certain requirements as workers that cannot be fulfilled

Paid work is not really an option for some single mothers. For example, without educational and vocational qualifications and with no work experience Susanne will probably not be likely to earn much more than she receives in state benefits, housing and child benefit. It makes no financial sense to enter paid employment. Moreover, there are hardly any opportunities and desirable jobs which pay enough for her and her daughters to live independently. Susanne is also not prepared to do just any job:

> It does not matter [that I have fun in my job]. I would even clean toilets. The most important thing is that the job pays well. Not that I only earn DM 1,500 (£667). Then I would still have to go to the benefit office. . . . That would mean that I remain a state benefit recipient. . . . You work in a factory, although that would not be a job for me, where the Kindergarten is next door, they do exist. . . . I think DM 2,500 (£1,100) is what you would need, to be able to get by with rent and everything.

Similarly, Conni, a White working-class single mother, lives in an unmodernized ground-floor one-bedroom flat with her mother and her two daughters in East Berlin. Paid work is also not really an option for her because it would be difficult to make enough for her and her daughters to live on:

I don't really want to go to work by all means but I would like to have more money in the house. It all more or less has to do with money. . . . I have not really worked properly apart from the two years in this apprenticeship. That is already lethargy more or less, I would say. I am used more or less to being at home, and you can get used to this. . . . I got used to being at home.

Because of her work experience and the type of work Conni thinks she would be able to get, non-financial gain from employment is difficult for her to imagine.

Another Susanne, White and lower-middle class, has one young son and lives in a modernized purpose-built old building in West Berlin. She has been trained as a clerk/administrator and identifies herself very much as a worker. She has been looking for a part-time job for a long time. Her self-esteem is running low because she has not been very successful in finding a job:

I have noticed that it is very difficult to find anything [a job] because I want to work part-time of course. Although I have one thousand fears whether I will be able to do it. Also job wise . . . when I read the adverts, you have to be perfect and flexible and and and. They are all things I have not got. I cannot be flexible. I am not perfect.

She is by now so frustrated that she cannot find an appropriate job that she does not necessarily resent unfriendly labour-market conditions but blames herself and her situation as a mother:

I would feel better if I had no child. That is a definite. . . . I had work. I had work in sales. When you are free and independent you can do all sorts of things. I could work in all sorts of areas. I could do night shifts, no problem.

Previous research has shown that education seems to be closely related with the degree of single mothers' self-satisfaction and self-esteem. Single mothers in the old Länder who have lower educational and vocational attainment view their situation negatively in comparison with single mothers who are more highly educated and may have a less traditional attitude and therefore feel less guilty. Moreover, the latter might also be less likely to be confronted with conservative attitudes or outright prejudice against single mothers within their social and familiar networks (Sander, 1993).

(iv) Redefinition and preparation for the future

For some of the single mothers I interviewed in East and West Berlin the birth of their child meant an enormous shift in their perception of responsibility.

Some women might not have had a clearly defined aim regarding education and other qualifications. However, the birth of their child had sometimes kick-started thoughts about their future.

As single mothers in the new Länder learn more about their rights and entitlements, my data show that they also feel less inhibited in receiving state benefits. In both the old and the new Länder, single mothers have used state benefits as a modest means to seek new orientations and options in life as well as an opportunity to rear their child. In this way the state is not merely a replacement for the patriarchal breadwinner.

In a study of part of West Berlin, Mädje and Neusüß (1994a, 1994b) also find that single mothers use state benefits as an enabler. Despite the poverty and social stigma attached to receiving benefits, most of these single mothers do not see state benefit dependency as a personal failure. Instead, they feel justified in receiving state benefits as a kind of reimbursement for rearing a child who would eventually become a working member of society. These single mothers feel further justified in placing responsibility for their lifestyle on society.

However, such views might also be a self-defence mechanism to justify dependency on state benefits. I would further suggest that it is quite a normal reaction for interviewees to appear more confident and secure than they actually feel. It can be taken for granted that most people justify the situation they are in. I have found in interviews that some single mothers in West Berlin use a 'moral superiority factor' for legitimating their situation. they see themselves as more deserving than, for example, asylum seekers.

Sabine is a good example of this 'enabler' attitude. She is a White middle-class woman who is a qualified nurse and lives in a modernized one-bedroom flat in East Berlin. She has given up her job as a nurse and is going to do the equivalent of 'A' levels at college. Sabine does not just identify herself as a mother but also recognizes her own need to do something satisfying. She accepts that she has to be state dependent for a while to be able to achieve this. She uses the child rearing time to redefine her life and has given herself another three years to think about what she wants to do in the future while she studies at college:

> I also prefer to do something that I enjoy, therefore I make the compromise of receiving money from the state and I have to defend it there instead of working for years and years in private nursing homes and getting dissatisfied. I have to judge for myself what is more important for me and how I can manage better.

Single mothers' individual decisions about whether or not to enter paid work are embedded within complex structures. The four discourses emerging from my study and described above, illuminate these decision-making processes.

7. Conclusion: Single Mothers in Unified Germany: Workers, Mothers, Dependants or Man Eaters?

In this chapter I have argued that Germany, although now one country, continues to show two national trends among single mothers relating to their composition, labour-force characteristics and participation rates.

I further showed that single mothers can be considered a residual social category. Although motherhood is initially encouraged and rewarded, ultimately single mothers are not catered for either as full-time workers or as paid carers. The German welfare state regime focuses on the male-breadwinner/female-home-maker model, which has been modernized by women working part-time only. However, social policy treats single mothers as dependants more than as mothers or workers. The German welfare state is content that single mothers remain in some form of dependency. It is prepared to replace the male-breadwinner role in part. In so doing the traditional conservative welfare state regime is not jeopardized.

However social policy regimes cannot entirely explain why single mothers act the way they do, because this typology ignores social contexts. Despite Germany's male-breadwinner/female-home-maker regime, single mothers are not only taking part in the labour force but also in full-time work, and more so than married mothers. This view assumes that inclusion of single mothers into employment is the means of social inclusion and equality. The kind of work undertaken (skilled or unskilled, menial or not) does not correlate with the gains experienced such as satisfaction. However, single mothers also remain poor and face a double burden.

It seems that single mothers are developing in an opposite direction to that intended by state policies. Therefore, it can be argued, there is a gap between individual attitudes and behaviour with regard to gender, and public gender attitudes and behaviour represented by welfare state regimes. In addition, socio-economic contexts and the cultural and historical backgrounds of the former two Germanies, as well as lifestyle discourses and individualization processes, have to be considered when analysing these phenomena. For example, there is the strong old Länder–new Länder divide as well as the strong rural–urban divide for single mothers.

However, data from my own research point to the fact that single mothers in the West can share similar sets of values and belief systems with those in the East. For example, both can identify themselves as not just either mothers or workers. Describing single mothers as either mothers (West) or workers (East) is too simplistic. Secondly, there is no major difference in attitudes towards employment on the part of the mothers in both East and West Berlin who at the time of interview were not in paid employment.

From my study four discourses became obvious. The first is that single mothers want to work but face obstacles such as insufficient child care. Secondly, there are single mothers who want to be full-time mothers for as long as they feel that the child requires it. Thirdly, there are mothers who want to be 'good' mothers as well as workers but face obstacles in combining these two, for example in finding part-time work.

The fourth discourse concerns single mothers who want to use their time as a state-dependent mother to redefine their lives or to educate themselves further to 'build a future'. Here the state becomes the acceptable breadwinner for a time. These mothers have realized that paid employment may be a means of social inclusion and equality. However, the other side of the coin is that single mothers also remain poor and are faced with the double burden of paid employment and unpaid domestic work. Sometimes further education becomes a way to exit the poverty trap, enhancing future prospects with motherhood. Sometimes full-time child-rearing time is used to help in seeking self-fulfilment.

In public discourse the notion of state-dependent single motherhood as a way of redefinition or 'escaping patriarchy' is beginning to be seen as a social threat by men who may feel left behind. It is to be seen whether this view will become more widespread and lead to single mothers being scapegoated for high public expenditure. However, Germany is considered to be a relatively stable conservative social market economy, in comparison with more 'liberal' welfare states such as Britain and the USA, which seek to dismantle the welfare state.

However single mothers in Germany, as in the USA and Britain, have to face a Catch 22: if they decide to rear their child they are discriminated against because they receive state benefits. If these women decide to enter paid employment they are disadvantaged because labour markets are gendered. It is difficult to live self-sufficiently especially with part-time work. Full-time work might jeopardize their role as mothers. Whatever choice a single mother makes she is stigmatized.

Note

1   The study was made possible by a Human Capital and Mobility Research Fellowship at the Gender Institute at the London School of Economics and Political Science and was funded by the European Union.
2   Few women responded to my advert in a daily free advertising paper (*Zweite Hand*) but most agreed to be interviewed when I explained my research to them in waiting rooms of state benefit offices of Reinickendorf borough council in West Berlin and in Friedrichshain council in East Berlin. Reinickendorf is a large and socially polarized suburb at the edge of the city with mediocre to good infrastructure. Friedrichshain is a deprived inner-city area with good infrastructure. The 14 interviewed single mothers in Friedrichshain tended to live in unmodernized or partly modernized one-bedroom flats in purpose-built houses built in the middle of the last century. The 15 interviewed single mothers in Reinickendorf tended to live in one-bedroom flats in modern council blocks or high rise flats on medium to large council estates. All interviewees were White with German nationality, with the exception of two Turkish single mothers who lived in Reinickendorf. Most of the

single mothers had educational qualifications comparable with the rest of the population but little work experience. Most only had one child which tended to be under four years of age. Unless otherwise noted all quotations from single mothers are from the author's interviews.

References

BECK, U. and BECK-GERNSHEIM E. (1990) *Das ganz normale Chaos der Liebe*, Frankfurt a.M., Suhrkamp.

BECK, U. and BECK-GERNSHEIM E. (1994) (eds) *Riskante Freiheiten*, Frankfurt a.M., Suhrkamp.

BEHREND, H. (1995) 'East German Women and the Wende' *The European Journal of Women's Studies*, **2**, pp. 237–255.

BERGER, H., HINRICHS, W., PRILLER, E. and SCHULTZ, A. (1993) 'Veränderungen der Struktur und der sozialen Lage ostdeutscher Haushalte nach 1990' Working Group Social Reporting, Wissenschaftszentrum Berlin für Sozialforschung, Paper P 93–105, Berlin.

BERGLER, R. (1964) *Kinder aus gestörten und unvollständigen Familien*, Weinheim, Julius Beltz.

BERTRAM, H. and DANNENBECK, C. (1991) 'Familien in städtischen und ländlichen Regionen' in Bertram, H. (ed) *Die Familie in Westdeutschland*, pp. 79–112, Opladen, Leske & Budrich.

BERTRAM, B. (1995) 'Die Wende, die erwerbstätigen Frauen und die Familien in den neuen Bundesländern' in Krappmann, L., Schneewind, K. A., Vascovics, L. A. and Wurzbacher, G. (eds) *Familie und Lebensverlauf im gesellschaftlichen Umbruch*, pp. 266–284, Stuttgart, Ferdinand Enke Verlag.

BIRG, H. and FLÖTHMANN, E. J. (1994) 'Erwerbsorientierung und Lebenslauf von jungen Frauen in unterschiedlichen regionalen Lebenswelten' *Beiträge zur Arbeitsmarkt- und Berufsforschung*, **179**, Sonderdruck, pp. 253–280.

BÖHM, T. (1993) 'Allein mit Kindern – eine Familienform' in Friedrich Ebert Stiftung, Referat Frauenpolitik *Alleinerziehende in den Neuen Bundesländern*, Heft 9, pp. 9–14, Bonn, Friedrich Ebert Stiftung.

BRAND, R. (1989) 'Single parents and family preservation in the Federal Republic of Germany', *Child Welfare*, LXVIII, 2, pp. 189–195

BRAUN, M., SCOTT, J. and ALWIN, D. F. (1994) 'Economic necessity or self-actualization? Attitudes towards women's labour force participation in East and West Germany' *European Sociological Review*, **10**, 1, pp. 29–47.

BRINCK, C. (1995a) 'Wo ist Vati?' *Focus*, **5**, pp. 137–142.

BRINCK, C. (1995b) 'Warum Väter zählen' *Focus*, **14**, pp. 212–217.

BRÜNING, N. (1996) 'Schlechte Moral – Für iminer mehr Kinder muß der Staat zahlen' *Focus*, **2**, pp. 21.

BUBA, H. P., FRÜCHTEL, F. and PICKEL, G. (1995) 'Haushalts- und Familienformen junger Erwachsener und ihre Bedeutung im Ablösungsprozeß von der Herkunfts-familie – Ein Vergleich in den neuen und alten Bundesländern' in Krappmann, L., Schneewind, K. A., Vaskovics, L. A. and Wurzbacher, G. (eds) *Familie und Lebensverlauf im gesellschaftlichen Umbruch*, pp. 119–136, Stuttgart, Ferdinand Enke Verlag.

BUNDESMINISTERIUM FÜR FAMILIEN, SENIOREN, FRAUEN UND JUGEND (1994) *Materialien zur Familienpolitik der Bundesregierung*, Bonn, Bundesministerium für Familien, Senioren, Frauen und Jugend, Referat Oeffentlichkeitsarbeit.

CIERPKA, A., FREVERT, G. and CIERPKA, M. (1992) 'Männer schmutzen nur! – Eine Untersuchung über alleinerziehende Mütter in einem Mutter-Kind Programm' *Praxis der Kinderpsychologie und Kinderpsychatrie*, **41**, pp. 168–175.

CLASEN, J. and GOULD, A. (1995) 'Stability and change in welfare states: Germany and Sweden in the 1990s' *Policy and Politics*, **23**, 3, pp. 189–201.

DANNENBECK, S., KEISER, S. and ROSENDORFER, T. (1995) 'Familienalltag in den alten und neuen Bundesländern – Aspekte der Vereinbarkeit von Beruf und Familie' in Krappmann L., Schneewind, K. A., Vaskovics, L. A. and Wurzbacher, G. (eds) *Familie und Lebensverlauf im gesellschaftlichen Umbruch*, pp. 103–118, Stuttgart, Ferdinand Enke Verlag.

DEACON, B. (1992) *The New Eastern Europe – Social Policy Past, Present and Future*, London, Sage.

DRAUSCHKE, P., STOLZENBURG, M., MÄDJE, E. and NEUSÜß, C. (1993) 'Ausdauernd, selbstbewußt und (noch) optimistisch' in Friedrich Ebert Stiftung, Referat Frauenpolitik, Alleinerziehende in den Neuen Bundesländern, Heft 9, pp. 21–42, Bonn, Friedrich Ebert Stiftung.

DRAUSCHKE, P. and STOLZENBURG, M. (1994a) 'Alleinerziehende Frauen in Berlin Ost – sie wohnen wie immer, nur anders' in Bundesforschungsanstalt für Landeskunde und Raumordnung (eds) *Wohnsituation Alleinerziehender II*, Heft 62, p. 85–96, Bonn Bundesforschungsanstalt für Landeskunde und Raumordnung.

DRAUSCHKE, P. and STOLZENBERG, M. (1994b) 'Zur Situation alleinerziehender Frauen in Berlin Ost auf dem Arbeitsmarkt' Sozialwissenschaftliches Forschungszentrum e.V., *Sozialreport*, 1,Gelsenkirchen, Sozialwissenschaftliches Forschungszentrum.

DUNCAN, S. (1995) 'Theorizing European Gender Systems' *Journal of European Policy*, **5**, 4,pp. 263–284.

EDWARDS, R. and DUNCAN, S. (1996) 'Rational economic man or lone mothers in context? The uptake of paid work' in Silva E. B. (ed) *Good Enough Mothering*, pp. 114–129, London & New York, Routledge.

ESPING-ANDERSEN, G. (1990) *The Three Worlds of Welfare Capitalism*, Cambridge, Polity Press.

Frankfurter Allgemeine Zeitung (1995) 'Nur ein Teil der Sozialhilfebezieher wäre von einer Reform betroffen', *Frankfurter Allgemeine Zeitung*, 26.1.1995, p. 14.

FRISE, M. and STAHLBERG, J. (1992) *Allein mit Kind – Alleinerziehende Mütter und Väter*, München, Piper.

GIDDENS, A. (1987) *Social Theory Today*, Stanford, Stanford University Press.

GUTSCHMIDT, G. (1986) *Kind und Beruf – Alltag alleinerziehender Mütter*, Weinheim, Juventa Verlag.

GUTSCHMIDT, G. (1989) 'Armut in Einelternfamilien' *Blätter derWohlfahrtspflege*, **11–12**, pp. 335–338.

GUTSCHMIDT, G. (1994a) 'Alleinerziehende und Sozialhilfe; Klischee und Realität' *Informationen für Einelternfamilien*, Verband Alleinerziehender Mütter und Väter e.V., 6–7, pp 1–4.

GUTSCHMIDT, G. (1994b) *Single mit Kind – Alleinerziehen – wie es die anderen machen*, Freiburg, Herder.

GYSI, J. (1989) (ed) *Familienleben in der DDR – Zum Alltag von Familien mit Kindern*, Berlin, Akademie-Verlag.

HAUSER, R., MÜLLER, K., WAGNER, G. G. and FRICK, J. (1991) 'Incomes in East and West Germany on the Eve of Union – some results based on the German Socio-Economic Panel', Discussion Papers, German Institute for Economic Research, 34, Berlin.

HAUSER, R. (1992) 'Germany' in Roll, J. (ed) *Lone parent families in the European Community – The 1992 report to the European Commission*, pp. 24–25, London, European Family & Social Policy Unit.

HAUSER, R., FRICK, J., MÜLLER, K. and WAGNER, G. G. (1994) 'Inequality in income: a comparison of East and West Germans before reunification and during transition'. *Journal of European Social Policy*, **4**, 4, pp. 277–295.

HEILIGER, A. (1993) *Alleinerziehen als Befreiung*, Pfaffenweiler, Centaurus-Verlagsgesellschaft.

HOBSON, B. (1994) 'Solo mothers, Social Policy Regimes and the Logics of Gender' in Sainsbury, D. (ed) *Gendering Welfare States*, pp. 170–187, London, Sage.

KAUFMANN, F. X. (1995) *Zukunft der Familie im vereinten Deutschland – Gesellschaftliche und politische Bedingungen*, München, Verlag C.H. Beck.

KLETT-DAVIES, M. (1996a) 'Single mothers in Britain: an underclass?' Paper presented at the annual British Sociological Association conference, 1–4 April, Reading.

KLETT-DAVIES, M. (1996b) 'Single mothers in Britain and Germany: An underclass?' Paper presented at the annual Social Policy Association conference, 16–18 July, Sheffield.

LAISNEY, F., LECHNER, M., STAAT, M. and WAGENHALS, G. (1993) 'Labour Force and Welfare Participation of Lone Mothers in West Germany' Discussion paper, Zentrum für Europäische Wirtschaftsforschung, 93–26, Mannheim.

LEIBFRIED, S. (1993) 'Towards a European welfare state?' in Jones, C. (ed) *New Perspectives on the Welfare State in Europe*, pp. 133–150, London, Routledge.

LEWIS, J. and OSTNER, I. (1994) 'Gender and the Evolution of European Social Policies' ZeS-Arbeitspapier, Centre for Social Policy Research, University of Bremen, 4, Bremen.

MÄDJE, E. and NEUSÜß, E. (1994a) 'Frauen im Sozialstaat: subjective Deutungen, Orientierungen und staatliches Handeln am Beispiel alleinerziehender Sozialhilfeempfängerinnen' Dissertation, Freie Universität Berlin, Fachbereich Politische Wissenschaft, Berlin.

MÄDJE, E. and NEUSÜß, C. (1994b) 'Lone mothers on welfare in West Berlin: disadvantaged citizens or women avoiding patriarchy?' *Environment and Planning A*, **26**, pp. 1419–1433.

McFATE, K., SMEEDING, T. and RAINWATER, L. (1995) 'Markets and States: poverty trends and transfer effectiveness in the 1980s' in McFate, K., Lawson, R. and Wilson, W. J. (eds) *Poverty, inequality and the future of social policy*, pp. 29–66, New York, Russell Sage.

MEYER, D. and STAUFENBIEL, N. (1994) 'Alleinerziehende im Vergleich zu verheirateten Frauen' in Bundesforschungsanstalt für Landeskunde und Raumordnung (eds) *Wohnsituation Alleinerziehender II*, Heft 62, pp. 97–105, Bonn, Bundesforschungsanstalt für Landeskunde und Raumordnung.

MEYER, S. and SCHULZE, E. (1989) *Balancen des Glücks – Neue Lebensformen: Paare ohne Trauschein, Alleinerziehende und Singles*, München, Verlag C.H. Beck.

MEYER, T. (1994) 'The German and British Welfare States as Employers: Patriarchal or Emancipatory?' in Sainsbury, D. (ed) *Gendering Welfare States*, pp. 62–82, London, Sage.

NAPP-PETERS, A. (1983) 'Geschlechtsrollenstereotypen und ihr Einfluß auf Einstellungen zur Ein-Elternteil-Situation' *Kölner Zeitschrift für Soziologie und Sozialpsychologie*, **35**, pp. 321–334.

NAPP-PETERS, A. (1987) *Ein-Elternteil-Familien – Soziale Randgruppe oder neues familiales Selbstverständnis?*, Weinheim, Juventa Verlag.

NAUCK, B. (1993) 'Frauen und ihre Kinder: Reginale und soziale Differenzierungen in Einstellungen zu Kindern, im generativen Verhalten und in den Kindschaftsverhältnissen' in Nauck, B. (ed) *Lebensgestaltung von Frauen*, pp. 45–86, Weinheim, Juventa.

NAVE-HERZ, R. and KRÜGER, D. (1992) *Ein-Eltern-Familien – Eine empirische Studie zur Lebenssituation und Lebensplanung alleinerziehender Mütter und Väter*, Materialien zur Frauenforschung, Bielefeld, Kleine Verlag.

NAVE-HERZ, R. (1992a) 'Ledige Mutterschaft; eine alternative Lebensform?' *Zeitschrift für Sozialisationsforschung und Erziehungssoziologie*, **6**, pp. 219–232.

NAVE-HERZ, R. (1992b) *Frauen zwischen Tradition und Moderne*, Bielefeld, Kleine Verlag.

NAVE-HERZ, R. (1994) *Familie Heute – Wandel der Familienstrukturen und Folgen für die Erziehung*, Darmstadt, Wissenschaftliche Buchgesellschaft.

NEUBAUER, E. (1993a) *Zwölf Wege der Familienpolitik inder Europäischen Gemeinschaft: eigenständige Systeme und vergleichbare Qualitiäten?*, Schriftenreihe des Bundesministeriums für Familien und Senioren, 22.1, Stuttgart, Kohlhammer.

NEUBAUER, E. (1993b) *Zwölf Wege der Familienpolitik in der Europäischen Gemeinschaft: Länderberichte*, Schriftenreihe des Bundesministeriums für Familien und Senioren, 22.2, Stuttgart, Kohlhammer.

NIEPEL, G. (1994a) *Alleinerziehende – Abschied von einem Klischee*, Opladen, Leske & Budrich.

NIEPEL, G. (1994b) *Soziale Netze und soziale Unterstützung alleinerziehender Frauen; eine empirische Studie*, Opladen, Leske & Budrich.

PEUCKERT, R. (1996) *Familienformen im sozialen Wandel*, Opladen, Leske & Budrich.

PFAU-EFFINGER, B. (1994) 'The gender contract and part-time paid work by women – Finland and Germany compared' *Environment and Planning A*, **26**, pp. 1355–1376.

QUACK, S. and MAIER, F. (1994) 'From state socialism to market economy – women's employment in East Germany' *Environment and Planning A*, **26**, pp. 1257–1276.

SACKMANN, R. and HÄUSSERMANN, H. (1994) 'Regional differences in female labour-market participation in Germany' *Environmental and Planning A*, **26**, pp. 1377–1396.

SANDER, E. (1993) 'Die Situation des Alleinerziehens aus der Sicht der betroffenen Mütter' *Psychologie in Erziehung und Unterricht*, **40**, pp. 241–248.

SCHENK, S. and SCHLEGEL, U. (1993) 'Frauen in den neuen Bundesländern – Zurück in eine andere Moderne?' *Berliner Journal für Soziologie*, **3**, pp. 369–384.

SCHNEIDER, N. F. (1994) *Familie und private Lebensführung in West- und Ostdeutschland*, Stuttgart, Ferdinand Enke Verlag.

SCHÖNINGH, I., ASLANIDIS, M. and FAUBEL-DIEKMANN, S. (1991) *Alleinerziehende Frauen – Zwischen Lebenskrise und neuem Selbstverständnis*, Obláden, Leske & Budrich.

SCHÜLEIN, J. A. (1994) 'Zur Entwicklung des famiären Zusammenslebens: Von der Überlebensgruppe zur individualisierten Beziehungsgemeinschaft' in Simsa, R. (ed) *Kein Herr im Haus*, Frankfurt a.M., Fischer.

SCHÜLEIN, J. A. and SIMSA, R. (1994) 'Zur Diskriminierung von Einelternfamilien in Gesellschaft und Forschung' in Simsa, R. (ed) (1994) *Kein Herr im Haus*, Frankfurt a.M., Fischer.

SCHULTHEIS, F. (1987) 'Fatale Strategien und ungeplante Konsequenzen beim Aushandeln "familialer Risiken" zwischen Mutter, Kind und "Vater Staat"' *Soziale Welt*, **38**, pp. 40–56.

SCHWARZ, G. and MIEDER, R. (1993) 'Identitäten von Alleinerziehenden', in Friedrich Ebert Stiftung, Referat Frauenpolitik, *Alleinerziehende in den Neuen Bundesländern*, Heft 9, pp. 21–42, Bonn, Friedrich Ebert Stiftung.

SORENSEN, A. and TRAPPE, H. (1995) 'The Persistence of Gender Inequality in Earnings in the German Democratic Republic' *American Sociological Review*, **60**, pp. 398–406.

STAAT, M. and WAGENHALS, G. (1993) 'The Labour Supply of Lone Mothers in the Federal Republic of Germany', Diskussionsbeiträge aus dem Institut für Volkswirtschaftslehre, 82, Stuttgart, Universität Hohenheim.

STAAT, M. and WAGENHALS, G. (1994) 'The Labour Supply of German Single Mothers: A Bivariate Probit Model' *Vierteljahrshefte zur Wirtschaftsordnung*, **1/2**, Deutsches Institut für Wirtschaftsforschung, pp. 113–118.

STATISTISCHES BUNDESAMT (1995) *Haushalte und Familien, Reihe 3*, Wiesbaden, Kusterdingen, Metzler Poeschel.

STATISTISCHES BUNDESAMT (1996) Unpublished tables from 1994 Mikrozensus data, Wiesbaden.

TIETZE, B. (1993) 'Alleinerziehende – Prüfstein für Familienpolitik', in Friedrich Ebert Stiftung, Referat Frauenpolitik, *Alleinerziehende in den Neuen Bundesländern*, Heft 9, pp. 15–20, Bonn, Friedrich Ebert Stiftung.

VOIT, H. (1993) 'Haushalte und Familien – Ergebnisse des Mikrozensus April 1991' *Wirtschaft und Statistik*, **3**, pp. 191–199.

WALTHER, U. J. (1992) *Wohnsituation Alleinerziehender*, Heft 43, Bonn, Bundesforschungsanstalt für Landeskunde und Raumordnung.

WILSON, M. (1993) 'The German welfare state: a conservative regime in crisis' in Cochrane, A. and Clarke, J. (eds) *Comparing Welfare States: Britain in international context*, pp. 141–171, London, Sage.

WONG, Y., GARFINKEL, I. and McLANAHAN, S. (1993) 'Single-Mother families in eight countries: economic status and social policy' *Social Service Review*, **67**, 2, pp. 177–197.

Chapter 8

Single Mothers in France: Supported Mothers and Workers

Nadine Lefaucheur and Claude Martin

1. Introduction

The generic term 'single-parent families' (*familles monoparentales*) was not used in France until the late 1970s. These families were previously either divided into narrower categories according to marital status and moral standards (unmarried mothers, widows, divorcees) or lumped together and mixed with step and 'absent' families into one large group referred to as 'dissociated families'. This chapter similarly uses single parents as the generic term.

Since the late 1970s, the proportion of single-parent families has increased by more than 50 per cent but, as we will see in section 2, the main changes concern the distribution of single parents by marital status. As race and ethnicity are not recorded in French statistics, we will infer these from nationality, place of birth or residence. Section 3 is concerned with the development of discourses around single motherhood in France prior to and after the introduction of the generic 'single parent' term. We show the importance of concern with declining birth rates in the development of attitudes and policies towards single parents. In section 4 we will examine the special benefits created for single-parent families during the 1970s in more detail, discussing how a pro-natalist stance has led to single mothers being supported both as mothers and as workers. But, in section 5, we will see that the situation of single parents varies greatly according to their previous commitment to a traditional breadwinner/home-maker conjugal way of life, and by regional labour markets. Finally, in section 6, we look at the lifestyle and social supports available to single mothers in different neighbourhoods.

2. Single Mothers in France

Numbers and characteristics

In 1990 (last census), there were approximately 1.2 million single parents bringing up 1.9 million children aged under 25[1] in Metropolitan France. In other words, single parents accounted for 13 per cent of families with children, with 11 per cent of all children living with just one of their parents. This is a significant increase from the 720,000 single parents (9 per cent of families with children), and 1,300,000 children (8 per cent) who lived with one parent in 1968 – although less of an increase than in other countries discussed in this book.

Beyond these increases in number and proportion, the main changes over the last three decades concern the distribution of single parents by marital status, and are related to demographical and legal changes. As the average life span is now close to 82 for women and 74 for men (up from 74 and 67 in the early 1960s) it is not surprising to find that the share of widows among parents with dependent children dropped from 54 per cent in 1968 to 20 per cent in 1990. Following the legalization of divorce by mutual consent in 1975, the number of divorces tripled. The marriage rate has also declined significantly and there has been a large increase in cohabitation rates. Thus, although birth rates have fallen since the early 1960s, there has been a dramatic growth in 'illegitimate' births (from 6 per cent to a third of all births). However, most unmarried parents of newborn children are cohabitating, and most children born out of wedlock are legally recognized by both their parents. Consequently, the proportions of single parents who are divorced or never married have increased, respectively, from 17 and 8 per cent in the early 1960s to 43 and 21 per cent in 1990. In 1968, three out of five children in single-parent families had only one 'legal' living parent. Today, almost four out of five have two legal living parents, although they live with only one of them on a daily basis.

As a result of these changes, single parents are younger. Most of them are currently in their thirties (32 per cent) or in their forties (36 per cent), and the proportion of single parents over the age of 50 has declined from 50 per cent in the early 1960s to 20 per cent in 1990. Single parents are also more likely to be women than men: 80 per cent of single parents in 1968 and 86 per cent in 1990 were women. The typical lone parent is still a single mother. In 1968, however, she was a widow in her fifties, whereas nowadays she is a divorcee in her late thirties or early forties.

Due to the declining birth rate, single parents have fewer dependent children: 1.6 on average in 1990, compared with more than 1.8 in 1968. These children are also younger: 15 per cent were under age seven in 1968, and 18 per cent in 1990. However, while single parents became younger as a whole, the proportion at the younger end, aged 19–24, decreased during the 1970s, whereas it has increased since the early 1980s. Young people now live for a longer time with their parents, mainly as a result of their sharply rising rate of unemployment.

Foreign and overseas single parents

'Race' and 'ethnicity' are not recorded by the French system of statistical data, as this could be seen as very 'politically uncorrect', 'anti-Republican' or even racist. These categories can only be inferred from place of birth or residence, or from nationality.

Single parents are less likely to be foreigners than partnered ones (6 per cent compared with 9 per cent), but they are slightly more likely to have acquired French nationality and, above all, are two or three times more likely to live in or be born in one of the four French overseas *départements*.[2] When they are foreigners, parents are less likely to be single if they are Europeans, Moroccans, Tunisians and, above all, Turks, while they are more likely to be single parents if they are Algerians or Black Africans. The proportions of men and/or of widows and widowers are higher among foreign single parents – and the lower the proportion of single parents for any foreign nationality, the more likely they are to be widowed and/or men. Foreign single mothers are very likely (much more than French single mothers) to be domestic employees, unskilled workers or unemployed.

In contrast, French single parents who live in, or who were born in, the overseas *départements* are less likely to be men and/or widowed than the other French single parents. In these *départments* (called DOM), single mothers are more often in their thirties than in their forties, and one out of four is under age 30. Most of them, independent of age, were never married: 51 per cent in Réunion, 66 per cent in Guadeloupe, 72 per cent in Martinique, and 80 per cent in French Guyana. The poverty rate is much higher in DOM than in Metropolitan France. Overseas parents are all the more likely to be single as they belong to underprivileged groups, and are more likely to be poor and on welfare as they are single (63 per cent, compared with just 24 per cent of single parents in Metropolitan France).

As a consequence of the high levels of poverty and unemployment in DOM, emigration from DOM is important and many Caribbeans, who are French by nationality, work in the public sector in Metropolitan France, mainly in hospitals. A quarter of the heads of families in Metropolitan France who were born in DOM are single parents; like those who still live overseas, they are younger and much more likely to have never been married than single parents who were born in Metropolitan France. Nonetheless, they are twice as likely to be divorcees and to have fewer dependent children than those who still live overseas. This is due partly to the fact that those who emigrate differ from those who stay in DOM, and partly to the fact that immigrants behave more like Metropolitans when they live in Metropolitan France.

Single mothers and paid work

Whereas partnered mothers' labour-force participation rates have rapidly risen in France over the last two decades – from 43 per cent in 1975 to 72 per cent in 1993 – those of single mothers have always been even higher: 72 per cent in 1975, and 82 per cent in 1993. Single mothers are more likely to be either employed or seeking employment than partnered mothers who have the same number of children in the same age groups. The only exception concerns mothers with only one child where this child is under three: in this group the rate for partnered mothers is a little higher than that for single mothers (74 per cent compared with 68 per cent).

Among single mothers, 92 per cent of divorcees and 85 per cent of those who were never married are employed or job-seekers, whereas this is the case for only 64 per cent of widows, who are more likely to be retired or non-working. There are great disparities according to age however: three out of four widows who have at least one dependent child under age 18 and are in their thirties or forties are either working or seeking employment.

Single mothers are not only more likely to work than partnered ones, they are also less likely to work part time (18 per cent compared with 29 per cent), especially when they hold a highly qualified job (8 per cent compared with 21 per cent). However, they are a little more likely to hold casual work, a fixed-term job or a subsidized job (6 per cent compared with 4 per cent).

Indeed, being in the labour force does not mean being employed, since unemployment rates have dramatically increased in the last two decades in France (up to 17 per cent of single mothers and 13 per cent of partnered mothers, in 1992). This depends also on age and marital status: among mothers with children under three, 26 per cent of single mothers and 11 per cent of partnered mothers are job-seekers. Never-married single mothers, who are more likely to be the youngest, are also more likely to be unemployed than the divorcees and, overall, than widows (24 per cent, compared with 15 and 10 per cent). A larger proportion of single mothers is nevertheless actually employed compared with partnered mothers (67 per cent compared with 58 per cent), especially among divorcees (77 per cent, compared with only 54 per cent of widows). As a consequence of high and increasing rates of French mothers' labour-force participation, seven out of ten divorcees or widows say that the divorce from, or the death of, their husband had no constraining consequences on their participation in the labour force; on the contrary, following these events, 5 per cent changed jobs, 17 per cent started working or working again, or working full time instead of part time, and only 7 per cent became unemployed or stopped working, temporarily or definitively.

Single parents, either men or women, are more likely than partnered ones to have higher education and to be an executive or a professional, especially when they are divorcees. But single fathers are twice as likely as single mothers to be in such a situation. Their own father was also more likely than partnered fathers' own fathers to be an executive or a professional. The same is true as regards single mothers compared with partnered mothers. However, single parents are also, in contrast, more likely than partnered ones not to have any qualifications and to be workers or low qualified employees.

3. Discourses Around Single Motherhood in France

Before the 1970s: 'Christian angelism' and 'pro-birth patriotism'

For centuries, the policies adopted in France with regard to women having children out of wedlock have largely been governed by the issue of illegitimate children being killed or abandoned, in accordance with two patterns that we have labelled 'Christian angelism' and 'pro-birth patriotism' (Lefaucheur, 1994, 1995a). To dissuade 'sinful' women from trying to suppress the fruit of their sin, according to the 'Christian angelic' view, they should be given the opportunity to abandon the child. Hospitals and homes for foundlings spread over the country from the sixteenth century onwards, while some hospitals offered 'girls big with child' and adulterous women a place to give birth clandestinely. The existence of such institutions, it was thought, removed all excuses for infanticide and justified the death sentence introduced by Henri II (1556) for women who concealed their pregnancy and whose child died before being baptized.

On the eve of the French Revolution, there was a growing concern about the growth of the population. Infant death, formerly seen as a 'lesser evil', was reformulated as a 'worst evil', on a par with abortion and infanticide. As for children conceived out of wedlock, a main objective was to ensure their 'preservation', as the country needed all its children, even bastards, to guarantee its military, colonial and economic strength. This 'pro-birth patriotic' objective seemed compromised by the then current practice of transferring care of the child to the community or to foster families. As a result, French Revolutionaries decided in 1793 to prevent children from being abandoned by providing assistance to unmarried mothers and establishing maternity homes.

In the post-Revolutionary period, the practice advocated by welfare authorities was that of the *tours* (revolving cylinders placed at the entrance to hospitals or foundling homes, enabling people to abandon children anonymously). This gave rise to fierce controversy throughout the nineteenth century. Most of the supporters and opponents of the *tour* system believed that the issue of illegitimacy was a threat to morality as well as to the public purse. Thus, in 1837 in Paris an allowance was introduced for unmarried mothers who did not abandon their baby when leaving Maternité hospital, this attempt to resolve the issue of foundlings with the minimum moral and financial cost to society was extended progressively to all French *départements*.

The question of depopulation became a political issue again in the context of the Franco-German conflicts of the late nineteenth and early twentieth centuries. In the 1890s, epidemiological evidence on the influence of the conditions of pregnancy and the type of feeding on infant mortality prompted the adoption of various protective measures aimed at the mother and the infant. These included the establishment of homes for mothers (where a secret pregnancy was generally possible) so as to enable unmarried or deserted mothers to rest at the end of their pregnancy and keep their child with them to feed it in the early months of its life. The emphasis was also put on vocational training and provision of employment to single mothers, for most of them were workers or servants and supposed to be able to return to work rapidly after giving birth. This pattern of 'supported mother and worker' prevailed during the Third Republic of the 1930s, applying also to working-class married mothers (Lefaucheur, 1995b). Setting up a home for lone pregnant women in each *département* to combat the abandonment of newborn children was made compulsory by the Family Code of 1943.

The question of illegitimacy and abandonment has also been bound up with another issue over the last hundred years; that of the effects of the parents' separation on children's socialization. This was especially developed by criminologists, sociologists and child psychiatrists from the last decade of the nineteenth century. Some relied on theories of heredity and some on theories of environment, but most established a 'scientific' link between family 'dissociation' and juvenile delinquency (Lefaucheur, 1996). These interpretations of the effects of family breakdown were challenged during the 1950s by work on institutionalization, attachment to the mother and maternal deprivation, which placed emphasis on the normality or the quality of the relationships within the family, not of the family structure itself.

At the same time as the notion of 'risks' associated with family breakdown dominated the field of juvenile delinquency and child psychiatry, a concept of an increased risk of impoverishment caused by the forming a family emerged. Thus, it became seen as appropriate to 'socialize' this risk through family allowances, enabling a horizontal redistribution of incomes between households (depending on the number of children) in order to increase the birth rate and encourage large families. A 1913 law provided state assistance to large, poverty-stricken families, and a 1932 law made family allowances compulsory for all salaried workers in industry and commerce with at least two children. In 1946, the Family Allowance Funds became part of the general Social Security system, and since 1975, all families have been eligible for family benefits.

The First World War had already led to a proliferation of charities and subsidies to assist widows and orphans. However, it was not until the 1930s that the notion emerged of a 'family risk' of poverty, linked to the absence or death of one of the parents, and affecting members of families which were not yet called 'one-parent families'. Some slight attempts were made to socialize this risk: from 1938, as with married couples where the wife did not work, families where the mother was solely responsible for household expenses received an increase in family benefits. Four years later, widows were allowed to retain the entitlement to family benefits acquired by their deceased husband. After the Liberation (in 1944/45), the first dispensation from the rules linking entitlement to family allowance with being in paid employment was granted to war widows, while the single-income benefit was extended to single mothers. Homes with creches (*hôtels maternels*) were also created in the 1960s to avoid fostering 'institutionalization' by sheltering and supporting working lone mothers with babies, so as to enable them to care for their children after work and be 'workers and mothers'.

Since the Second World War, different associations of 'women heads of households' (either with dependent children or not) have been set up, following a hierarchy of marital status and moral standards. Associations of widows were created first: war widows in 1945, and civilian widows some years later. Some associations of divorced or separated women were formed during the 1960s. Never-married mothers, often feeling uncomfortable in these associations even when they were labelled 'associations of women heads of family', created specific groups in the early 1970s. At the same time groups of separated fathers claiming custody were also formed. For most people, it was then still unthinkable to put war widows, unmarried mothers, deserted wives and custodial fathers into the same category.

The turning point of the 1970s: 'single parent-families' and 'family crisis'

During the late 1970s, the expression *familles monoparentales* was introduced in France by feminist academics who sought to promote recognition of the fact that women were 'extremely capable of raising their children alone' (Michel, 1978). They argued that the single-parent family (regardless of the sex and marital status of single parents) was a 'real family'; a life-style as respectable as, and even more 'modern' than the usual type of conjugal family. The term was generally embraced by policy makers, social workers, and the media. Its success can be analysed as an indication of a growing social anxiety about a mounting 'family crisis'. This crisis was marked by changes in demographic trends, in moral and legal standards regarding sexual and conjugal life and by the 'new poverty' resulting from the rise in unemployment that began in the early 1970s. Regarding all single-parent families as constituting a separate and single category permitted the crystallization of most social representations linked to these 'crises'. Thus conservatives and familialists could judge the likelihood of poverty among single-parent families as a perverse effect of, even a punishment for, the growing sense of independence among women, and the associated increase in divorce and single parenthood. Liberals and feminists, in contrast, could denounce this connection as another indication of intolerable discrimination against women in the labour force (Lefaucheur, 1986).

Since the early 1960s, many civil laws concerning family relations have been reformed, especially during the period between 1965 and 1975. In particular, 'parental authority' replaced 'paternal power' in 1970; family laws were rewritten in 1972, in such a way that married fathers could legally recognize their illegitimate children, and almost all legal inequalities between legitimate and illegitimate children were suppressed. Similarly, laws on divorce by mutual consent and on free termination of pregnancy were passed in 1975.

These numerous changes in conjugal life and family law, combined with demographic changes in death rates and birth rates, have had a considerable impact on the rate of growth of single-parent families, and on their distribution by marital status, age and gender.

4. The French Welfare State Regime

In the discussion about the different types of welfare-state regimes, France appears in very different positions, depending on the author concerned (see Esping-Andersen, 1990; Lewis, 1992; Ferrera, 1996 for a discussion; see also Martin, in press). For example, it is difficult to classify France in the conservative, Catholic/corporatist model along with Germany, as Esping-Andersen suggests. This narrowly considers France on the basis of its corporatist range of insurance measures, ignoring the importance of social assistance in the development of French social welfare, as discussed in section 3. The history of post-war 'French-style' social security demonstrates that it did not really choose between the major Conservative Bismarckian or Beveridgian models, that were then available. For this reason, it is usual to present the French welfare state as a mixed, intermediate type that had been influenced by both Bismarck and Beveridge, and that has tried to enjoy the benefits offered by both approaches. The Bismarckian model was very influential until the late 1980s, but since then the Beveridgian trend has gathered strength with the project to use taxation to fund certain risks (such as the 'family risk' and the 'dependence risk') and the attempt to expand into a universal scheme, with a stronger role assumed by the state.

Nevertheless, Jane Lewis (1992) has recently proposed a 'gendered welfare state' classification, in which France assumes a much clearer position. From a gendered perspective, she suggests, France has developed a 'parental model', by concentrating more on the child than on women in social welfare measures – particularly in the field of its explicit family policy – or at least by recognizing women both as ungendered parents and workers. This perspective is much more helpful in analysing the situation of single mothers in France.

Single-parent benefits

The 1970s were marked by the creation of two social benefits targeted at supporting single parents. This development, however, did not take into account the important changes in demographic trends and conjugal life mentioned in section 3, or changes that were beginning to take place in the labour market. The reference framework was still that of the 1950s or 1960s – a time when single parents were mainly widows and deserted unmarried mothers, who confronted serious obstacles if they had no previous work experience once they suddenly found themselves widowed, pregnant or deserted and alone with dependent children. However, it was also a time of full employment, when one could easily find a job without prior experience, and when policy-makers could think that single parents mainly needed temporary financial support while searching for more permanent financial security through paid work.

The first benefit, created in 1970, called *allocation d'orphelin* (orphan allowance), was intended to provide unsupported single parents with a permanent support to compensate for the other parent's absence. It was available to the guardians of children whose parents were either dead or legally unknown (full benefit) or to the parent of children whose other parent was either deceased or legally unknown (partial benefit). Following two reforms in 1973 and 1975, this allowance, which was formerly means tested, became available to all single parents who did not receive any support from the absent parent, regardless of income. (This ran contrary to the general evolution towards means-testing in matters of family benefits.) The *allocation d'orphelin* was renamed *allocation de soutien familial* or ASF (family support allowance) and reformed again in 1984. It was made available also to single parents who did not receive any child support from the non-custodial parent for two months, as an advance on the alimony set by the court. This amounts to approximately 10 per cent of the guaranteed minimum wage (SMIC) and is now paid to about 470,000 single parents: 30 per cent for orphans, 50 per cent for children who have only one legal parent, and 20 per cent for children deserted by an absent parent (only about half of those who actually apply) (Martin, 1995).

The second benefit, called *allocation de parent isolé* (lone parent allowance) or *API* was created in 1976. It is a differential and transitory benefit which rounds up the income of single parents or pregnant single women to a certain subsistence level (about 53 per cent of SMIC for a lone parent or a lone pregnant woman, plus about 18 per cent of SMIC per dependent child), for one to three and half years, depending on the child's age. It is available during pregnancy, for the first year after the separation of a couple, and/or until the youngest child reaches the age of three.

API was originally designed to enable 'about 35,000' widows or deserted mothers to become rapidly (one year at the most) self-sufficient by working. Unfortunately, because of the dramatic rise in both unemployment and single parenthood, its results fell well short of its expectations. Many more single parents qualified for API and had many more difficulties in securing a stable form of employment. About 14,000 single parents (12 per cent of all single parents) were eligible in 1992. Among them, less than two per cent were actually widowed; this was partly a consequence of the declining rate of widows and widowers among single parents and partly a result of the creation, within the social insurance system, of another benefit intended to support widowed single parents (*assurance veuvage*).

In creating API, parliament made it available also to single fathers, but principally to single pregnant women and to mothers with children under three, regardless of the duration of their 'single' status. Their objectives were to prevent a decline in birthrate and an increase in abortions (the law on free termination of pregnancy had been passed the previous year), and to allow young, single mothers to stay at home and care for their children before they entered nursery school. The main aim in this latter case was to prevent what experts identified as 'emotional deficiency' – delinquency or other problems which were commonly associated with children raised in single-parent households, especially those of unmarried mothers. It was not expected that young mothers, mainly unmarried, would constitute such a large share of recipients as they do today, when most recipients are either pregnant (7 per cent) or responsible for at least one child under three (71 per cent).

Congruent with the dramatic increase in the number of beneficiaries of API and in young single mothers 'on welfare', a discourse on the 'perverse effects' of API, regarded as a disincentive to work and to establishing conjugal life, has become prevalent among social workers. The criticisms were not levelled at API granted to mothers with children over the age of three who became single through divorce, marital separation or widowhood: it was still seen as legitimate to provide temporary assistance (one year at the most) to help them in adapting to their new situation. However, the never-married and formerly cohabiting single mothers with young children were frequently accused of living off welfare for three years instead of striving for financial independence through obtaining employment or improving their skills to qualify for the job market. They were also accused of attempting to become pregnant at an interval of every three years, precisely coinciding with the moment their benefit was to terminate, as well as concealing the cohabiting father or rejecting him in order to continue receiving benefits. However, in the 1980s, research has tended to allay these suspicions by showing that the deterrent effects of API were both difficult to prove and probably limited (Ray et al., 1983; Ray, 1985), and that the rate of fraud or 'recidivism' cases was lower than generally estimated (ACT, 1984).

Moreover, a subsistence allowance, the *revenu minimum d'insertion* (minimum guaranteed income for social integration) or *RMI*, was created in 1988 (its amount is worth about three-quarters of API). Again, it soon became apparent that many more persons were also eligible than originally expected, and that single parents constituted a large share: 138,000 in 1993, or 12 per cent of all single parents (slightly above the proportion eligible for API), amounting to 20 per cent of all beneficiaries of RMI. It became evident that supporting single mothers for a limited period with API was not enough to enable them to become rapidly self-sufficient. Although some still accuse single mothers of wanting to live on handouts, it is gender inequalities within the labour market, the increasing difficulties in finding a job, and the 'two-tierization' of society (the 'social fracture' that Chirac denounced during his 1995 election campaign) that are more often the real issues at hand. Nevertheless, as part of the current planned reform of social security, some policy-makers propose either to suppress API (its recipients would be entitled to RMI) or to diminish its amount down to the RMI levels and also to make it compulsory for its recipients to be on a training course or an 'integration' programme (following the model of special training programmes for single mothers set up in the 1980s, where those who were registered as job-seekers received priority for attending paid vocational 'integrating' programmes).

Single parents are of course entitled to general family benefits (for families with at least two dependent children), housing benefits, handicapped or young children benefits. Nevertheless, about ten per cent of those who have at least one child under age 18 do not benefit from any family allowance because they have only one child, aged over three, and because their income is above the poverty level. However, if single parents' income is large enough to be taxable, they get a special reduction.

Single parents' children do not have any legal priority on the waiting lists for *crèches* (except those run by maternity homes) or for nursery schools. Nevertheless, those under three[3] whose mothers work are more likely to be cared for in *crèches* or to go to nursery school before their third birthday than are partnered parents' children whose mothers work (respectively 18 and 11 per cent for single parents and 13 and 9 per cent for partnered parents); they are almost as likely to be cared for by a relative or a childminder (respectively 25 and 23 per cent, and 23 and 25 per cent), but are much less likely to be cared for by their own mother (11 compared with 19 per cent).

The increase in the number of single parent families and the fact that a quarter of them are entitled to one of the 'social minima' (API or RMI) are frequently seen as a symbol of the two-tierization in French society. It is indeed true that the position of single parents in the labour force and their living conditions are, in general, disadvantaged ones compared with those of coupled parents. But, as single parents do not actually form a whole, these positions and circumstances also vary considerably according to gender, age and marital status, as well as class, place of residence, ethnic group (as discussed earlier), individual attitudes and strategies.

5. Single Mothers in Labour Markets

Effects of commitment to traditional conjugality on labour market commitment

Gender is obviously a major dimension of labour markets. It is also a major dimension of single-parenthood: 86 per cent of single parents are women, and single fathers differ from single mothers in many aspects. However, single fathers differ also differ from partnered fathers, and single mothers differ from partnered mothers. These numerous disparities cannot be uniqely explained by gender. Some are also related to differences in age, marital status, number and age of dependent children, and these in turn follow disparities in stages within the life course and commitment to a traditional conjugal way of life.

Compared with partnered parents, single parents are indeed likely to be either at an earlier stage (never married), or at a later stage (divorced or widowed) of the parental life course. Single mothers are hence more likely than partnered mothers to be over 40, or (to a lesser extent) under 25, and to have fewer dependent children (1.6 on average, compared with 1.9). Contrary to a common perception that portrays single mothers' children as babies, their children are also more likely to be aged over 12 (60 per cent as opposed to 49 per cent for partnered mothers). Single fathers, who are much less likely to have never been married, and much more likely to be widowed than single mothers, are hence more likely to be over 40, and to have dependent children over age 12, because men more easily claim or gain custody when children are older.

These differences in age, in marital status, and in size of family are also associated with unequal levels of commitment to a traditional conjugal way of life. Such a way of life implies a division of labour between partners, which can be more or less important but which usually means that women put their 'family duties ' before their own working career and are complemented by male partners who are more committed to the breadwinner role. Obviously, never-married single parents (and, to a lesser extent, divorced ones) have generally been the least committed to this conjugal life-style, while widows (and, to a lesser extent, those who are deserted or separated) have usually been more deeply involved in such a way of life and for a longer time. These disparities in the duration and intensity of such a commitment result in different employment patterns, and in unequal levels of employment, wages and circumstances, and account for the main differences between single mothers according to their age and marital status. Most French mothers work – all the more when they are single. But the more and the longer single mothers had been previously committed to a gendered, conjugal way of life, the less likely they usually are to secure a good position in the labour market, while the contrary is true for single fathers. In contrast, the more and the longer single parents, either men or women, had been previously committed to a conjugal way of life, either highly gendered or not, the more likely they are to have accumulated assets and goods, especially housing.

It must nevertheless be mentioned that age groups are also generation groups whose members share certain values and must cope with particular situations: the oldest single parents are not only the most likely to have been involved for a long term period in a conjugal way of life, they are also the most likely to have been committed to a lifestyle characterized by low rates of uptake of paid work by mothers. If younger mothers are likely to be the least committed to such a lifestyle, they must also cope with a state of high unemployment, especially for young people and women, and are most likely to experience or to have experienced great difficulties in securing stable employment. Those who are in their late forties belong, on the contrary, to a generation of women that are more likely to have chosen salaried work when they were young and who entered a labour market that was characterized by full employment.

One must also keep in mind the fact that about half of single parents repartner within five years, and that the population of single parents is not composed of all the parents who became single but only of those among them who have not repartnered. This helps exlain why the mean salary of the never-married single mothers in their late forties is the highest of all groups of single mothers by age and marital status: they are very likely to be the least committed to a traditional conjugal lifestyle. They are less likely to have lived in a couple for a long time before becoming a single mother, and gave priority to their working career by choice or obligation, as they did not want to or could not repartner.

The mean monthly net salary of single parents who work full time is slightly higher than that of partnered parents who are the same sex, that of women being worth three-quarters that of men. Among salaried single parents, divorcees earn the highest mean salary, independent of sex, but those who never married earn the lowest mean salary among fathers while they do almost as well on average as the divorcees among mothers. With regards to wage expectations, having been married and highly committed to traditional conjugality is usually to men's advantage, but to women's disadvantage.

The effects of previous commitment to a traditional conjugal way of life are interwoven with other important differences: in the values, attitudes and practices, which we discuss in section 6, as well as those we turn to now: the constraints and opportunities in regional labour markets.

Regional labour markets and single mothers' labour-force participation

Single parents are unequally dispersed over metropolitan France, and their geographical distribution is associated with gender, age and marital status. The highest proportions can be found in larger cities, like Lyons, Bordeaux, Toulouse and Marseilles, on the Mediterranean coast, and particlarly in the Paris region: 56 per cent of single parents live in agglomerations of more than 100,000 inhabitants, where they constitute 17 per cent of all the families with children, and one out of four Parisian families with children is a single-parent one. The more parents are single in a given region or area, the more single parents are women (except in the Paris region) and the less they are widowed.

Constraints and opportunities upon single parents within local labour markets have not actually been documented in France, perhaps because of the French tradition of administrative centralization. Comparing the employment rates and the occupational distribution of parents by marital status and sex, for the different administrative regions or *départements* of France can nevertheless provide some insights into these issues, as the geographical distribution of single parents is correlated with qualification and occupation, as well as with disparities in their employment and circumstances.[4]

Single parents, especially mothers, are less likely than partnered parents to come from a farming family or to be a farmer. Since farming frequently implies a highly gendered division of labour and a traditional conjugal way of life, farming parents are less likely to separate or divorce. They are less able to continue farming when they become single – all the more so when they are women, whose role is more likely to be considered that of a helper. Hence, single mothers are four times less likely than partnered mothers, and five times less likely than single fathers, to be farmers. Among single parents, the widowed are three times (fathers) or six times (mothers) more likely to be farmers than other single parents. The situation for other forms of self-employment or non-salaried work is largely similar to farming. However, single fathers are more likely than single mothers (and also than partnered fathers) to be an employer or a self-employed artisan or shopkeeper. This perhaps is a result of fathers being more likely to get custody rights when they are in such occupations.

This situation explains in part why, in rural areas, single parents are less numerous and why they are more likely than in other areas to be widowed, men, self-employed or out of the labour force. This is particularly the case in the more rural west and centre of France and, above all, in the Massif Central. In the *département* of Aveyron, for example, where 23 per cent of all heads of households are self-employed or non-salaried (compared with 10 per cent on average in the whole of metropolitan France), single parents represent less than 8 per cent of families with children. Among them 29 per cent are widowed, 16 per cent never married (compared with 19 and 24 per cent on average in the whole of metropolitan France), and 10 per cent self-employed (twice the average), while a third of single mothers and a fifth of single fathers are not in the labour force (compared with 18 and 13 per cent on average).

In the peripheral *département* of Morbihan in Britanny (main town Lorient), proportions of farmers and other self-employed people are also above average. There are more single-parent families, but fewer widows and never-married single parents than in Aveyron. However, because of the greater development of an industrial sector (canning industry, food processing, shipbuilding) and services in Morbihan, twice as many single mothers are workers in the *département* than in Aveyron and fewer stay out of the labour force. Nevertheless, because of the current industrial crisis, many more are unemployed and registered as job-seekers.

Aveyron and Morbihan are located in the eight administrative regions of the west, centre and south west of France, where the share of farmers, self-employed and retired heads of household is higher than in other regions. In this 'traditional' France, the working rate of partnered mothers is above average, mainly as a result of high rates of self-employment, which usually means 'conjugal employment' (farming, food retailing, shopkeeping, hotel business, and so on). The working rate of single mothers, who are less likely to be self-employed, is slightly above that of partnered mothers but below the average for single mothers in the whole of France. On the contrary, their unemployment rate is above average and almost twice that of partnered mothers: they are more likely to search for a job or register as job-seekers than to be entitled to training courses or social programmes.

A very different pattern can be found in the industrial regions of the north and east of France that have gone through a dramatic economic crisis. In these regions, the working rates of mothers, single or partnered, are the lowest in mainland France. In the region of Nord-Pas de Calais, for example, one out of two mothers is not employed. When unemployed, four out of five partnered mothers are not registered as job-seekers as they are not entitled to unemployment benefits – either because they have never worked or, more often, because they have 'chosen' (in the face of job shortage) to stay home and take care of their children. Such a 'choice' is not really available to single mothers: among those who do not work, one out of two is registered as a job-seeker and the other is very likely to benefit from API or RMI. However, there are great disparities among single mothers depending on their marital status: in Nord-Pas de Calais, two out of three divorcees, but only two out of five widows or never-married mothers, are actually employed. Twelve per cent of widows, 22 per cent of divorcees, and 33 per cent of never-married single mothers are registered as job-seekers, while 13 per cent of divorcees, 25 per cent of unmarried mothers, and 42 per cent of widows are neither working nor job-seekers, although they are not retired.

Another very different pattern again is found in the Ile-de-France, the Greater Paris Metropolitan area, where the highest rates of employment can be found, especially as regards single mothers (80 per cent, compared with 67 per cent for the whole of metropolitan France). The latter are more likely than elsewhere in metropolitan France to be unmarried, salaried and highly qualified employees or professionals. Only four per cent of divorcees and six per cent of never-married single mothers are neither employed nor job-seekers. As elsewhere, unmarried mothers are more likely to be unemployed and less likely to hold a highly qualified job than divorcees; however 14 per cent only are unemployed while 28 per cent are professionals or highly qualified employees.

A similar pattern, although less marked (especially for never-married single mothers), can be found in the cities and surrounding areas of Bordeaux and Toulouse (the only areas in the south-west where single parents are quite numerous, less likely to be men and widowed, and where the single mothers' activity rates are above average), as well as in Lyons, Marseilles and their surrounding regions.

In the south-eastern and Mediterranean regions, rates of non-farming self-employment are above average and the share of highly qualified or professional jobs is one of the largest in France, after the Paris area. Contrary to the situation in the south-western regions, single mothers' working rates are much higher than those of partnered mothers, all the more so when they are divorcees. In the *département* of Rhône (main town: Lyons) for example, where the proportions of single parents (and of women among them) are above average, 74 per cent of single mothers are actually employed (compared with 59 per cent of partnered mothers). Of all those who actually work, 32 per cent of single mothers and 35 per cent of partnered mothers (but as much as 50 per cent of single fathers) are senior or middle-ranking executives or professionals.

Finally, the share of executives, professionals and employees is below average in the industrial/agricultural regions of northern and eastern France, where single mothers are more likely to be farmers or workers, and where rates of single parenthood are below average. In the two eastern regions of Burgundy and Franche-Comté, mothers' employment and unemployment rates are average, which means that those of single mothers are both about 10 per cent higher. In the northern region of Champagne-Ardennes and the western regions of the Loire and Basse-Normandie, single mothers' employment rate is below average, while that of partnered mothers is above average, which means that they are very close. However, single mothers are twice as likely to be job-seekers as partnered mothers.

Basse-Normandie is the only French region where partnered mothers are on the whole more likely to be actually employed than single mothers. In the *département* of Calvados (main town: Caen), as many single as partnered mothers are working (61 per cent) – three out of ten in industry (mainly electronics, metal-working and motor industry). However, the proportion of job-seekers, only 9 per cent for partnered mothers, climbs to 23 per cent for single mothers (and as high as 40 per cent for those who are never-married).

6. Single Mothers in Neighbourhoods

Single mothers' living conditions and lifestyle

Even if, as detailed earlier, single mothers earn a higher average salary than partnered mothers, the size-adjusted disposable family income of the latter is higher, mainly because they benefit from the salary of their partner (which is likely to be higher than their own). In contrast, the mean size-adjusted disposable income of single fathers' families is higher than that of partnered parents' households, all the more so when single fathers are divorced or separated. Consequently, a larger proportion of single mothers than single fathers earn an income that is below the poverty level (defined as half the size-adjusted disposable average family income, including benefits). However, even if single fathers are not as likely as single mothers to be poor, their poverty rate has been on the rise for the last decade. Nevertheless, among parents who have more than one dependent child, the poverty rates of those who are single are quite similar to those of partnered-parent households where the female partner does not work.

Single parents are more likely than partnered parents to live either in working-class districts or, on the contrary, in the well-off areas. In the latter case, they are more likely to be men or to be never-married or divorced mothers over the age of 40. Single parents' living conditions are, on average, worse than those of partnered parents. The former are half as likely as the latter to own their place of residence (31 per cent compared with 61 per cent), and to live in single-family housing (38 per cent compared with 66 per cent). Whereas they are slightly more likely to have all basic modern conveniences, they are less likely to possess a freezer (38 per cent against 59 per cent) or a dish-washer (28 and 51 per cent). They are also more dissatisfied with their environment and with levels of noise pollution (32 and 21 per cent), and with their accommodation in general (14 against 7 per cent). Single parents are also less likely to go on vacation or to spend evenings out. While fewer have a car (69 compared with 95 per cent), they are more likely to live in the centre of a big city and they usually live closer to their work, their children's school and shopping centres. They move more frequently than partnered parents, but they usually move within the same town or *département*.

Disparities in living conditions within the single-parent population are related to differences in consumption practices and in the accumulation of assets and household goods, which vary with age and generation of single parents, with their degree of commitment to traditional conjugality, and, consequently, with their marital status. The youngest and the never-married single parents are less likely than the older and the widowed to own their place of residence, to live in single-family housing, to have a phone, a freezer or a washing-machine, and more likely to live in HLM (local authority) housing or in the centre of a big city, especially if they are women. Divorcees in their forties are the most likely to own a dish-washer or a car, to go away on holiday or to go out in the evenings.

Age and generation factors intertwine with gender and level of previous commitment to a conjugal lifestyle in such a way that they allocate single parents to different, and generally opposite, positions with regards to their labour-market position, housing and other living conditions.

The level of their previous commitment to a traditional conjugal life as a vital factor was shown in a study of single mothers' housing and life histories (Lefaucheur, 1987). The five never-married interviewees, who lived in very difficult conditions in a housing estate near Rouen (Normandy), were on the whole more satisfied with their living conditions than the five divorced interviewees who lived in Lorient (Brittany) – despite the fact that the living conditions of the latter group were clearly better. The former decided to leave their violent partners after a rather short period of common life. They were young workers or unemployed mothers of foreign or disadvantaged origins, whose childhood and youth had been very disturbed. They considered that becoming a single mother offered them some advantages, and that they received significant help either from social services or from their friends or colleagues, or even from their boss.

In contrast, the Lorient group were clerks in their forties. They had married marines or navy workers (Lorient is a military harbour, with an arsenal and a submarine naval base), who volunteered to move frequently in order to be more rapidly promoted and buy a house. Hence they were obliged to leave their job many times to follow their husband in metropolitan France or overseas, and could not always find employment in the bases where he was transferred. In as much as they had put the 'building of a home' before a personal career, they felt severely deceived when their husband left for another woman (or when they discovered that he was unfaithful, and decided to leave him because their own commitment to conjugal life had been wrecked by his infidelities). When interviewed, they proved to have a very negative perception of their situation as single mothers. Their parents actually provided them with a high level of support after the separation, housing them and their children for some months or even for one or two years, but they considered that they received almost no help and that people treated them as if they were *filles-mères* (the expression used in the nineteenth-century to refer to never-married mothers and which became very pejorative). They felt ashamed to live in public housing, as though they had 'come down' the social ladder.

Support from family and friends

A survey about support given by relatives and friends to single parents was conducted in 1990 among 336 mothers who were divorced or separated for more than four years, and received, or had previously received, benefits from the Family Allowance Fund (Martin, 1994, 1996) in the *département* of Calvados in Normandy (main town: Caen). Here single mothers are as likely as partnered mothers to be working, but are more likely to be job-seeking. The survey showed that support varies a lot according to age and qualifications: the most qualified mothers (those who were at least holders of the French baccalaureate) were twice as likely as the less qualified ones (those who had no diploma) to get child support from the absent father (70 per cent compared with 35 per cent) and the amount of the child support received by workers was less than 60 per cent of that received by executives or professionals. Of mothers who had a higher education, 37 per cent considered that the absent father was still a member of the family, half of their children met him at least once a month and only 13 per cent never met him, but the corresponding figures for those who had no diploma were respectively 15, 30 and 50 per cent.

The social networks of the less qualified mothers were mostly family ones: 36 per cent of them met their own parents daily, and most of those who had grandparents or siblings met them at least twice a month, while one in two said that they had no close friends, and only one in six claimed more than five friends. In contrast, the most qualified mothers' social networks were highly friendship based: four out of ten claimed more than five close friends and only one said that she had no close friends. They were the most likely to say that they got some support from their friends (60 compared with 21 per cent). Moreover, while they saw their family half as frequently as the less qualified they also said they got some support from their own parents (79 as opposed to 51 per cent) or siblings (58 and 28 per cent). Overall, they were much less likely than the non-qualified to feel that they were 'lonely' (20 as against 50 per cent) and much more likely to feel that their social network was 'rich, wide, and complex' (60 and 25 per cent). Non-qualified mothers were indeed more likely than qualified mothers to meet only relatives, and less likely to be repartnered (14 per cent as opposed to 45 per cent), all the more so as they were older.

Different patterns of after-divorce or separation support emerged from the survey. Non-qualified separated or divorced mothers, who previously had little or no work experience and were highly committed to a marital lifestyle, got support from their own family (if they got any at all), and were likely to feel lonely and dependent, all the more so as they were older. Qualified and working mothers were more likely to repartner rapidly when they were in their thirties, and more likely to 'choose' to be self-sufficient when they were in their forties – living alone but supported by a wide network of friends and, possibly, a 'living apart' partner.

This 'two-tierization' of social networks and support for single mothers according to qualifications was also found in a survey conducted in 1992 by Arlette Gautier among 158 single mothers living in a working district of Reims, the main town of Marne (a *département* in the Champagne region, where unemployment rates are above average and mothers are more likely to be workers or hold unqualified jobs). Only one in five single mothers had achieved the French baccalaureate or received a higher education. Twelve per cent were full-time home-makers (10 per cent had never worked) and 24 per cent job-seekers, but only 9 per cent were entitled to API and 4 per cent to RMI; 20 per cent did not get any benefit and 10 per cent received ASF, while 35 per cent got child support from the absent father (more likely if they were more qualified).

Three out of ten never met their parents, usually because they were deceased, and half the children never met their father. Those who had good or close friends had made their acquaintance at work or during childhood, but a third of single mothers had found good friends in the neighbourhood. Only one out of ten had a living-apart regular partner.

Thirteen per cent of mothers were never invited to visit by relatives or friends, 23 per cent never invited anybody to their house, and 16 per cent invited only or were invited only by their parents. A third of single mothers were thus very isolated: they were more likely to be unqualified and unemployed, to be in their twenties or fifties, to have at least three dependent children, not to go away on holiday, to suffer from loneliness, to feel afraid and dissatisfied with their housing and environment, and to wish to move to another district.

In contrast, one in four single mothers was well supported, met relatives and friends at least once a week, had good relationships with the absent father, had supportive close friends, went away on holiday, had a car, received support from parents as regards child care or financial aid when things got rough, appreciated her housing and environment, and did not feel lonely but planned to repartner some day. She was very likely to be qualified and employed, and to have only one or two children.

7. Conclusion

In France, illegitimacy has been seen for centuries as a threat to morality, and because of the frequent abandonment of children born out of wedlock, a threat to the public purse. Family breakdown is also widely considered to be a major cause of juvenile delinquency. However, these issues have generally been regarded more as social problems than as the social threats they are assumed to pose in Britain and the USA. The policies adopted in France have mostly been targeted at preventing the risk of infanticide associated with illegitimacy and/ or that of infant mortality associated with abandonment, by the creation of foundling hospitals and maternity homes. During the last century, the pro-birth orientation of family policies led to support for single mothers so as to enable them to be 'mothers and workers'.

The 1970s were a turning point as regards family law, conjugal life and demographic trends, as well as policies towards single-parent families, which placed them in one overall category – regardless of marital status – and entitled them to special benefits. API, a differential and transitory benefit, has been designed to enable single parents to become rapidly self-sufficient by working, at the latest when their youngest child reaches the age of three. However, the dramatic rise in unemployment in the 1990s has made this much more difficult, so that the number of single mothers with children aged over three entitled to RMI (general minimum guaranteed income) is now as great as those who benefit from API. A reform of API is currently under discussion, with the aim of improving the integration of single mothers into the labour force.

There are 1.2 million single parents with children under age 25 in France, that is to say 13 per cent of households with children. The typical single mother is a divorcee in her early forties, whereas thirty years ago she was a widow in her fifties. Foreigners are less likely to be single parents than those who are French by birth, whereas parents who were born in the overseas *départements* are much more likely to be single and never-married than those who were born in metropolitan France.

There are many differences between single parents and partnered parents, as well as between single mothers and single fathers. They cannot be explained only by gender, but are also related to differences in age, marital status, number and age of dependent children that follow disparities in stages within the life course and degrees of commitment to a traditional conjugal way of life. Most French mothers work, all the more when they are single: 58 per cent of partnered mothers and 67 per cent of single mothers are employed, whereas 9 per cent of the former and 17 per cent of the latter are registered as job-seekers. Few mothers work part time.

The mean salary of single parents who work full time is slightly higher than that of the partnered parents who are the same sex – that of women being worth three-quarters of that of men. However, the mean size-adjusted disposable income of single-parent families is lower than that of two-parent families. One single parent out of four is 'on welfare'. Single parents' circumstances are on average poorer than those of partnered parents. However, there are great disparities between single parents, whose standards of living and own assessments of their achievements are influenced, sometimes in conflicting ways, by their previous commitment to a traditional conjugal lifestyle.

Apart from the overseas *départements*, the highest porportions of single parents can be found in the larger cities, the Mediterranean coast and particularly the Paris region. Geographical distribution of single parents is correlated with qualification and occupation, as well as with disparities in their employment. As they are less likely than partnered parents to be farmers or self-employed, all the more so if they are women, they are less numerous (and more likely to be widowed) in rural areas and in the regions of the west, centre and south west, where single mothers' working rates are below average and where they are more likely to be registered as job-seekers.

Very different patterns can be found in the depressed industrial regions of the north and east, where the working rates of mothers, single or partnered, are the lowest in mainland France. Patterns are different again in the Paris region, where employment rates are the highest. This is especially the case for single mothers in the Paris region, who are much more likely there than elsewhere in France to be unmarried, salaried and highly qualified. In the south-eastern regions, where the share of highly qualified or professional jobs is also above average (although less than in Paris), single mothers' employment rates, especially divorcees', are much higher than those of partnered mothers.

Surveys of the support received by single mothers from relatives, friends and neighbours have been conducted in two rural and industrial regions in northern France. They show that disparities within the single-mother population are as important for social support as they are for qualification, employment, income and standards of living: the less single mothers are qualified, the less they are likely to have rich, wide, complex and supportive social networks.

To sum up, in France, single mothers have long been supported as mothers by public policies aiming to prevent infanticide and abandonment, and to safeguard morals or the birth rate. Today, however, they are more supported as parents. As 'normal' parents, they are entitled to the same family benefits and child-care support received by all parents. As custodial parents, 40 per cent of them benefit from a guaranteed child support (ASF). As single parents, those who are liable to income tax (about 60 per cent) benefit from special tax deductions, and, for a while, as poor single parents, 12 per cent benefit from a transitory single-parent guaranteed income (API). As parents, they are also supposed to be workers: when they are entitled to a specific support as single parents, it is usually so as to enable them to become rapidly self-sufficient by working. However, due to the dramatic increase in unemployment and poverty, single parents are more and more supported as poor and 'excluded' people: as many are now entitled to RMI (guaranteed minimum *insertion* income) as to API. This will probably lead to a reform to bring API into line with RMI – that is to say supporting single mothers more as 'excluded' poor people than as deserted or 'isolated' mothers and workers.

Notes

1   Until 1990, in the French censuses 'children' were defined as umarried people under 25 living with one or both parents, and 'single parents' as parents living without a partner with at least one unmarried child under 25. Unless we state that we are using other definitions, we use these in this chapter. (But note, for family benefits 'children' are usually defined as under age 18.) Most data in this chapter come from the 1990 Census.
2   There are 22 administrative regions and 96 administrative *départements* in metropolitan France, plus five *départements* overseas: one in the Indian Ocean: La Réunion, and four in America: Guyana, Martinique, Guadeloupe and Saint Pierre and Miquelon. We do not take the overseas departments into account in this chapter unless otherwise stated.
3   Almost all children aged three and above (and a third of 2-year-old children) go to nursery school in France, whether their mother works or not, or is single or not.
4   The *département* and regional data on employment rates, marital status and occupational distribution of single parents and partnered mothers have been especially calculated for this chapter from the 1990 Census.

References

ACT (1984) *Recherches sur l'efficacité économique et sociale de l'Allocation de Parent Isolé*, Paris: Caisse nationale d'allocations familiales.

ESPING-ANDERSEN, G. (1990) *The Three Worlds of Welfare Capitalism*, Cambridge: Polity Press.

FERRERA, M. (1996) 'The "southern model" of welfare in social Europe', *Journal of European Social Policy*, **6**, 1, pp. 17–37.

GAUTIER, A. (1992) *(Se) vivre à Croix-Rouge*, Reims: Union départementale des associations familiales de la Marne and Association des familles monoparentales de la Marne.

LEFAUCHEUR, N. (1986) 'How the one-parent families appeared in France', in Deven, F. and Cliquet, R. L. (Eds) *One-Parent Families in Europe*, pp. 73–81, The Hague/Brussels: NIDI/CBGS.

LEFAUCHEUR, N. (1987) *Les familles monoparentales: une catégorie spécifique?*, Paris: Plan Construction.

LEFAUCHEUR, N. (1994) ' "At risk families" and "family risks": a brief history of social welfare provision for single parent families in France', in MIRE – Maison

Française d'Oxford (Eds) *Comparing Social Welfare Systems in Europe*, pp. 449–69, Oxford: Maison Française.

LEFAUCHEUR, N. (1995a) 'La sociéte française et le traitement des naissances hors mariage: de l'angélisme au patriotisme', in Lefaucheur, N. and Martin, C. (Eds) *Qui doit nourrir l'enfant dont le père est "absent"? Rapport de recherche sur les fondements des politiques familiales européennes (Angleterre, France, Italie, Portugal)*, pp. 125–43, Paris: Caisse nationale d'allocations familiales.

LEFAUCHEUR, N. (1995b) 'L'article 9 de la loi de 1892 et la question de l'assistance aux femmes en couches', in Auslander, L. and Zancarini-Fournel, M. (Eds) *Différence des sexes et protection sociale (XIX*ᵉ*–XX*ᵉ *siècles)*, pp. 165–82, Saint-Denis: Presses Universitaires de Vincennes.

LEFAUCHEUR, N. (1995c) 'French policies towards lone parents: social categories and social policies', in McFate, K., Lawson, R. and Wilson, J. W. (Eds) *Poverty, Inequality and the Future of Social Policy: Western States in the New World Order*, pp. 257–89, New York: Russell Sage Foundation.

LEFAUCHEUR N. (1996) 'Dissociation familiale et délinquance juvénile, ou la trompeuse éloquence des chiffres', in Le Gall, D. and Martin, C. (Eds) *Familles et politiques sociales*, pp. 179–95, Paris: L'Harmattan.

LEFAUCHEUR, N. and MARTIN, C. (1993) 'Lone parent families in France: situation and research', in Hudson, J. and Galaway, B. (Eds) *Single Parent Families: Perspectives on Research and Policy*, pp. 31–50, Toronto: Thompson Educational Publishing.

LEWIS, J. (1992) 'Gender and the development of welfare regimes', *Journal of European Social Policy*, **2**, 3, pp. 159–73.

MARTIN, C. (1994) 'Diversité des trajectoires post-désunion. Entre le risque de solitude, la défense de son autonomie et la recomposition familiale', *Population*, **6**, pp. 1557–84.

MARTIN, C. (1995) 'Father, mother and the welfare-state. Family and social transfers after marital breakdown', *Journal of European Social Policy*, **5**, 1, pp. 43–63.

MARTIN, C. (1996) *L'après-divorce. Rupture du lien familial et vulnérabilité*, Rennes: Presses Universitaires de Rennes.

MARTIN, C. (in press) 'Social welfare and the family in southern Europe', *South European Society and Politics*, M. Rhodes (Ed.), Special issue on Southern European Welfare States.

MICHEL, A. (1978) *Sociologie de la famille et du mariage*, Paris: Presses Universitaires de France.

RAY, J. C., CARVOYEUR, L. S. and LIMAN TINGUIRI, M. K. (1983) *Allocation de Parent Isolé et désincitation au travail*, Nancy: LASARE, Université de Nancy.

RAY, J. C. (1985) 'L'allocation de parent isolé désincite-t-elle au travail?' in Commissariat général du Plan (Ed.) *Evaluation des politiques sociales*, pp. 75–112, Paris: La Documentation Française.

Chapter 9

Single Mothers in Sweden: Supported Workers Who Mother

Ulla Björnberg

1. Introduction

In international comparisons of the economic situation of lone mothers,[1] Swedish lone mothers have been presented as being in an advantageous social and economic situation because of their high labour-force participation in combination with a high level of support from the welfare state (Lone Parent Families, 1990; Wong, Garfinkel and McLanahan, 1993; Hobson, 1994). Until recently, there has also been a commonly held belief in Sweden that lone mothers are not different from married mothers in terms of their participation in the labour market. Further, lone mothers have usually been seen as one homogeneous group.

In contrast, this chapter will examine the situation for different categories of lone mothers, and compare lone mothers with married mothers, in order to shed some light on systematic differences between them in terms of labour market position and orientation. The intention is also to study the changes that have occurred since the economic recession in 1990, which brought with it a steep rise in unemployment. Have the changes occurring during the 1990s affected lone mothers in similar ways to married mothers? During the last 15 years industrialized countries have also experienced the so-called 'feminization of poverty'. This is linked to the development of lone motherhood and the varying possibilities of lone mothers supporting themselves by paid labour. Is this type of development also discernible in a social democratic welfare state such as Sweden?

Section 2 describes lone motherhood in Sweden, focusing on demographic trends and employment position. This is followed by an overview of current political discourses on lone motherhood and divorce (section 3) and a description of the policy regime in Sweden and its implications for lone mothers and their roles as supporters of their children (Section 4). Section 5 goes on to examine variability in labour-market participation by ethnic origin and the regions where mothers live. Finally, section 6 considers how being a mother at work is perceived by lone mothers compared with married mothers.

The basis for this section is an interview study of mothers, carried out in 1992. In the final section, I present my conclusions about lone motherhood and paid work in Sweden.

2. Lone Motherhood in Sweden

Lone-mother families

Statistical information on the demographic characteristics of lone parents is scarce in Sweden. This fact is in itself an indication of the public view of lone parenthood as an accepted and normal family form. Given increasing divorce and separation, the number of families with lone mothers has increased in Sweden in recent decades. In 1990 lone mothers with children aged under 18 amounted to 16 per cent of all households with children (*Folk-och Bostadsräkningarna*, 1990). The share of families with lone fathers has also increased, but still this family form is relatively unusual – only around 3 per cent of all households with children.

In Sweden as in most other Western countries, divorce and separation are the most common reasons for lone motherhood. In 1990 divorced and separated married mothers accounted for half of all lone mothers (Table 9.1). While the category of never-married lone mothers is increasing, this group consists of both separated (ex-partnered) cohabitees and single (never-partnered) women, and is mainly constituted by the former. In Sweden, almost 50 per cent of children are born outside marriage. Most of these children have cohabiting parents and their families are regarded in principle as normal nuclear families both legally and statistically. It is relatively unusual for women to choose to have children without co-habiting with the father of the child.

Recent statistics suggest that the likelihood of divorce and separation is related to socio-economic circumstances. Low levels of education and unemployment increase the risk for divorce for both women and men (*Skilsmässor och Separationer*, 1995) and lone mothers have lower educational levels compared with married mothers[2] (Table 9.2).

	1985 (%)	1990 (%)
Single and separated cohabitees	39	46
Separated married/divorced	55	50
Widowed	6	4
Total	100	100
N =	151,368	158,099

Source Folk-och Bostadsräkningarna, 1985; unpublished figures from *Folk-och Bostadsräkningarna*, 1990. Calculations by Björnberg.
Table 9.1 Lone mothers with children under 18 by marital status: Sweden, 1985–90

	Level of education			
	Basic (%)	Higher (%)	University (%)	Total (%)
Lone mothers	25	53	22	100
Married mothers	16	49	35	100

Source Arbetskraftsundersökningarna, 1994. Calculations by Björnberg.
Table 9.2 Lone mothers and married mothers with children under 18, by level of educational attainment: Sweden, 1994

The age distributions of married and lone mothers are fairly similar, although a somewhat higher proportion of lone mothers (8 per cent as opposed to 3 per cent) is to be found among the younger mothers under 24 year of age. Compared with married mothers, lone mothers have fewer children; 63 per cent have only one child compared with 37 per cent of married mothers. The age distribution of the children, however, is fairly similar in both groups (Björnberg and Eydal, 1995a).

Lone mothers and employment

The labour force participation[3] of lone mothers in Sweden has, over the last decade, remained almost as high as that for married mothers – above 80 per cent.[4] Since 1991, however, the rate of participation by all mothers has diminished by almost 10 per cent. This is mostly a consequence of the growth in unemployment and an increase in persons attending education – factors which affected the whole working population (there are very few full-time housewives in Sweden). In 1994, the participation rate for lone mothers was 70 per cent, and that for married and cohabiting mothers 79 per cent.[5]

	Part time*		Full time	
	1991 (%)	1994 (%)	1991 (%)	1994 (%)
Mothers with pre-school children				
Married mothers	51	48	43	46
Lone mothers	44	46	51	49
Mothers with school-age children				
Married mothers	46	42	51	54
Lone mothers	29	31	69	66

Note * part time is defined as 20–34 hours per week (long part time); full time as over 35 hours per week
Source Arbetskraftsundersökningarna, 1991 and 1994. Calculations by Björnberg.
Table 9.3 Percentage of employed lone and married mothers (aged 25–44 years) working full time and part time by age of children: Sweden, 1991 and 1994

In Sweden short part-time work (1–19 hours work per week) is quite uncommon. For instance, in 1994 only 4–5 per cent of mothers with children under 17 years worked short part time. The part-time pattern has remained relatively stable between 1991 and 1994. The differences between mothers at different educational levels are small, but the lower the education the higher the share of short part-time workers – with the exception that married mothers with pre-school children tend to have higher rates of short part-time work. Long part time (20–34 hours work per week) is more prevalent among married mothers.

In 1994 about 48 per cent of mothers worked full time (more than 35 hours). The differences in rates of full-time paid work relate to the age of the child and the educational level of the mother. Having school-age children and higher education increases the propensity to work full time, in particular for lone mothers. The higher the level of education, the higher the share of full-time working mothers among married as well as lone mothers. Table 9.3 suggests that there has been a decrease in the rates of full-time work among mothers since 1991. In many workplaces women have been offered part-time work instead of being made redundant. An interesting observation is that the proportion of married mothers working full time has increased, whereas it has decreased among lone mothers, in particular among the highly educated groups. This might be explained by the increased rate of underemployment among lone mothers.

In the Labour Force Surveys the category 'underemployment' is based on a question about whether the person wants to work more hours than currently. Among women, the rate of underemployment increased considerably between 1991 and 1994 (in absolute figures it more than doubled). In 1994, between 6–18 per cent of women declared that they would like to work more hours. Lone mothers in general had higher shares of underemployment in 1994, especially mothers with higher edcuational levels. This is an indication that a wish to work full time is not only a matter of money but a matter of career. It is also an indication of the more precarious situation of lone mothers.

Unemployment among mothers aged 25–44 rose from 2 per cent to 7 per cent between 1991 and 1994. Among the younger groups (20–24 years) unemployment among married mothers increased from 2 to 17 per cent, and among lone mothers from 7 to 29 per cent. The gap between the two categories has increased considerably during the economic recession. Unemployment rates among lone mothers, although low before 1992 (1–3 per cent) were twice as high as that for married mothers. In 1991 and 1994, lone mothers were three times more likely to be unemployed than married mothers (see Table 9.4 below).

In Table 9.4, the 'risk' of unemployment (expressed as disparity ratios[6]) has been calculated for lone mothers compared with married mothers in relation to the age of children. Mothers with pre-school children run twice as high a 'risk' compared with mothers of older children. The figures show that mothers with young children have a higher probability of being unemployed

	1991	1994
	Disparity ratios	
Civil status		
Married mothers	1.00	1.00
Lone mothers	3.01	2.63
Mothers with pre-school children		
Married mothers	1.00	1.00
Lone mothers	3.53	2.62
Mothers with school-age children		
Married mothers	1.00	1.00
Lone mothers	2.79	2.90
All mothers		
With school age children	1.00	1.00
With pre-school children	1.46	1.43

Source Arbetskraftsundersökningarna, 1991 and 1994. Calculations by Björnberg.
Table 9.4 Unemployment among lone and married mothers aged 25–44 by age of children: Sweden, 1991 and 1994

than mothers with school-age children, which suggests that both marital status and age of children have an independent effect on the rate of unemployment.

Level of education is the most important dimension behind unemployment among mothers, and the risk of unemployment falls with increased education. Thus, mothers with a basic education were four times more likely to be unemployed as mothers with a university education, and unemployment is considerably higher the lower the level of education among both lone and married mothers (see Figure 9.1). However, the figures suggest that lone mothers have the more precarious labour market situation, and with the same educational attainment the 'risk' of unemployment is double for lone mothers. Thus, the differences between the groups cannot be explained simply because of lone mothers' lower levels of education than married mothers.

In 1991 lone mothers at university level and with school children were seven times (and in 1994 six times), more likely than married mothers in the same group to be unemployed. Thus, to be a highly educated lone mother does not seem to produce a better bargaining position (there is no reason to believe that lone mothers with university education would prefer to register as unemployed to a higher extent than married mothers). The unemployment 'risk' for lone mothers with basic education and with school-age children also increased considerably between 1991 and 1994. The pattern of unemployment rates suggests that lone mothers have a weaker bargaining position in the labour market.

The picture of lone mothers having a weaker position in the labour market is underlined by data on 'temporary employment'. This is somewhat higher among lone mothers, in particular for those with pre-school children and with

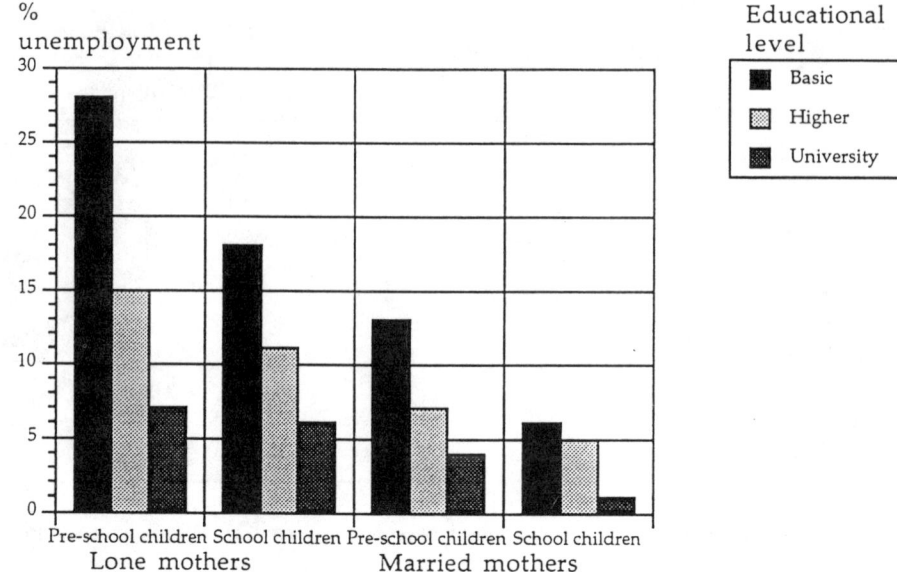

Source: *Arbetskraftsundersökningarna*, 1991 and 1994. Calculations by Björnberg.
Figure 9.1 Rates of unemployment among lone mothers and married mothers (aged 25–44) by age of children and educational attainment: Sweden, 1994

	Educational Level		
	Basic (%)	Higher (%)	University (%)
Mothers with pre-school children			
Married mothers	13	9	10
Lone mothers	15	16	17
Mothers with school-age children			
Married mothers	9	11	7
Lone mothers	10	11	13

Source *Arbetskraftsundersökningarna*, 1994. Calculations by Björnberg.
Table 9.5 Percentage of lone and married mothers with temporary employment by education and age of children: Sweden, 1994

higher education. The general pattern is that the proportion of temporary employment increases with the degree of education. See Table 9.5.

Summary

The situation for lone mothers has deteriorated considerably since the late 1980s, both relatively and absolutely. In 1988, 35 per cent of children of lone mothers lived in low-income households, but this figure rose to 60 per cent by the beginning of the 1990s. Equivalent figures for children in two-parent households were 15 per cent and 25 per cent. (*Ojämlikheten i Sverige*, 1988; Sjöberg, 1995). The explanations behind this development can partly be found in the data presented in this section. It can also be explained by reductions in social benefits and by increased costs of living (*Ensamföräldrarna – en utsatt grupp?*, 1996).

Could lone mothers' greater precariousness in the labour market be a result of processes starting with the economic recession in 1991, or did the reasons exist earlier? The information presented in this section suggests that this precariousness existed, but was less pronounced, in 1991 because levels of unemployment were lower than in 1994. In 1991 unemployment for lone mothers was twice as high as for married mothers, regardless of level of education and age of the mother. Having small children and being a lone mother, or having low educational attainments, already entailed a high 'risk' of job insecurity. By 1994, however, levels of precariousness had increased substantially (except for the most precarious group of lone mothers with pre-school children and basic education only, where unemployment was already 15 per cent in 1991). Even full-time work has decreased for lone mothers, in all educational groups, since 1991. Meanwhile underemployment has also increased considerably. This suggests that large numbers of mothers, and in particular lone mothers, have been forced to reduce their working hours.

The conclusion to be drawn is that the recession in the Swedish economy has contributed to a higher level of precariousness in the labour market for lone mothers. However, there were already systematic differences between married and lone mothers in 1991. Thus it seems likely that the policy regime at the national level is not a sufficient tool to promote self support by lone mothers.

3. Swedish Discourses Around Lone Motherhood

In the 1960s and 1970s the laws on marriage and parenting in Sweden were changed in accordance with changing family patterns. All adult, non-pensioner individuals, male and female, are supposed to contribute to the financial support of the nuclear family. Divorce has been made easier, cohabiting has been harmonized with marriage and lone parenthood has become accepted as a social phenomenon. Parenting is stressed to a much higher extent than partnership in the Swedish political context. Social policies and family laws tend to emphasize the living conditions of children and to equalize these, regardless of family form or family conditions (Björnberg, 1992; Björnberg and Eydal, 1995b).

While open stigmatization of lone parenthood or lone mothers is rare, some political parties emphasize the role of 'the family'. The major right-wing party, the Moderates, and the more rurally based Centre Party, both favour the nuclear family (although usually without much emphasis on a traditional female 'home-maker' role). The peripheral Christian Democrat Party goes further in arguing for benefit payments to allow mothers to stay at home as housewives (quite in opposition to dominant discourse and practice). All political parties, however, express concerns about the rate of divorce; but the general approach is pragmatic rather than moralistic including a desire to diminish the negative social effect of divorce and separation.

In the public sphere there has been a tacit effort to avoid the stigmatization of lone motherhood. It is symptomatic that public statistics for lone parents in Sweden are lacking and that there has been little research on lone mothers, and even less on lone fathers. Lone mothers do, however, at times complain of 'having an eye kept on them' by various groups in their neighbourhoods – such as school teachers, social workers, tenants, neighbours and even relatives. They often want to show that they can manage on their own and try to resist professional support. Lone mothers also tend to avoid living in neighbourhoods where they are subject to such informal social control (Björnberg, 1981).

Nevertheless, there is a growing awareness of the heterogeneity of the category of lone mother – some being well off and managing very well and others being less well off, in particular those with low levels of education and an insecure position in the labour market (in other words, along the lines of social class). Recent reports suggest that many lone mothers belong to those groups which have been most affected by the recession and by changes in welfare provision (*Ensamma Mammor*, 1994; *Ensamföräldrarna – en utsatt grupp?*, 1996). Recently there has been much discussion about the role of fathers, and considerable effort has been put into increasing general awareness of the importance of active fatherhood for the relationship between fathers and children. There is a strong conviction that the father–child relationship should continue after divorce. This means not only that fathers should pay child maintenance, but also that they should share custodial responsibilities with the mother. One means of accomplishing this has been the introduction of joint legal custody as the norm in divorce. The shared parental responsibility grants the child the right to have access to both his/her parents, and this means that both parents retain their legal responsibility for the child. However, this does not necessarily mean that the child lives with both parents on a commuting basis, which could be a quite demanding lifestyle for the child. (Although evidence suggests that children, under certain circumstances, may adapt to this situation, see Andenaes, 1996). State support of child maintenance through advance payment (see section 4) has been another way of strengthening the parental role after family rupture.

The cost to the state of the system of child maintenance advances has increased considerably during the last decade. The amount subsequently recouped by the state from fathers is low, and there is perceived need to reduce costs. A recent investigation suggests that some mothers receive this benefit without really needing it (*Bidragsförskott*, 1995). The government have recently put forward new proposals to deal with this problem, and these stress the financial responsibilities of both fathers and mothers.

In conclusion, over the last decades lone motherhood has been regarded as an unavoidable phenomenon within overarching processes of social change. Individuals' free choice of lifestyles has been promoted, or at least not opposed. More recently, however, concern about the children of lone mothers has been expressed, who are regarded as victims of cuts in welfare provision both in terms of individual support and social services. Duncan and Edwards (see chapter 3, this volume) classify discourses on lone motherhood into four types: lone mothers as a social threat, as a social problem, as a lifestyle change and finally as escaping patriarchy and the control of men. Following this categorization, the national discourse on lone mothers in Sweden could be interpreted as moving from an emphasis on lone mothers as part of lifestyle change, towards lone mothers as a social problem. Lone mothers are increasingly portrayed as one of the groups that have fared less well than others during the restructuring of the economy in Sweden since the 1980s.

The Swedish Welfare Regime and Lone Mothers

It has become a popular exercise among social policy researchers to classify welfare states in terms of regime types. In many of these schemes the concept of citizenship is important, which refers to the relative dependency of individuals for their social support on markets and on how states intervene in this. Some classification schemes refer to policy profiles within the framework of major political ideologies, such as liberalism, conservatism and socialism (or rather social democracy). One example of this approach is represented by Esping Andersen (1990). In this work, social citizenship is characterized by its degree of decommodification – the extent to which an individual is dependent on the market for survival. Access to social insurance of different kinds contributes to relative independence from markets. In Esping-Andersen's scheme Sweden is classified as a social democratic regime type, characterized by universal entitlement, emphasis on individual benefits and a support system largely financed by taxes.

Other classification schemes classify states according to the position of women with regard to what is essentially a male model of citizenship. In these schemes citizenship is conceptualized in terms of the relative autonomy for individuals within economic, social and political life (Orloff, 1993; Lewis and Ostner, 1994). These attempts to classify welfare regimes or gender regimes have been criticized on a number of grounds. For instance, Duncan (1995: 273) criticizes 'the theoretical assumption that gender relations operate at the national scale alone, and the use of national averages in presenting empirical differences'. He argues that local and regional differences should be incorporated into the analyses of gender regimes. In addition few classifications of welfare regimes consider the provision of social services as parts of the general welfare system (an exception is Anttonen and Sipilä, 1995). Social services, education in a wide sense, and labour market policies are often constructed on a local basis and thus provide locally based differences in options and living conditions. Local policies are influential in administering social insurance benefits. For instance, in Sweden, sick leave is combined with individual programmes of rehabilitation, which are regarded as obligatory. Such programmes are developed locally. Other scholars propose a differentiated set of criteria with which to evaluate the relative position of target groups within the welfare systems (see e.g. Hobson, 1994). Similarly, social democratic, liberal or conservative regime types vary according to historical circumstances and place. For instance, the Sweden of 1996 is a different type of social democratic welfare state compared with 1976. As a gendered welfare state Sweden had a quite different profile in 1950 compared with 1990 (Hirdman, 1994). These arguments point to the complexities in constructing welfare states and put a question mark over the utility of classifying regimes.

The welfare regime for lone mothers has changed considerably in Sweden over the years and they have been incorporated into a universal system of benefits and services (Lilja, 1989; Björnberg, 1994). The general aim has been to equalize mothers, regardless of their marital status. In addition, since the 1960s there has been a political majority in favour of full employment for both men and women, regardless of marital or parental status. Public attitudes favour labour-force participation, and both social policies and labour market policies are aimed at encouraging employment. Examples of this endeavour are the ambitious programmes for labour market policies, which have been developed in order to maintain a high rate of employment. Social benefits for persons not in work are tied to demands that the recipients should be registered at the Employment Office (*Arbetsförmedlingen*). In order to receive social insurance benefits people have to be available for work and they cannot turn down offers of jobs without the risk of losing their registration. Social security and pensions are tied to employment in the sense that benefits are constructed as income compensation (often 75–80 per cent of loss of income is covered). The amount received on a universal basis is very low and most cases below the poverty level.

The children of lone parents are given priority for public child care in most municipalities (*kommuner*). This principle has been established partly to give lone parents the ability to support their families by wages, and partly to give children the social and educational stimulation that child care can offer. The fees that lone parents pay for child care are set at an affordable level related to income.

Table 9.6 shows the relative use of child care by children living with a lone parent compared with those living with two parents. Almost half of children with two parents use municipal child care compared with three-quarters of children of lone parents.

Despite a relatively high level of employment among lone mothers, many of them receive public support in order to manage daily living. This need for

	With municipal day care* (%)	Number
Children living with two parents	47	703 000
Both parents working or studying	53	376 000
One parent on parental leave	26	186 000
One parent unemployed	11	37 000
Children living with lone parent	76	94 000
Parent working or studying	70	66 000
Parent on parental leave	11	10 000
Parent unemployed	17	16 000

Note * includes public nurseries and municipal childminders
Source Barnomsorgsundersökningen, 1994.
Table 9.6 Municipal day care for children aged 3 months to 6 years, by family type and economic status: Sweden, 1994

support is related to the low incomes of these women. In 1985, public transfers of different kinds accounted for 40 per cent of the net income of lone mothers, compared with just 8 per cent for families with two breadwinners. In 1993, 70 per cent of lone mothers received allowances or transfers of some sort, compared with 22 per cent of couple households, excluding child allowance (*barnbidrag*) which is a universal benefit (Gustafsson, 1993).

Very few educational and labour market programmes specifically target lone mothers as a group. In general, benefits are universal – in other words, no specific benefits for lone parents exist except for child maintenance advance (*bidragsförskott*), paid regularly from the Social Insurance Office (*Försäkringskassan*). There is a certain minimum to which a child is entitled (as a social citizenship right). This amount was roughly £130 per child per month in 1995. The money advanced is claimed from the other parent (almost always the father of the child). This system liberates mothers from searing conflicts over money with their ex-husbands.

All mothers, regardless of marital status, are entitled to parental leave with 75 per cent cover of loss of income (gradually lowered from 90 per cent in 1994). Entitlement is granted to persons who have either been employed or available for employment for 240 days before the birth, and who have been registered at the Social Insurance Office. The minimal level of earnings qualifying as employment is about £600 a year (at 1995 levels). Unemployment does not disqualify a person from parental leave if they are registered at the Employment Exchange. Those who do not qualify receive only the small amount of £6 a day, which is far from enough for subsistence. The economic recession of the 1990s means that it has become more difficult for young women to qualify for parental insurance benefits because of low labour demand.

Overall Sweden can be classified as a 'parent-worker, citizen model' (Hobson, 1994). As such, benefits are linked to participation in the labour market and parenting. Within this system, lone mothers are targeted as a group in two ways: firstly, in being allocated priority in child-care provision, and, secondly, through the system of state support for children's maintenance payments. The regime overall supports women as working mothers. Lone mothers, as well as other citizens, are supported with benefits which take low-earning women out of poverty. They are provided with child care by the state and they pay fees for this according to their income levels. Children of lone mothers have priority for child-care places even in cases where the mother is not in paid work. The weakness and the strength of the system is that it presupposes that lone mothers also are able to obtain a paid job. However, recent figures suggest that labour markets for lone mothers have become considerably smaller over the last few years. In addition, the costs of child care have increased and so have many other social costs for health, social insurance and housing. Benefits have also been reduced, and in some municipalities lone mothers no longer have priority for child care if they are not employed. Recent investigations suggest that the proportion of lone mothers with financial problems has increased considerably since the 1980s (Sjöberg, 1995).

5. Lone Mothers in Labour Markets: Ethnicity and Location

The regional dimension

As discussed in section 4, the comparative welfare state literature tends to assume uniformity within welfare states. This is unlikely to be the case, and in this section I consider the importance of regional and ethnic differences in the economic position of lone mothers in Sweden. For the purposes of this study, Sweden has been divided into three regional types: 'Metropolitan' (Stockholm, Göteborg and Malmö); 'Forest' which comprises rural and peripheral regions; and 'Other' which are the more densely populated and urbanized areas outside the metropolitan regions. Comparing distributions of lone mothers across the regional types we find a somewhat higher proportion of lone mothers in the 'metropolitan' area – three per cent more in 1994. At this level of aggregation, regional differences do not seem to be important in terms of the probability of the formation of mother-headed families. However, in the peripheral regions the proportion of mother-headed families has increased by three per cent (more than 6,000 households) between 1991 and 1994, which is considerable. The proportion of lone mothers is catching up in these areas.

Is there a regional dimension to be found in the pattern of labour market participation among lone and married mothers in Sweden? For this specific population, the peripheral areas have lower rates of labour market participation. However, the same is true for married mothers – both rates follow general regional trends and at first sight there seems to be no discernible regional effect on the employment rates of lone mothers compared with married mothers.

Nevertheless, women in the 'Metropolitan' areas tend to work part time

	Metropolitan regions (%)	Forest regions (%)	Other regions (%)
Mothers with pre-school children			
Married mothers	39	49	54
Lone mothers	41	50	49
Mothers with school children			
Married mothers	37	42	46
Lone mothers	27	28	35

Note * part time is defined as long part time (20–34 hours per week)
Source Arbetskraftsundersökningarna, 1994. Calculations by Björnberg.
Table 9.7 Lone and married mothers (aged 25–44 years) working part time* by age of children and regional type: Sweden, 1994

to a smaller extent than in the other areas – a gap of about 10 per cent (Table 9.7). Rates of underemployment and temporary employment are also considerably higher among lone mothers in the 'forest region', especially among mothers with pre-school children where 25 per cent are underemployed. This supports the contention that the more marginal employment position of lone mothers is exacerbated if they live in the more economically peripheral 'forest' regions.

In explaining this relatively undifferentiated employment pattern it is important to understand the role that local policies such as employment policy, social policy and urban and regional policy have in Sweden. During the 1960s, regional policy emphasized the restructuring of local industries, and the labour force was encouraged, via welfare policies, to move to those parts of Sweden where new industries were developing (predominantly in the metropolitan areas: Elander, 1978). During the 1970s, educational programmes were developed in order that people should adapt to new jobs within manufacturing, and in services. Similarly, as jobs within manufacturing diminished, the public sector expanded and made jobs available for women. In a study on local variations in women's employment the most important explanatory factor turned out to be type of local labour market, that is the types of jobs available for women (Friberg and Ohlander, 1987). A large public service sector had a positive impact on job opportunities for women, and crucially child-care services were also developed during this period. Living in peripheral areas was not, in itself, important and the proportion of lone mothers had only a small impact on female employment, which explains the low variation of figures on mothers' employment given above.

Other studies have given support for a hypothesis that the relative degree of influence of women in local councils has a positive influence on the level of public social services (Hedlund, 1994). Thus, we can probably expect a circular effect between the political influence of women and female employment, which would lend support to the idea of local 'gender contracts' (see Duncan, 1995).

253

Educational programmes have also been used as means to keep unemployment at a low level. Adult education (*komvux*) has expanded vastly during the last ten or fifteen years. It is an established part of local labour market policy for those persons with only a few years of obligatory schooling, or no secondary school education at all. It is also used by persons needing new vocational training because of unemployment or work injury, where the caring occupations (one of the more important work areas for women) are emphasized. In a recent study of a regional area with a tradition of mining (Bergslagen) the author presents *komvux* as an important aspect of the local culture, run and financed by local authorities. In order to facilitate participation in adult education among parents, one parent per household was entitled to an extra (taxed) child allowance of 990 SEK (£100) per child below 16 years. This child allowance was abolished in 1995 and it is assumed that many lone mothers have been prevented from attending adult education because of this (*Ensamföräldrarna – en utsatt grupp?*, 1996).

The ethnic dimension

In 1994 immigrant headed households made up 13 per cent of all households with children. Divorce is relatively more frequent among immigrants. Reflecting this, the proportion of mother-headed households is also higher – 5 per cent more than among Swedish origin households.

Available statistics in Sweden on immigrant women and their family and economic status are scarce, and crude in categorization. The ethnic dimension is simply categorized according to country of origin. In 1995 309,050 women born outside Sweden, aged 25–64, lived in Sweden. Over 40 per cent came from the Nordic Countries, 31 per cent from the rest of Europe (more than two-thirds of whom were from former Eastern Europe) and 17 per cent had been born in Asia (predominantly Iran, Turkey, Iraq and Libya). The origins of the remaining 12 per cent were spread in small numbers over the rest of the world (*Bakgrundsfakta*, 1995: 4).

For the purpose of this study, the ethnic dimension has been assessed by dividing women into three groups: born in Sweden; born in OECD countries; born in the rest of the world – labelled as 'other countries'. Comparing countries of origin, we find considerable differences on all the measured dimensions of labour market position. Labour-force participation is highest among married women born in Sweden and it falls with social and ethnic distance from this norm. The lowest rate of activity is found among lone mothers who were born outside the OECD area and have pre-school children (38 per cent) and the highest is among Swedish married mothers with school-age children (93 per cent). Labour-force participation for women born in Sweden was 89 per cent compared with 77 per cent for women born in the OECD, and 46 per cent for those with origins outside the OECD countries.

The reason behind the low labour-force participation among non-Swedish born women is partly due to higher rates of enrolment in education, and partly due to a wish to be full-time mothers. It could also be a sign of mistrust of ever being offered a job after long periods of unemployment. The rates of unemployment are very high among non-Swedish born women (see Figure 9.2). The situation is quite serious for women from 'other countries' where 30 to 40 per cent of these mothers are unemployed – and this applies to both married and lone mothers from 'other countries'. The pattern of difference between married and lone mothers, however, is similar to that for Swedish born – married mothers seem to fare better as far as employment is concerned.

I have not yet considered educational level in this analysis. Levels of education are lower among women born outside Sweden, including those for Nordic countries and Europe. Considerably more women from Asia have only a basic education (*Bakgrundsfakta*, 1995). Thus, the higher rates of unemployment among mothers born outside Sweden can partly be explained by their level of education. Cultural discrimination is also an explanation of the structural differences in employment opportunities, a factor also affecting men of non-Swedish origin. Thus, being born outside Sweden brings a greater likelihood of unemployment, especially among women born in countries outside Europe. The 'risk' for this group has increased since 1991, and was almost six times higher for mothers from countries outside the OECD-bloc than for Swedish mothers.

When we compare the relative 'risk' of unemployment within these groups, we find that for women born in other countries the 'risk' does not increase as much with lone-parent status as for women born in Sweden or in

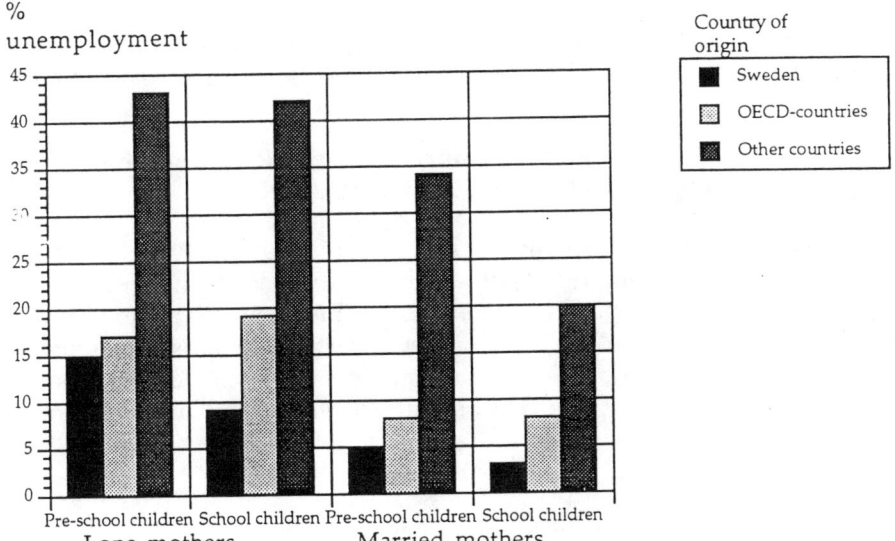

Source: *Arbetskraftsundersökningarna*, 1994. Calculations by Björnberg.
Figure 9.2 Unemployment for lone and married mothers (aged 25–44) according to country of origin and age of children: Sweden, 1994

OECD countries. This is an indication that it is already a sufficient handicap to be born outside the OECD. For women born in Sweden and in OECD countries though, it does make a great difference whether mothers are married or lone, and whether they have young children or not. This pattern supports the hypothesis of cultural discrimination against mothers of 'non-Western origin'.

Disparities in employment between lone and married mothers is even more pronounced when comparing rates of part-time and full-time work for the ethnic groups. Full-time work is quite rare among mothers from the 'other countries', but the differences between mothers born in Sweden and mothers born in OECD countries is not so pronounced. Comparing lone mothers with children under seven years, only 6 per cent of mothers from 'other countries' work full time, compared with 34 per cent of lone mothers with Swedish or OECD origin. There is a similar pattern among married mothers. In other words, the labour-force participation of mothers from 'other countries' is low on every aspect. Rates of short part-time work are twice as high for mothers with pre-school children among women from 'other countries'.

Considering the second indicator of precariousness in the labour market – 'underemployment' – the differences between the groups takes the same direction. Fewer Swedish mothers are underemployed compared with women of other national origins. Again, this is the pattern noted in section 2 – that lone mothers are underemployed to a higher extent than married mothers. The differences between the ethnic groups are quite small.

The third indicator, 'temporary employment', shows similar discrepancies between groups. Temporary employment is more common among women born in 'other countries' – a difference of about 5–10 per cent. Among women born outside Sweden, however, temporary employment is more common among married mothers, whereas the picture is reversed for Swedish mothers.

6. Lone Mothers in Neighbourhoods: Work Orientation, Social Support and Social Constraints

In this section, lone mothers' orientation towards work and family will be examined, drawing on the results of a study (carried out by myself in 1992) concerning the reconciliation of work and family life among employed parents with 5-year-old pre-school children. The whole study comprised 670 individuals, randomly sampled, with 149 lone mothers. The sample area was the Swedish west coast, centred on Göteborg and including both urban and rural areas.

Orientations towards employment

The results suggest that lone mothers have a high orientation towards employment. In the sample almost 70 per cent of the lone mothers worked full time compared with 30 per cent of the married mothers. Lone mothers also had two jobs to a higher extent than did married mothers. Compared with the general figures presented in section 2 on rates of part-time and full-time work, lone mothers from the sample were more likely to work full time and married mothers to work part time. This different pattern cannot be explained by occupation, since the two groups have similar occupations. Rather it seems likely that local factors have a differentiating impact; for instance in the area studied there might be a higher rate of small business. In such households married mothers have a lower rate of full-time occupation (Björnberg and Bäck-Wiklund, 1990). Parts of the area studied have a long tradition of high female employment with low salaries. Furthermore, Göteborg has a higher proportion of lone mothers, where full-time employment is also more prevalent, including the employment of lone mothers. This may explain the higher rates of full-time employment among lone mothers.

Lone mothers' relatively precarious position in the labour market is reflected in their attitudes towards job security. Lone mothers considered themselves to have less secure jobs compared with married mothers.[7] Furthermore, lone mothers reported less understanding attitudes among their work colleagues and employers when they had to stay at home with a sick child, than did married and cohabiting mothers. Indeed, 20 per cent of lone mothers, compared with 5 per cent of married mothers, reported no understanding from employers in such situations.

Work and family identity

Mothers were asked to indicate the importance of family versus professional life for their self-identity on a five-point scale. It was expected that the work orientation of mothers with pre-school children would be rather weak. This was confirmed by the study. Very few women held the view that work was the most important locus of their self-identity, and a majority considered family as the most important ingredient. However, in comparison with married mothers, lone mothers tended to emphasize work as being more important to their self-identity: 47 per cent had higher orientations towards work compared with 36 per cent for the married mothers.

Work orientation was also measured by a question where mothers were asked to rank the three most important reasons why they were in employment. The breadwinner role was judged the most important reason for work among all women (70 per cent). But within this, comparing lone mothers with married mothers, there are some interesting differences. For lone mothers, the ranking order for job motives were breadwinning, self-esteem and economic independence. For married mothers, however, the rank order was breadwinning, social contact and self-esteem. Altogether, these results suggest that lone mothers are strongly motivated to be self-supporting and to take on a role as working mother.

Ulla Björnberg

Balancing work, family and children

The act of balancing family and paid work was measured on the basis of a set of questions asking mothers if they had made any adaptations in their working conditions for the sake of their children, which had resulted in less or more work. Almost all women, regardless of marital status, had adapted their working conditions to meet the needs of their children, most commonly by reducing their working hours. This option is built into the parental leave system in Sweden. Parents are allowed to reduce their working hours until their children have reached eight years of age. The reduction of working hours can attract state benefits if the parents choose to work part time as part of parental leave. However, the majority of parents do not use parental leave to finance part-time work; they prefer to take a complete break from paid work during the child's first year. Adaptations in working conditions for the sake of children were found to have been practised by married mothers more often than by lone mothers. Lone mothers had also put more effort into their jobs than married mothers. For instance, 21 per cent had changed to a better-paid job compared with only 8 per cent of married mothers; 14 per cent had taken an extra job compared with 8 per cent of married mothers; and twice as many worked over-time compared with married mothers (11 per cent as against 6 per cent). Again, the lone mothers turned out to be more job-oriented.

Mothers were also asked about job advancement: did they perceive obstacles to this, and if so, did these result from work or family? Married mothers expressed disadvantages related to their own selves, to their children and their partner. Thus, in terms of making a career, the family or the self would create the main obstacle for most women. More lone mothers judged disadvantages relating to themselves, but in general there were no remarkable differences between mothers living in different family forms as to what they judged would be disadvantageous.

In response to a direct question about their evaluation of how they managed to reconcile work and family, an overwhelming majority (75 per cent) of the mothers thought that they managed quite well. However, lone mothers experienced greater problems than married mothers: 34 per cent compared with 25 per cent – a significant difference.

More than half of the lone mothers considered that the disequilibrium occurred at their own expense, 38 per cent at the expense of their children and 16 per cent at the expense of their job. The differences with married mothers were substantial on all indicators. It seems that women in general consider that any lack of balance between work and family lives results in personal damage and is family-related rather than job-related.

This personal damage could be in relation to the mothers' health. Lone mothers reported themselves as less healthy compared with married and cohabiting mothers, indicating that lone mothers are under greater pressure. On every health indicator, lone mothers reported negative values more frequently than married mothers. As many as a quarter of the lone mothers said that they often had feelings of 'inadequacy' and 'aches in the body'. They were often tired, which is surprising because the lone mothers sampled were younger than the married mothers.

Social support

Research on lone mothers' organization of their everyday lives suggests that feelings about their situation are connected to the adaptation targets they adopt. A significant starting point is whether they define their situation as temporary or long term. On the one hand, those who do not want to accept their situation as a lone mother have a hard time settling down and starting a new life, and thus in adopting coping strategies. In such cases, life becomes a continuous 'temporary' occurrence. On the other hand, those who accept their situation, and see themselves as independent and self-supporting, have better preconditions for building up their own lives; they start educating themselves, obtain jobs, build up stable social networks and develop their own interests (Moxnes, 1992; Bastard and Cardia-Vonèche, 1990). The different strategies which lone mothers develop, and the ways in which they experience their family situation, depend on a number of factors that are related to how the family form developed and the external conditions under which the mother and her children live, such as the economy, social contacts, discrimination, and external threats such as violence by ex-partner or new male partners. Most important is the educational level; the higher the level the more successful the adaptation. In a similar way local social networks are of major importance for successful adaptation strategies (Mayer and Schultze, 1989; Cochran et al., 1990; Lassbo, 1992).

An important factor in a lone mother's social support network is her relationship with the father of her children. The better the co-operation of the former spouse around parenting, the better the situation of the children in terms of psychological well-being and school work (Sandquist, 1993; William-Olsson, 1991). In my study, lone mothers were asked whether they had problems in relation to the father of their children. Only 13 per cent stated that they did not have any contact at all, while 42 per cent stated that there were problems and just as many had no problems at all. For those who did have problems, these were related to relationships – conflicts regarding visits, children getting involved in conflicts between the former spouses, and everyday matters of practical custody. More than 50 per cent of mothers complained that the fathers took too little responsibility for their children (see Table 9.8).

The figures indicate that maintenance and custody, as such, are not a problem concerning many lone mothers. This is in stark difference to lone mothers in other countries. While only 10 per cent of Swedish lone mothers have complaints concerning child maintenance and custody, around 60–70 per cent of West German and Polish lone mothers have such problems[8] (Björn-

Range of problems	%
Have no contact	13
Have no problems	42
Have problems	42
Conflicts about child support	12
Conflicts about parental responsibility	10
Conflicts about visiting rights	32
Conflicts between ex-partner and myself	30
The children become part of our conflicts	25
My ex-partner takes too little responsibility for the children	52
Other	29
	n=149

Source author's survey 1992

Table 9.8 Problems experienced by lone mothers with the father of their children: west Sweden, 1992

berg, 1994). It is likely that the Swedish system of state-supported maintenance and the principle of joint custody create fewer problems of this kind. Nevertheless complaints among Swedish mothers about fathers taking too little responsibility for their children are as frequent as in other countries.

The purpose of this section has been to examine the problems in reconciling work and family life for lone mothers compared with married mothers. The systematic differences in the labour market positions of lone and married mothers presented in section 2 raised questions about the underlying reasons for these. Could it be that lone mothers have less motivation to work? Could it be the precarious situation of lone mothers, as mothers, which make them less attractive to the labour market? The west coast survey provides clear evidence that lone mothers are motivated to work in order to be self-supporting and to gain self-esteem and economic independence. In combining family and work, lone mothers tend to emphasize work at the expense of their own health. A majority of lone mothers, as well as married mothers, consider that they manage to balance family and work fairly well, although lone mothers feel that the stresses of everyday life make them tired. The data also suggest that the economic situation of lone mothers has deteriorated in the past few years and that many lone mothers have worries about the precariousness of their situation. They worry about losing their jobs, and many feel that employers and colleagues disapprove when they have to stay at home with a sick child. Supportive networks are important in coping with this situation, and a lot could probably be gained by increased co-operation over parental responsibilities between the ex-partners.

7. Summary and Concluding Remarks

In this chapter I have analysed the labour market position and work orientations of different categories of lone and married mothers in Sweden. I have also examined whether there have been any changes since the economic recession that started in 1991. The results suggest that there are systematic differences between categories of lone mothers. Lone mothers in general have a more precarious position in the labour market than married mothers, including those with higher education. However, lone mothers born outside Europe and other OECD countries have the most precarious situation, as do very young lone mothers, those with lower education and with pre-school children. On all three variables of unemployment, temporary employment and underemployment, the situation for lone mothers is less favourable compared with married mothers. The results also suggest that the position of lone mothers in general deteriorated during 1991–94, the years of economic hardship in Sweden.

The data suggest that many Swedish lone mothers and their children live in a stressful and insecure situation. Economic stress is currently increasing, due to changes in the economic conditions and the social infrastructure, unemployment, the increased cost of living and of child care. Since my own study, carried out 1992, many child-care institutions have been forced to reduce staff and raise costs. There are reasons to suspect that the situation for lone mothers and their children has deteriorated, with new rules being introduced in some local authorities which remove the priority access to child-care places while parents are unemployed. In the political debate in Sweden it has sometimes been argued that social assistance benefits for non-working individuals are as high as the low salaries paid in certain sector of the labour market, and that this might act as a disincentive to taking these low-paid jobs. There is, however, no research supporting this contention (see Oswald, 1995). Rather, the evidence from my study suggests that lone mothers take on extra jobs and work extra hours in order to solve their financial problems, and also for social reasons.

In the Swedish context, however, the results are surprising for different reasons. There is a general view that lone mothers are working on similar premises as married mothers. There are many reasons for this supposition: one is that child care is available for lone mothers at costs which are adapted to their ability to pay. Another is the general effort to neutralize the attitudes toward lone motherhood and to regard mothers as equal, regardless of their marital status. Furthermore, the logic of the benefit system is that employment for all groups is the norm and social support is of a temporary character. Female employment is built into the welfare system and is linked to most kinds of social benefits. But the figures on the labour market position of lone mothers suggest that they are subject to systematic discrimination in the labour market, in particular if they have pre-school children. It makes little difference if the children of lone mothers have access to high-quality child care and that lone mothers are motivated towards paid work. This pattern has been present latently since the 1980s, but became openly apparent with the economic recession. As long as the rates of unemployment remain high, discrimination against lone mothers will probably remain.

The political context of lone motherhood in Sweden was described as being generally neutral or even favourable towards lone mothers. Since the 1960s and the 1970s, women in general (regardless of their marital status and family situation) have been encouraged to contribute to the support of their family on an equal basis to men. In particular, different child-care policies have been developed in order to facilitate combining work and family life, and lone mothers were favoured in access to public child-care places for their children. Labour market policies and regional policies were applied to reach the goal of full employment. Of particular importance was the expansion of the public service sector during the 1970s and early 1980s, which created many jobs for women in areas such as health services, care, cleaning and education. Regional policy was deliberately used to create balanced regions in terms of social welfare, with equality in social service provision regardless of regional type. This development is one reason why we find relatively equal labour-market participation among women in 'metropolitan' areas, peripheral 'forest' areas and 'other' densely populated areas. At higher levels of regional disaggregation – for instance municipalities – we would probably find greater disparities in patterns due to variations in local labour markets and political context. The data presented in this chapter suggests that lone mothers have a more precarious position in the labour market in all three regional types, giving reason to believe that local labour markets with different opportunities would be less favourable to lone mothers. At present severe restructuring processes are affecting the economy, but the full effects of such changes remain to be studied.

Some reasons for the difficulties faced by lone mothers can be suggested, but it has to be pointed out that these are only hypotheses. One suggestion concerns the increased demands on the labour force in workplaces. Over the last few years there have been many rationalizations and reorganizations in several sectors and organizations. For women working in the health services, for instance, there has been an increase in stress over the last decade (Szulkin and Tåhlin, 1994). It may be that employers think that the demands on lone mothers at home are higher than those for married mothers, and that the total work capacity of lone mothers is lower (in other words that lone mothers are not able to make a satisfactory work input). In general there is mistrust of mothers as a workforce, in the sense that mothers have the burden of responsibility for both home and work. Some employers believe that this double burden reduces mothers' capacity for paid work (Kugelberg, 1993).

It may also be that employers are afraid that lone mothers will take more days off to care for sick children than married mothers do, since lone mothers have no one to share these responsibilities. Parents in Sweden are entitled to 120 days of leave altogether to take care of a sick child until the child is twelve. We know from statistics that men are taking leave to care for sick children, but we have no exact information about if and how divorced and separated parents cooperate on such custodial matters.

It is obvious that further research is required to shed light on the different mechanisms behind the labour-force participation of lone mothers, and which need to be understood in order to evaluate the long-term consequences. We already know that economic deprivation is far greater among lone-mother households than for other households, and that it has increased considerably since the 1980s. Comparisons with Denmark are interesting from a Swedish perspective, since female employment and welfare support systems have many similarities with Sweden. Similar tendencies have been observed in Denmark, where high rates of unemployment were already established in the 1980s (*Uden Arbeide*, 1992).

We lack clear knowledge about the distribution of periods of unemployment for lone mothers compared with married mothers, except that married mothers are in a better position than lone mothers. The data presented in this chapter, however, indicate that the 'feminization of poverty' is now emerging as a phenomenon in Sweden as it has in many other countries. Low-paid jobs are a part of this picture, as is increased precariousness of lone mothers in the labour market and discrimination against them – in particular against those with small children. Increased costs for public social services and housing add to the economic problems of many lone mothers.

Behind the patterns described lies a patriarchal value system which has become reactivated in the wake of the economic crisis. A woman who is living with a man is attributed a higher labour market value than a woman who lives alone. The data also suggest that there is increasing ethnic polarization in Swedish society. Women (but also men) of non-European origin are becoming marginalized on the labour market (Gustafsson and Ekberg, 1995). It does not seem likely that this group will become integrated in the labour market unless strong measures are taken in order to integrate them into mainstream Swedish society.

To improve the situation for lone mothers policies are needed that are explicitly tailored for their situation. Local educational programmes of general character are not sufficient. In order to improve the bargaining position of unemployed lone mothers, additional programmes are needed at a local level. For these to be profitably tailored to actual circumstances more research is needed, since variability in the social and economic positions of lone mothers is, apparently, extensive.

Acknowledgements

The Labour Force Survey data was calculated with assistance from Gudny Björk Eydal and Tómas Bjarnarson at the Department of Sociology, Göteborg University. They have also made valuable critical comments on this chapter as a whole.

Notes

1   Lone mothers are defined as a category of mothers heading households with children but without a male partner, regardless of previous marriage or cohabiting experiences. This term is preferred to 'single mothers' which is also used to refer to never-married/partnered mothers.

2   In this chapter the category married mothers does not include cohabiting mothers.

3   Participation in the labour force is a measure which indicates the numbers who want to work or would be working if not prevented by sickness, parental leave or other leaves of absence. It includes those in employment, temporarily absent from employment or unemployed. It excludes those who are in education, retired persons or those who do not want to, or are not able to, work. It is calculated on the basis of national representative samples. In the tables all the figures are significant at a 95 per cent level of confidence.

4   The Labour Force Surveys are carried out on a regular basis by Statistics Sweden, using national representative samples. In this text figures are yearly averages.

5   For the purpose of this chapter I have made a secondary analysis using data which are not included in the standard publications from the Labour Force Surveys. I compare figures in 1991 with those in 1994 because an ethnic dimension was not included earlier. Similarly, earlier labour market surveys did not treat different categories of lone mothers consistently.

6   The disparity ratio is a measure of the probability of being exposed to a problem. In Swedish practice the measure is labelled 'odds' and it describes here the probability of lone mothers being unemployed compared with the standard for married mothers. The score for married mothers is set at 1.00 and the 'odds' of lone mothers is the ratio of the two groups (Vuksanovic, 1994; Eriksson and Goldthorpe, 1992).

7   The distribution of different types of jobs among single mothers does not reveal any striking dissimilarities. Also the distribution of education is fairly equal in the sample.

8   The study referred to was part of a co-operative international study on the reconciliation of work and family among parents with pre-school children (Björnberg, 1994).

References

ANDENAES, A. (1996) 'Challenges and solutions for children with two homes in the Nordic countries', in Brannen, J. and Edwards, R. (Eds) *Perspectives on Parenting and Childhood: Looking Back and Moving Forward*, London: South Bank University.

ANTTONEN, A. and SIPILÄ, J. (1995) 'Five regimes of social care services', unpublished paper, Department of Social Policy and Social Work, University of Tampere.

Arbetskraftsundersökningarna (1991, 1994) (Labour Force Surveys), Stockholm: Statistika Centralbyrån (Statistics Sweden).

Bakgrundsfakta till Arbetsmarknads-och Utbildningsstatistiken 1995: 4 Utbildningsnivå för Utrikes födda – Rapport från Enkätundersökning Våren 1995 (1995) (Backgrounds Facts for Labour Market and Educational Statistics. Level of Education for Individuals Born Outside Sweden) Stockholm: Statistika Centralbyrån.

Barnomsorgsundersökningen 1994 Förskolebarn (3 månader-6 år) (1994) *Statitistiska Meddelanden* (Child Care Investigation. Pre-school Children Three Months – Six Years), Stockholm: Statistika Centralbyrån.

BASTARD, B. and CARDIA-VONÈCHE, L. 'One parent families facing economic problems. A study of fifty households in France', in Björnberg, U. (Ed.) *One Parent Families – Lifestyles and Values*, Amsterdam: SISWO.

Bidragsförskott – Effektivitetsrevision av ett Statligt Stöd till Barnfamiljer (1995) (Child Maintenance Support – Efficiency Review of a Public Benefit for Families with Children), Stockholm: Riksrevisionsverket.

BJÖRNBERG, U. (1981) *En sextiotalsförort mot åttiotalet. En studie av livsformer och samhällsliv mot backgrund av regionala förändringar på arbetsmarknad och i bosättningsmönster* (A Suburb of the Sixties in the Eighties) Research report No. 66, Department of Sociology: Göteborg University.

BJÖRNBERG, U. and BÄCK-WIKLUND, M. (1990) *Vardagslivets Organisering i Familj och Närsamhälle* (Organisation of Everyday Life in Family and Locality), Göteborg: Daidalos.

BJÖRNBERG, U. (1992) 'Tvåförsörjarfamiljen i teori och verklighet' (The dual earner family in theory and in reality) in Acker, J. et al. *Kvinnors och Mäns Liv och Arbete* (Life and Work of Women and Men), pp. 153–218, Stockholm: SNS Förlag.

BJÖRNBERG, U. (1994) 'Ökad press på alltfler ensamstående mödrar' (Increased pressure on single mothers), *Kvinnovetenskaplig Tidskrift* **15**, 2, pp. 12–25.

BJÖRNBERG, U. and EYDAL, G. (1995a) 'Why and how do lone parents work? national report on Sweden', unpublished paper prepared for European Observatory on National Family Policies, Department of Sociology, Göteborg University.

BJÖRNBERG, U. and EYDAL, G. (1995b) 'Family obligations in Sweden' in Millar, J. and Warman, A. (Eds) *Defining Family Obligations in Europe*, Bath Social Policy Papers No. 23, Bath: University of Bath.

COCHRAN, M., HENDERSON, C. JR, LARNER, M. and GUNNARSSON, L. (Eds) (1990) *Extending Families. The Social Networks of Parents and their Children*, Cambridge: Cambridge University Press.

DUNCAN, S. (1995) 'Theorizing European gender systems', *Journal of Social Policy*, **5**, pp. 264–83.

DUNCAN, S. and EDWARDS, R. (forthcoming) 'Lone mothers and paid work: neighbourhoods, local labour markets and welfare state regimes'.

EKBERG, J. and GUSTAFSSON, B. (1995) *Invandrare på Arbetsmarknaden* (Immigrants in the Labour Market), Stockholm: SNS Förlag.

ELANDER, I. (1978) *The Necessary and Desirable: A Study of Social Democratic Ideology and Regional Policy 1940–72*, Arkiv for studier i arbetarrörelsens historia, Stockholm.

Ensamma Mammor. En rapport om ensamstående mödrars hälsa och livsvillkor (1994) (Lone mums. A Report on the Health and Living Conditions of Lone Mothers), Stockholm: Folkhälsoinstitutet.

Ensamföräldrarna – en utsatt grupp? (1966) (Lone Parents – a Group at Risk?), Välfärdsprojektet, Stockholm: Socialdepartementet.

ERIKSSON, R. and GOLDTHORPE, J. (1992) *The Constant Flux. A Study of Class Mobility in Industrial Societies*, Oxford: Clarendon Press.

ESPING ANDERSEN, G. (1990) *The Three Worlds of Welfare Capitalism* Cambridge: Polity Press.

Ulla Björnberg

Folk-och Bostadräkningarna (1975, 1985, 1990) (Population and Housing Census), Stockholm: Statistika Centralbyrån.

FRIBERG, T. and OHLANDER, L-O. (1987) *Kvinnors Lönearbete* (Women's Paid Work) ERU-rapport 49, Östersund: Institute for Regional Development.

GUSTAFSSON, B. (1993) 'Economic well-being and family policy', unpublished paper, Research Program at the Department of Economics, Göteborg University.

GUSTAFSSON, B. and EKBERG, J. (1995) *Invandrare på Arbetsmarknaden* (Immigrants in the Labour Market), Stockholm: SNS Förlag.

HEDLUND, G. (1994) 'Women and cut back management', in *Politics: a Power Base for Women?* Örebro Womens Studies No 3, Örebro: University of Örebro.

HIRDMAN, Y. (1994) *Women – from Possibility to Problem? Gender Conflict in the Welfare State – the Swedish Model*. Research Report No. 3, Stockholm: The Swedish Centre for Working Life.

HOBSON, B. (1994) 'Solo mothers, social policy regimes, and the logics of gender', in Sainsbury, D. (Ed.) *Gendering Welfare States*, pp. 170–87, London, California, New Delhi: Sage Publications Ltd.

KUGELBERG, C. (1993) 'Kvinnor och män, mammor och pappor på en arbetsplats' (Women and men, mums and dads in a work place) in Agell, A., Arve-Parès, B. and Björnberg, U. (Eds) *Om Modernt ffmiljeliv och ffmiljeseparationer – En Antologi från ett ffrskarseminarium* (On Modern Family Life and Family Separations), pp. 71–86, Stockholm: Socialvetenskapliga Forskningsrådet.

LASSBO, G. (1992) 'I get by with a little help from my friends', in Björnberg, U. (Ed.) *One Parent Families*, pp. 57–70, Amsterdam: SISWO.

LEWIS, J. and OSTNER, I. (1994) *Gender and the Evolution of European Social Policies*, ZeS-Arbeitspapier Nr 4/94, Bremen: Zentrum für Sozialpolitik, Universität Bremen.

LILJA, E. (1989) *Välfärdsskapandets dilemma. Om människan och hennes behov i kommunal socialvårspraktik* (The Dilemma of Providing Welfare. On Human Needs in the Practice of Municipal Social Service), Stockholm: Nordiska Institutet för Sammhällsplanering.

Lone-Parent Families. The Economic Challenge (1990) Social Policy Studies No. 8, Paris: OECD.

MAYER, S. and SCHULTZE, E. (1989) *Balancen des Glücks. Neue Lebensformen: Paare ohne Trauschein. Alleinerziehende und Singles* (Balancing Happiness. New Ways of Life: Unmarried Couples, Lone Parents and Singles), München: Beck'sche Reihe.

MOXNES, K. (1992) 'One parent family strategies', in Björnberg, U. (Ed.) *One Parent Families*, pp. 57–70, Amsterdam: SISWO.

NORMAN, K. (1996) 'Tillhörighet i Smedjebacken. Sociala relationer och kulturell identitet i en bergslagskommun' (Belonging to Smedjebacken. Social relationships and cultural identity in a municipality of Bergslagen), in Ekman, A-K. (Ed.) *Bortom Bruksandan. Föreställningar om Kultur, Historia och Utveckling i Bergslagen* (Beyond the Spirit of the Factory Village. Images of Culture, History and Development in Berglsagen), Stockholm: Fritzes.

Ojämlikheten i Sverige. Levnadsförhållanden, no 51 (1988) (Inequality in Sweden), Stockholm: Statistska Centralbyrån.

ORLOFF, A. S. (1993) 'Gender and the social rights of citizenship: state policies and gender relations in comparative research', *American Sociological Review*, **58**, 3, pp. 303–28.

OSWALD, A. J. (1995) 'Bitar i arbetslöshetspusslet' (Pieces in the unemployment jigsaw), *Arbetsmarknad & Arbetsliv*, 1, pp. 5–30.

SANDQVIST, E. (1993) *Pappor och Riktiga Karlar. Om Mäns- och Fädersroller i Ideologi och Verklighet* (Dads and Real Men. On the Roles of Men and Fathers in Ideology and Reality), Stockholm: Carlssons.

SJÖBERG, I. (1995) 'Klarar mamma maten?' (Can mummy provide the food?) *Välfärds Bulletinen*, 5, pp. 4–7.

Skilsmässor och Separationer V – Bakgrund och Utveckling (1995) (Divorces and Separations – Background and Development) Demografiska Rapporter, Stockholm: Statistiska Centralbyrån.

SZULKIN, R. AND TåHLIN, M. (1994) 'Arbetets utveckling' (Development of work) in Fritzell, J. and Lundberg, O. (Eds) *Vardagens Villkor. Levnadsförhållanden i Sverige under Tre Decennier* (Living Conditions in Every Day Life), pp. 87–116, Stockholm: Brombergs.

Uden Arbjede (1992) (Without work), Copenhagen: Social Commission.

VUCSANOVIC, M. (1994) 'Om logit regression' (On logit regressions) in Fritzell, J. and Lundberg, O. (Eds) *Vardagens Villkor. Levnadsförhållanden i Sverige under tre decennier* (Conditions of Everyday Life. Living conditions in Sweden), pp. 270–72, Stockholm: Brombergs.

WONG, Y.-L. I., GARFINKEL, I. and MCLANAHAN, S. (1993) 'Single-mother families in eight countries; economic status and social policy' in *Social Service Review*, 67, 2, pp. 177–97.

WILLIAM-OLSSON, I. (1991) *Barns Vardag med Skilda Föräldrar* (Everyday Life of Children with Divorced Parents) Stockholm: HLS Förlag.

Single Mothers – Mothers Versus Workers or Mothers and Workers

Simon Duncan and Rosalind Edwards

The chapters in this book, if they show nothing else, certainly make the point that single mothers' lives, experiences and actions are varied and diverse. This is not just the result of the different roles played by national policy regimes in positioning single mothers as mothers or workers, although as the chapters show this is important. Policies towards single mothers reflect the diverse expectations and goals of, for example, 'mother Ireland', the Japanese-style welfare society', 'pro-birth natalism' in France or the worker-citizen model in Sweden's 'people's home'. But in addition, single mothers' understandings of their position and prospects are substantially informed by conditions in local labour markets and neighbourhoods. It is quite different to live in the Nerima-ku district of Tokyo than elsewhere in the city, to live in Dublin rather than rural areas of Ireland, or in Calvados or Morbihan rather than Paris or Marseilles. These variable external conditions are not only material – such as benefit levels, the supply of jobs or child care – they are also attitudinal, in terms of national and local discourses about gender, the role of women and the status of single mothers.

Fundamentally, however, it is not just national and local conditions of life, whether material or attitudinal, that vary. Rather single mothers themselves hold varied understandings and beliefs about what is right for them and their children, and how they might best act given the variable conditions in which they find themselves. These discourses about the role of women and nature of motherhood vis-à-vis paid work, negotiated and subscribed to by single mothers, do not necessarily vary merely according to national welfare regime type. For example, German single mothers in old and new Länder, for many years, experienced different welfare state policy conditions, but both can share similar sets of values and belief systems, as well as there being variations between single mothers in a single Land.

Theorizing and Researching Variability

This overall situation of variability, in single mothers' conditions of life and in their understandings and motivations, has considerable implications for theory, research and policy.

In theoretical terms, as Crow (1997) discusses, awareness of the diversity of welfare states and their vulnerability to reversal or retrenchment has led to growing disillusionment with general functionalist theories of *the* welfare state and convergence, and renewed interest in comparisons of different welfare states within Europe, as well as attention to other welfare states outside Europe, such as Japan. Esping-Andersen's (1990) work, which we discussed in our Introduction, is an example of a theoretical framework that attempts to highlight this diversity. However, this only addresses variability at the level of nation states. As Crow (1997) also points out, growing theoretical debates around 'globalization' have also been accompanied by renewed awareness of regional and local variations, and a questioning of the extent to which national governments can direct and influence what goes on within their borders. Globalization and the rise of both political and business supra-national organizations have meant the withering of national states. Many of the countries represented in this book are members of the European Union, which is now effectively formulating its own policy frameworks. Global spatial divisions of labour, largely bypassing national states, have been mapped out on regional and local levels (Massey, 1995). The effects of particular welfare state policy regimes on the economic behaviour of single mothers is thus shaped by the opportunities and constraints provided by these influences.

In research terms, we now have plenty of information about single mothers and employment at the level of nation states, although this is not always fully comparative. (See Bradshaw et al., 1996, for an attempt to summarize this information for 20 countries.) This can be considered 'extensive' information, to use Sayer's term (1992), where the emphasis is on aggregate description at the categorical level of all single mothers or single parents. With information at this level it is almost inevitable that national policy emerges as the only effective factor in explaining variability and difference between single mothers. However, the discussions in this book point towards the importance of gaining more 'intensive' in-depth knowledge about the *processes* by which different groups of single mothers become, to various degrees, workers as well as mothers. To understand how and why single mothers act as they do demands an understanding of the contexts for their actions, where, as we mentioned above, local labour markets and neighbourhoods are equally important as influences as national policy. In addition, and crucially, we also need to understand the motives for single mothers' actions. In more formal terms, an understanding of the processes producing variable outcomes demands research on generative (causal) mechanisms in context. Thus, overall, comparative research needs to draw on both extensive (usually quantitative) and intensive (often qualitative) data for a fuller understanding of the situation and actions of single mothers vis-à-vis paid work within and across national contexts. (Similar points are made in relation to other areas of comparative social science research by Ragin, 1987; Rueschemeyer et al., 1992).

This conclusion also holds policy and political implications. For in drawing on the 'extensive' categorical and aggregate research tradition, it is all too easy to see single mothers and their actions in 'black box' terms – the category 'single mother' means a particular social behaviour and outcome within particular myopic political views. A comparative analytic approach, however, can challenge the uniform black box approach, for to admit difference calls into question both the assumptions about 'single mothers' so easily made, and the lack of attention to how and why behaviour might vary and outcomes be different. This myopic tendency is given a particular twist in the Anglo-American 'underclass' debate, where contrasting moral attitudes are categorically given to 'traditional' and single-parent families. It is by delving into the black box 'single mother', however, that we can discover social cause, and this may well have little correspondence with the aggregate categories of parenthood status. For example, research in both Sweden (Lassbo, 1994) and Britain (Burghes, 1994) indicates that it is not parenthood status per se that determines the quality of children's lives, measured as emotional and social development. Rather, the causal mechanisms reflect children's emotional resources as provided within family relationships (more amorphous concepts, such as love, discipline, support and esteem), as well as the material resources provided by family income. These factors vary within all parent types and disadvantaged outcomes can occur in all. But to appreciate these mechanisms demands progressing beyond the simple black box, categorical approach.

Single Mothers and Paid Work

What can we conclude about the position of single mothers as workers? Again the conventional wisdom is to argue that an increase in paid employment means a decrease in single mothers' poverty and improvements in the quality of life for them and their children. This assumption is more and more reflected in national policies, as most chapters show. Even in Ireland, where for so long mothers were supported to stay at home as full-time carers and domestic workers, policy steps are now in place to increase the uptake of part-time work by single mothers. This assumption, which also reflects something of a black box approach, seems misplaced on three grounds.

First, it is necessary to disaggregate what employment means. In Britain, for instance, policies aimed at expanding single mothers' uptake of part-time paid work do little to increase income levels, where the bulk of this work is badly paid. All that might happen is that there will be a transfer from benefits to earned income around an already low income level. Single mothers' conditions of life may even deteriorate given the insecurity of many such jobs in an increasingly deregulated labour market. Certainly, the evidence in this book shows that it is simplistic to equate employment levels with income levels. In Japan, for example, 90 per cent of single mothers are in employment, but most are also in poverty, with average incomes at only 39 per cent of two-parent families; in the USA, 60 per cent of single mothers now have paid work, but 30 per cent of these employed mothers still had incomes below half the national average in 1991 (Bradshaw et al., 1996). In both countries this is because the preponderance of single mothers hold low-paid, short-time and insecure jobs. Indicatively, the evidence shows that, by and large, it is not that single mothers earn much less than other women in couple families (although some exceptional groups, such as young and poorly educated single mothers, do earn less). Rather, single mothers share the employment situation of mothers as a whole, but do not have recourse to a compensating male income which is likely to be both higher and more secure. The policy implication is clear. It is the nature of the jobs supplied, and the distribution of work between men and women (and this must include unpaid domestic work) which needs to be changed if single mothers are to improve their situation by taking up paid work. Equipping them better to enter a sex-segregated and badly rewarded labour market will hardly improve matters.

Secondly, the national examples in this book point to the inadequacy of an approach based simply on employment. In Sweden, 70 per cent of single mothers are in employment, and only 3 per cent have incomes below half the national average. This outcome, in terms of material disadvantage, is strikingly different to the cases of Japan and the USA quoted above. Partly, this is because nearly all Swedish single mothers have full-time or 'long' part-time jobs (20–34 hours per week). But in turn, this high 'density' (as well as level) of labour-market participation is allowed by a pervasive, publicly funded child-care system, and where long parental leave, the provision of paid leave to be with sick children, and the right for parents of young children to a shorter working day, all make it easier to combine motherhood with paid work and career. This points to the folly of a government of one nation-state simplistically adopting particular aspects of another national welfare state's approach to encourage or force single mothers into the labour market without considering the wider policy context. The relative success of the Australian JET scheme, for example, has attracted the attention of British policy makers. Yet in Britain it is proposed to introduce the job training and counselling aspects of the package without its child-care assistance element or any publicly funded increase in child-care resources generally (Lister, 1996).

Moreover, only 10 per cent of the minority of Swedish single mothers without paid work have incomes below half the national average, compared with 80 per cent in Britain and 85 per cent in the USA (Bradshaw et al., 1996). This indicates the importance of social transfers to single mothers' living conditions – where in Sweden state-advanced maintenance provides the appropriate maintenance income for children in single-parent families irrespective of the non-resident parent's ability to pay it (and also regardless of the state's ability to recoup it). A second policy implication, therefore, is that social transfers to compensate for the costs of parenting should be an essential part of any reform package. It is no good expecting children to be raised on the cheap (and for many single mothers this will be very cheap) and then bemoaning the consequences.

Finally, the simplistic employment-based assumption for reform falls into the trap of seeing single mothers, dichotomously – as either mothers *or* workers, rather than both. It also tends to assume that sufficient income is an adequate resource for good parenting. As we mentioned earlier, the quality of family relationships and outcomes for children only partly connects with income. (In Britain, the example of Prince Charles bemoaning his unhappy childhood is instructive.) Emotional resources are equally important and time is a crucial factor in their provision. The US sociologist Etzioni's (1993) crude claims about a 'parenting deficit', whereby 'parents' are assumed to be spending less time with their children because *mothers* go out to work, have been attractive to those arguing for a return to 'traditional' values and the 'traditional' family (not least by those on the left looking for a 'third way' between the New Right and Socialism). There is actually little comparative evidence to support ideas of this deficit. Studies in Britain and Sweden, for example, show that mothers in full-time work (and, in Sweden, fathers) now spend more time with their children than the full-time housewives of three decades ago (Gershuny and Robinson, 1988; Nilsson, 1992; Lassbo, 1994). Similarly, if anything, parental employment can enhance the quality of parenting (Murray, 1995). While in the USA parents may indeed be spending less time with their children, this is likely to be the result of weak social support for parenting mentioned above, and the resultant stresses on home life which make it a less attractive place to spend time than the workplace (Hochschild, 1996. (See Fraser and Lacey, 1993; Campbell, 1996 for general critiques of the 'new communitarianism'.) Nonetheless, despite this rejection of Etzioni's prescriptions, and those of his interpreters, time is still an important resource in parenting, and the employment assumption of social policy reform neglects this at its peril. As with the debate on the underclass, an inability to tackle issues outside the remit of categorical description will leave the field to reactionary prescriptions.

The example of Sweden may be instructive here. As we have seen from the contributions to this book, Sweden has gone a long way (like France and other Scandinavian countries) in removing single mothers' poverty. This is partly because Sweden has gone furthest, at least in the formal sense of equal opportunity, in removing inequality between men and women. Nevertheless, a pervasive criticism by Swedish feminists is that this has been achieved (as far as it goes that is, for women are still not equal – and some areas, like informal power or male violence, are left relatively unchanged) by changing women's role but not men's (Acker, 1992; Holter, 1992). In other words, women have been enabled to become second-rate men. What is necessary, they argue, is a balance of power between men and women, involving a deeper change in the male role, including as a parent, rather than gender-neutral equality. This would, therefore, enable a recognition of differences between men and women – such as differences between motherhood and fatherhood – without reproducing inequality. Presumably, if this was achieved there would be as many single fathers as there are single mothers, with both having equal labour-market and domestic work participation rates. As single fathers usually have higher incomes than single mothers, the material results for the latter could be dramatic in many countries.

However, even if gender inequality were removed in this way, single parents – whether as mothers or fathers – would still suffer from a time deficit in comparison with the situation where (potentially at least) two parents are available. As Kamerman and Kahn note, 'when single mothers work, time pressures that are already severe for working mothers become worse' (1989: 31). All our contributors show that single mothers – from the mainly full-time mothers in Ireland through to the mainly full-time workers in Sweden – value their family lives and mothering. Perception of the amount of time parents should or need to spend with their children is both culturally variable and differs between mothers and fathers (with it being socially sanctioned for 'good' fathers to spend less time with their children than for 'good' mothers). Nevertheless, the issues of time and space remain for those single mothers who are in paid work to interact with their children on the more emotional level, while still working enough hours to earn an adequate household income. As things stand, single mothers need both to work more for the same income as coupled parents, and to spend more time with their children where the father is totally or partially absent – a physical impossibility. (And this is to say nothing of any leisure and personal time for single mothers.) As several of the contributors to this book reveal though, single mothers in some social groups and neighbourhoods, especially those where their status is not perceived as a stigma (such as the Black single mothers living in inner-city Britain or the young single mothers in the Near West Side of Cleveland, USA) are more likely to be able to draw on the emotional and practical support of their social networks in helping them to parent, or sharing the responsibility of bringing up their children. Few, if any, national policies address this aspect of single mothers' lives. Diversity in the availability of social and emotional support for employed single mothers in coping with time deficits in their child rearing leads us to the conclusion that child rearing needs to be socially valued and shared, and to be recognized as work. What it does not do is force us into the situation whereby single mothers have to position themselves as either mothers or workers, but not as both.

References

ACKER, J. (1992) 'Reformer och kvinnor i den framtida välfärdstaten', in J. Acker, A. Baude, U. Björnberg, E. Dahlström, G. Forsberg, L. Gonäs, H. Holter and A. Nilsson *Kvinnors och Mäns Liv och Arbete*, Stockholm: SNS Forlag.
BRADSHAW, J., KENNEDY, S., KILKEY, M., HUTTON, S., CORDEN, A., EARDLEY, T., HOLMES, H. and NEALE, J. (1996) *The Employment of Lone Parents: A Compari-*

son of Policy in 20 Countries, London/York: Family Policy Studies Centre/Joseph Rowntree Foundation.

BURGHES, L. (1994) *Lone Motherhood and Family Disruption: The Outcomes for Children*, Occasional Paper 18, London: Family Policy Studies Centre.

CAMPBELL, B. (1996) 'Old fogeys and angry young men', *Soundings*, **2**, pp. 47–64.

CROW, G. (1997) *Comparative Sociology and Social Theory: Beyond the Three Worlds*, Basingstoke: Macmillan.

ESPING-ANDERSEN, G. (1990) *The Three Worlds of Welfare Capitalism*, Cambridge: Polity Press.

ETZIONI, A. (1993) *The Spirit of Community: The Reinvention of American Society*, New York: Crown.

FRASER, E. and LACEY, N. (1993) *The Politics of Community: A Feminist Critique of the Liberal-Communitarian Debate*, Hemel Hempstead: Harvester Wheatsheaf.

GERSHUNY, J. and ROBINSON, J. (1988) 'Changes in the household division of labour', *Demography*, **24**, p. 4.

HOCHSCHILD, A. (1996) 'The emotional geography of work and family life', in L. Morris, and E. S. Lyon (Eds) *Gender Relations in Public and Private: New Research Perspectives*, Basingstoke: Macmillan.

HOLTER, H. (1992) 'Berättelsre om kvinnor, män, samhälle: kvinnoforskning under trettio år', in J. Acker, A. Baude, U. Björnberg, E. Dahlström, G. Forsberg, L. Gonäs, H. Holter and A. Nilsson *Kvinnors och Mäns Liv och Arbete*, Stockholm: SNS Forlag.

KAMERMAN, S. B. and KAHN, A. J. (1989) 'Single parent, female-headed families in Western Europe: social change and response', in International Social Security Association, *International Social Security Review*, Vol. 1, Geneva: International Social Security Association.

LASSBO, G. (1994) 'Enförälderfamilj – utvecklingsmiljö', *Social-Vetenskaplig Tidskrift*, **1**, 2–3, pp. 130–46.

LISTER, R. (1996) 'Blurring the vision', *The Guardian*, 3 July.

MASSEY, D. (1995) (2nd edn) *Spatial Divisions of Labour*, Basingstoke: Macmillan.

MURRAY, L. (1995) 'The politics of attachment', *Soundings*, **1**, pp. 65–76.

NILSSON, A. (1992) 'Den nye manen – finns han redan?', in J. Acker, A. Baude, U. Björnberg, E. Dahlström, G. Forsberg, L. Gonäs, H. Holter and A. Nilsson, *Kvinnors och Mäns Liv och Arbete*, Stockholm: SNS Forlag.

RAGIN, C. (1987) *The Comparative Method: Moving Beyond Qualitative and Quantitative Strategies*, Berkeley: University of California Press.

RUESCHEMEYER, D., STEPHENS, E. H. and STEPHENS, J. D. (1992) *Capitalist Development and Democracy*, Cambridge: Polity Press.

SAYER, A. (1992) (2nd edn) *Method in Social Science*, London: Routledge.

Notes on Contributors

Martha de Acosta is a research scientist at the Urban Child Research Center, Maxine Levin College of Urban Affairs, Cleveland State University. She holds a PhD degree in Educational Policy Studies from the University of Wisconsin, Madison and has over 25 years experience as a social science researcher, particularly in the area of sociology of education. Her current research focuses on home–community–school links and community-based approaches to building children's resilience. She has published on these topics in *The School Community Journal, Collaborations* and the *Journal of Teacher Education*.

Ulla Björnberg is Professor of Sociology at Göteborg University. She runs a programme on gender and family relations in contemporary family forms. She has been engaged in several international projects on family policy and family life in Eastern and Western Europe. Her studies have focused on reconciliation of employment and family life, child care, lone mothers, social problems and welfare.

Simon Duncan is Reader in Applied Social Studies at the University of Bradford, UK, and Associate Fellow at the Gender Institute, London School of Economics. He has researched on the local state and central–local government relations, housing provision in Britain and Europe, and on European gender systems. He is co-author of *The Local State and Uneven Development* (Polity, 1987), *Success and Failure in Housing Provision: European Systems Compared* (Butterworth/Heineman, 1992), and editor/contributor to *The Diverse Worlds of European Patriarchy* (Pion, 1994). He is Chair of the European Science Foundation network 'Gender Inequality and the European Regions', and is currently working on lone mothers and paid work in Britain and Europe, and on the politics of urban regeneration.

Rosalind Edwards is a Reader in Social Policy at the Social Sciences Research Centre, South Bank University. She has particular interests in motherhood and families, as well as feminist methodologies, on which she has published widely. She is currently researching lone mothers' uptake of paid work, parenting and step-parenting after divorce/separation, and children's understanding of parental involvement in their education. Her major publications include *Mature Women Students: Separating or Connecting Family and Education* (Taylor & Fancis, 1993) and (with David, Hughes and Ribbens) *Mothers and Education: Inside Out?* (Macmillan, 1993).

Martina Kett-Davies is a Research Fellow in the European Gender Research Laboratory at the London School of Economics and Political Science. Since her MA in Sociology at the Freie Universität Berlin in 1989, she has been a researcher at Kingston University and Goldsmiths College, University of London. She has published on small business financing and on the service sector and equal pay. Her current research focuses on lone motherhood in Germany and Britain, family sociology, gendered welfare states and paid employment.

Nadine Lefaucheur is a sociologist and researcher at the Centre National de la Recherche Scientifique, Paris. Her work is concerned mainly with the socio-political treatment of maternity outside wedlock and single-parent families. She is author of many articles, some of them published in *A History of Women* (Duby, Perrot and Thebaud, Eds, Belknap, 1994), *Poverty, Inequality and the Future of Social Policy* (McFate, Lawson and Wilson, Eds, Russel Sage, 1995) and *Single Parent Families: Perspectives on Research and Policy* (Hudson and Galaway, Eds, Thompson, 1993).

Marilyn McHugh is a research assistant at the Social Policy Research Centre, University of New South Wales, writing and researching in various social security and welfare areas. Her special interest is in sole-parent families. She is a co-author of *At the End of Eligibility: Female Sole Parents Whose Youngest Child Turns 16* (Sydney, 1994) and has collaborated on a Canadian comparative study of sole-parent policies in ten countries (forthcoming). Her current work is with the Budget Standards Unit at the SPRC: 'Determining Indicative Budget Standards for Australia'.

Eithne McLaughlin has held the Chair of Social Policy at the Queen's University of Belfast since 1995. Her research interests include equal opportunities and employment policies, unemployment and social security provision, community and informal care, and cross-national research on the nature of welfare regimes. She has published a number of books and articles in these areas, including *Understanding Employment* (Routledge, 1992); *Paying for Care – Lessons from Europe* (with C. Glendinning, HMSO, 1993); *Women, Employment and Social Policy in Northern Ireland* (Ed. with C. Davies, PRI, 1991) and *Work and Welfare Benefits* (with J. Millar and K. Cooke, Avebury, 1989).

Claude Martin is Chargé de Recherche at the Centre de Recherches Administratives et Politiques (CNRS, Rennes), and Associate Professor of Sociology at the National School of Public Health (Rennes) and at the University of Montréal, Québec, Canada. He is editor of *Home Based Care: The Elderly, the Family and the Welfare State* (University of Ottawa Press, 1993) and *Families et Politiques Sociales* (L'Harmattan, 1996). His most recent publications in English are 'Father, mother and the welfare state', *Journal of European Social Policy* (1995) and 'Social welfare and the family in Southern Europe', *South European Society and Politics* (in press). He is co-editor of the Franco-Canadian journal *Lien Social et Politiques*.

Jane Millar is Professor of Social Policy at the University of Bath. Her main research interests are in the policy areas of social security, family support and employment, and in the links between these. With Jonathan Bradshaw she was responsible for the first national survey of lone parents in the UK, *Lone Parent Families in the UK* (HMSO, 1991) and her most recent research, with A. Warman, is a cross-national study of 16 European countries, examining how family obligations are defined in law and policy, *Family Obligations in Europe* (Family Policy Studies Centre, 1996).

Ito Peng is Assistant Professor in the Department of Social Welfare, Hokusei Gakuen University, Sapporo, Japan. Her research interests focus on women, family and social policies in Japan, Britain and Canada. Her most recent publication in English is 'Welfare states in east Asia? Peripatetic learning, adaptive change and nation building' (co-written with R. Goodman) in G. Esping-Andersen (Ed.) *Welfare States in Transition.* (Sage, 1996). She is currently working on a project on social welfare regimes in Japan, Taiwan and Korea, and a project on community care and chronic care insurance systems in Japan.

Paula Rodgers is the Social Policy Officer of Save the Children (NI). She was formerly a Research Fellow in the Department of Sociology and Social Policy, Queen's University of Belfast. Her research interests include the sociology of voluntary aid agencies, policies towards disabled people, poverty and qualitative research methodologies. She is co-author of *Crime in Ireland 1945–1993* (NIO, 1996), and her research for the Standing Advisory Commission on Human Rights on the experiences of disabled people in Northern Ireland was published in the Commission's 1994 *Annual Report* (HMSO).

Index